Conscious Parenting

Also by Gabriel Cousens, MD

Conscious Eating

Depression-Free for Life

Tachyon Energy (with David Wagner)

Rainbow Green Live-Food Cuisine

*Spiritual Nutrition: Six Foundations for Spiritual Life
and the Awakening of Kundalini*

Creating Peace by Being Peace

There Is a Cure for Diabetes

Torah as a Guide to Enlightenment

Also by Leah Lynn (with Michael Chrisemer)

Baby Greens: A Live Food Approach for Children of All Ages

Conscious Parenting

The Holistic Guide to Raising and Nourishing Healthy, Happy Children

**Rabbi Gabriel Cousens, MD,
and Leah Lynn**

Forewords by
George Malkmus, Ruby Roth, and Will Tuttle

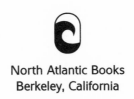

North Atlantic Books
Berkeley, California

Published by
North Atlantic Books
Berkeley, California

Cover photo ©Sergey Novikov/Shutterstock.com
Cover design by Nicole Hayward
Book design by Suzanne Albertson

Conscious Parenting: The Holistic Guide to Raising Joyful and Happy Children is sponsored and published by the Society for the Study of Native Arts and Sciences (dba North Atlantic Books), an educational nonprofit based in Berkeley, California, that collaborates with partners to develop cross-cultural perspectives, nurture holistic views of art, science, the humanities, and healing, and seed personal and global transformation by publishing work on the relationship of body, spirit, and nature.

DISCLAIMER: The creators of this text disclaim any liabilities for loss in connection with following any of the practices, exercises, and advice contained herein. To reduce the chance of harm, the reader should consult a professional before undertaking this or any other mental, physical, or spiritual health program. The instructions printed in this text are not in any way intended as a substitute for medical, mental, emotional, or spiritual counseling with a licensed physician, healthcare provider, or spiritual advisor.

North Atlantic Books' publications are available through most bookstores. For further information, visit our website at www.northatlanticbooks.com or call 800-733-3000.

Library of Congress Cataloging-in-Publication Data

Cousens, Gabriel, 1943–
    Conscious parenting : the holistic guide to raising joyful and happy children / Rabbi
    Gabriel Cousens, MD, Leah Lynn.
        pages cm
    Summary: "Lays out the connections between conscious nutrition for families and spiritually oriented parenting including health advice and easy, child-friendly vegan recipes"— Provided by publisher.
    ISBN 978-1-58394-996-2 (paperback) — ISBN 978-1-58394-997-9 (ebook)
    1. Children—Nutrition. 2. Veganism. 3. Vegan cooking. 4. Parenting—Religious aspects—Judaism. I. Lynn, Michaela, 1975– II. Title.
    RJ206.C784 2015
    641.5'636—dc23   2015001736

1 2 3 4 5 6 7 8 9 UNITED 20 19 18 17 16 15

Printed on recycled paper

It's a good feeling to know you're alive.

—Mr. Rogers

Contents

Authors' Acknowledgments

Leah (Michaela) Lynn's Acknowledgments

To the Divine within all there is, who parents all with grace, compassion, love, patience, guidance, and discipline, I give thanks, and dedicate this book to you. May the words that fill these pages point to you and glorify you. May the sacred life that you have given to all beings be blessed, protected, and supported.

To my trusted rabbi, doctor, counselor, coauthor, and friend, Gabriel Cousens, thank you for seizing every opportunity to support my physical, mental, social, emotional, and spiritual development. Without your partnership, medical advice, spiritual teachings, and deeply wise feedback, this book could not have been as comprehensive as it is.

To Quinn and Levi, I really love being your mama. What a privilege! Thank you for your exuberant joy and enthusiasm, strength, perseverance, and forgiveness. Thank you very much for telling me which of my recipes were bookworthy and which were not. I love to listen to your thoughts and ideas. I am scrumptiously more humble, happy, and alive because of you!

To my wonderful father, Ed Lynn: Dad, it is a tremendous blessing to have a *health minister* as a grandpa to Quinn and Levi! Thank you for your loving care of the children, which has enabled me to write. I am very inspired by your yearly forty-day juice fasts! Thanks for the superfoods for the kids at Christmas time, for the Vitamix for my birthday, and for planting extra kale and stocking up on spirulina when we're coming to visit! Although the contents of this book may not always reflect your personal beliefs, thank you for your steadfast love and support for my personal growth and quest for an authentic relationship with God.

To my beautiful Mother Peggy Lynn: Thank you for giving birth to me naturally, for choosing to breastfeed even though it meant the countering of culture, and for making us "weird" food when all of my peers were eating Froot Loops. Thank you, Mom and Dad, for raising us with scripture, with devotional music, and with prayer. These continue to be a lamp unto my feet and a light unto my path. I am blessed to be your child.

Thank you Michael Chrisemer, for your partnership in the raising of our two delightful children. Thank you for your example to them as an organic farmer, and as one who gives quiet attention to matters of the spirit.

Thank you to Ms. Anna Maria, Quinn's preschool teacher. The way that you received each parent and child with light and love, sincerity and depth, each and every day, continues to be an inspiration to me.

Rabbi Dr. Gabriel's Acknowledgments

I want to acknowledge HaShem *(God)*, who told us to be fruitful and multiply and has empowered me as a coauthor of this book, which I believe will empower many parents and grandparents to help raise alive and conscious children and grandchildren. I want to acknowledge Leah Lynn for getting the work started on the book, for making a much-needed contribution of support to parents with her prior book as well as her insight to entice me to get fully involved with this book as a coauthor.

I want to acknowledge my children, Raf and Heather, for giving me such a great experience of parenting, and the templates to fully understand myself through parenting, and for bringing forth my grandchildren, Rhea (from Raf), and Katja and Anise (from Heather). They have been a personal inspiration for the writing of this book, and for the idea of supporting parents to create healthy, alive, conscious children and grandchildren.

I want to acknowledge Nora Pearl for participating in the creation of our children and grandchildren, and my wonderful wife, Shanti Golds Cousens, and her mother, Emma Golds, for being great inspirations for the meaning of mothering, grandmothering, great-grandmothering, and great-great-grandmothering, to help me gain a deeper insight into the awakening process from a grandparent's, great-grandparent's, and great-great-grandparent's view.

I wish to acknowledge Yehoshua Kalev Sedam for his diligent work as research and production editor, and for bringing this project to fruition as the main person for supporting the overall production of the book.

I also want to acknowledge North Atlantic Books, Emily Boyd, Hisae Matsuda, and Mary Buckley for encouraging Leah and me to get this book done in a timely manner to bring it to the world.

Thank you,
Rabbi Gabriel Cousens, MD, MD(H), DD

Foreword by George Malkmus

"Train up a child in the way he should go." says the Bible in Proverbs 22:6. Sadly, I was raised nutritionally in the way I should not go—on the Standard American Diet—with lots of meat and sugar. This diet resulted in a diagnosis of colon cancer at age forty-two. Rather than accept traditional medical treatments for my cancer, I adopted the diet Dr. Cousens promotes in this book. Within a year my cancer was gone and here I am forty-plus years later and in my eighties. I have been on this one hundred percent plant-based diet for forty years and I still have a strong and healthy body. This book contains the information you need so you can raise healthy children who have been brought up eating "the way they should go" so they can live a long and healthy life, free of physical problems.

Reverend George Malkmus, founder of Hallelujah Acres
July 2015

Foreword by Ruby Roth

Standing in line at the grocery store with my ten-year-old stepdaughter, Akira, our eyes pass over the racks of magazines, their covers filled with the names of growing movements in health and nutrition: *yoga, paleo, meditation, vegetarian, grass-fed, humane....*

"'Sustainable Meat?'" she reads from a headline, "Yeah right ... they just never want to change."

I feel good. She was born and raised vegan, taught to think critically, locally, and globally. I don't worry about her: she's a little warrior, well-equipped to handle the sly nature of this world. *Conscious Parenting* is a gift that will help us continue to expand our vegan global awareness at a vital time.

Today, plenty current movements and practices encourage health, eco- or spiritual consciousness, sustainability, or personal peace of mind, but do not offer the *holistic* approach we need today to address our problems, the most pressing issues of health and well-being the world has ever seen. Often, what seems like a promising shift toward positive change only parallels the evasive nature of destructive habits. For example, on a micro level, consuming grass-fed, organic bison feels "revolutionary" compared to eating factory-farmed meat. But on a macro level, such "sustainable" choices require the same amount of resources (often even more so because the animals live longer); perpetuate pollution and the violent spilling of blood; continue systematic impregnation of animals (known as cross-species sexual perversion) as well as tail-docking, dehorning, tattooing, udder-singeing, and the use of bullrings; and ultimately leaves intact our anthropocentric view of the world, the belief that humans are the center of all reality. This self-serving and distorted belief is the root of the health, ecological, and even economic crises we find ourselves in today.

There should be no confusion about which of today's altruistic movements is comprehensively effective for both personal and planetary health and sustainability—veganism. In its broad reach it offers a revolution, not an illusionary feel-good modification of degenerative anti-life patterns.

Never before has there existed such radical health and ecological dysfunction from all sorts of chronic diseases, diabetes, and obesity, to the prevalence of vaccinations and environmental toxins and widespread ecological devastation. In the span of human history, this breakdown has happened so fast that most people are still blind to the normalization of destructive practices.

Conscious Parenting is a direct answer to these burning issues. It is a call to collectively think, eat, and live differently—to raise our standards of life and reach the potential inherent in ourselves and our kids. It calls for a new approach, which brings kids on board with health and wellness—in a both micro *and* macro senses. Dr. Cousens and Leah Lynn masterfully answer all the anti-vegan scare tactics and present new and compelling information on the safety and health benefits of raising vegan children. The mind-blowing conclusions in this book make it an essential guide and resource for every person who knows a child. It is the long-awaited scientific, holistic, and spiritual resource many vegan and health-conscious parents have been waiting for to safely and successfully raise vegan kids. Luckily for everyone, the transformative practices in this book are joyful for everyone in the family.

Through my own work introducing children to vegan choices, I find that when we give kids the information they need to make educated choices, they choose wisely—and often with much more diplomacy than adults. They are eager to take part in solutions that protect animals and the earth. It makes utter sense to them. *Conscious Parenting* will help the next generation approach life, informed by the connections between the physical body, cognition, society, ecology, and spirit—in the context of uplifting ourselves, our children, and the whole living web of life on the planet.

I'm encouraged that *Conscious Parenting* has fallen into your hands. Each book sold is a crack in the system, through which power will be unleashed by parents and children who long for a better world by all counts and measures—people who love all of existence from the vantage point of the present and future to come.

Ruby Roth, author of *V is for Vegan*
July 2015

Foreword by Will Tuttle

As parents, we wield enormous influence. We model a lifestyle that our impressionable child will naturally emulate. By consuming and modeling healthy, sustainable, and organic vegan foods and products, we sow seeds of awareness and sensitivity in our children. Our greatest delight is in feeling, connecting, awakening, caring, loving, and creating, and it begins with the daily ritual that we all participate in, our most intimate connection with the created world, that we call eating.

In this important and much-needed volume, Gabriel and Leah weave insights gleaned from decades of clinical research as well as from deep immersion in respected ancient wisdom traditions, and build a foundational understanding for holistic parenting that is as liberating as it is healing. By practicing the methods outlined here, we can confidently create a more just, sane, and joy-filled world for our children that respects and celebrates the web of life by which we are nourished and to which we all contribute.

This pioneering book is perhaps the first to address the important issues surrounding nutrition and parenting in a deep and holistic way. It offers parents fresh wisdom to help inspire a quantum leap in our capacity to be more conscious, loving, and healthy as children, families, and culturally as well.

Will Tuttle, PhD, author of *The World Peace Diet*
July 2015

Introduction

We cannot always build the future for our youth, but we can build our youth for the future.

—Franklin D. Roosevelt, Great Speeches

In our current time of global crises, there is an alternative to being consumed and negatively affected by the culture of death—a way of life that puts accumulative materialism, power over others, name, and fame at the center of life. It creates a way of life that leads to personal and planetary ecological destruction, acute and chronic disease, cruelty violence, suffering, and poverty. The bottom line of the culture of death is the effective production of material goods, which maximizes the accumulation of money and power for a few; it is a way of life that sacrifices the health of the many for the wealth of the few.

None of this is needed to create a healthy, happy, abundant world for everyone. There is an alternative—a natural way of life in harmony with the living planet and the network of life. We call it *"the culture of life and liberation."* It is a way of life that puts the Divine, and the spiritual evolution of our soul and the planetary soul, as the central purpose of our life. There is a subtle and perennial demand for this way of life that is gently sweeping across our planet, like a fresh breeze dispersing stagnant air and bringing relief from the oppressive heat of the culture of death.

The culture of life and liberation is a sacred lover, wooing us into prayerful, openhearted communion with the Divine, and with the living planet as an expression of the Divine. It is living life as love and harmony with all creation, honoring all life on the planet. Its bottom line is to elevate all souls and maximize love, kindness, compassion, generosity, and caring for humanity and the Earth in a way that creates abundance for all. It is an awake and conscious way that brings peace, abundance, love, joyous life, liberty, and pursuit of happiness to the world's population. It is successful conception after many years of barrenness, and a birthing woman's breath as she opens to love while in the throes of stretching beyond what we typically deem possible.

The culture of life and liberation is the light of a newborn baby's emergence after the energies of pregnancy and labor have come to completion. It is a miracle of creation, come to elevate all of creation. It is the smile on a grandparent's face when they see their alive and conscious grandchildren. The culture-of-life-and-liberation child is the pre-toddler who doesn't know the words, "It's no use," and who, having seen the possibility of standing, continues to get up and go for it, time and time and time again—but who's counting? He *will* get up and walk.

The culture of life and liberation is the happy child who asks us to pleeeeeease come out and splash in the rain, squish the mud, savor snowflakes, hide in leaf heaps, see illustrations in the clouds, climb up trees, slide down banisters, and to *stop everything* to take in deeply the scent of a flower or the sight of a six-legged speck traversing our path. It is a joyful child inviting us to hum the familiar song held in the collective heart. In other words, we are being summoned to fully live our lives. It is a way of life for our children and grandchildren that activates their potential to support this joy of life.

This way of life is reestablishing the joy, love, and ecstasy of the Divine in the center of our lives and that of our children, grandchildren, and families. It is celebrating the mystery of the Divine in the entire material plane. A profound and most difficult question in this materialistic modern world is: How do we as parents and grandparents remember to maintain the Divine in the center of our lives, and to protect and/or establish that sacred and holy space and awareness in our children and grandchildren? How do we inspire them to stay attuned and to keep going even when the numbing pressures of the culture-of-death values seem so overwhelming in their lives? The aim of this book is to provide safe, sound, and time-tested tools, advice, and inspiration for all of us who trek this magnificent human journey of parenthood, grandparenthood, and other vital child-nurturing roles.

Alive parenting speaks to a yearning within each parent's heart—a deep yet sometimes hidden yearning to guide, protect, teach, and nurture as a natural expression of one's fullest aliveness. What is one's fullest expression of aliveness? It is said, in Hebrew tradition, that the biblical Sarah was *alive* all the 127 years of her life. In other words, Sarah lived out her many years in the state of intimate, alive awareness of the Divine. While the stories, metaphors, and guidelines may vary from culture to culture, the yearning for full human aliveness is universal. Parental and grandparental love for one's child or grandchild is also universal. *Conscious Parenting* is devoted to the support of the awesome unfolding journey of aliveness that resides as a potential within each and every parent/ grandparent and child.

With the intention to support parents, grandparents, and others in the holistic care of children, our focus is primarily from birth to puberty—but we do include some basic issues of teen years and their brain/mind development into early adulthood. This book has been organized according to five domains of human development: physical, emotional, social, mental, and spiritual. But first, we delve into what it means to be in the roles of alive parent or grandparent and alive child, and how to create an *alive and conscious* environment of support for both of these roles. In the process, we elaborate a subtheme throughout the book, which is the importance of protecting our children's brain, mind, and consciousness on multiple levels—from vaccines and GMOs to the negative effects of excessive, undermining media exposure. We use a range of data, from science-journal articles to epidemiological telephone surveys and opinions by authorities.

Unfortunately, people on all sides of all discussions tend to expand their conclusions or, in some cases, as highlighted by the Centers for Disease Control and Prevention (CDC) exposés, simply falsify the data to make their egocentric or politically directed point. We have tried to create a balance by citing a variety of studies. Our motivation is to protect our children and grandchildren, so we have had to take a hard look at what is considered "normal and safe" for our children's brains and minds and to share the potential probable outcomes based on the limited studies and information available worldwide.

In some cases, we are giving preventative and protective information without waiting until it is definitely proven. It took thirty years, for instance, to definitively prove that smoking causes lung cancer—but we choose not to wait that long. Thirty years from now, our children will be grown up and it will be too late. For this reason, although we are trying to be accurate, even if we are sometimes wrong we choose to be inaccurate on the safe side, for the protection of our offspring. For this reason, we will be highlighting not only hard facts but also suggesting trends relevant to the protection of our children.

One special creative aspect of this book is the play of Rabbi Dr. Gabriel Cousens as grandfather, psychiatrist, family therapist, director of the Boston Teen Center and Petaluma People Services Center and teen program, mental health director of Sonoma County's Head Start program, family practice holistic physician, scientist, spiritual teacher in multiple cultural and family traditions including Native American sundancer, Spiritdance clan chief, yogi, and ordained rabbi, and of Leah Lynn as mother, Montessori teacher, and spiritual student/practitioner with a Christian background.

One role of the parent and grandparent is as keeper and carrier of the traditions, legacy, stories, and hidden treasure chest of a family, and its generational protector. Grandparents have a particular gift to offer in raising conscious and alive children because they are free to love and guide the young as wise elders without having to take daily responsibility for them. They can be the bridger of generations in supporting the highest evolution of the parents and children. They are free to share life's secrets and the healthy holistic perspectives that come with time and experience.

This active, multitraditional parenting and teaching experience of Leah and Rabbi Dr. Gabriel gives a unique multigenerational grounding to the parenting support and perspective in this book; it may be a support to single parents without access to such advice but with a sincere desire for the holistic healthy development of their children. Although this book has plenty of science to back its positions, its power, perspective, and love comes from the position of concerned parents and grandparents playing out their most important role in a healthy society—the raising of healthy, alive, and conscious children.

May we all be blessed with alive and conscious children and grand-children dancing in love.

—**Rabbi Gabriel Cousens, MD**
and Leah (Michaela) Lynn

A Grandfather's Blessing and Wisdom Advice to Parents

Dear parents of this wonderful child,

May you be blessed to know the subtle parental teaching of Malachi 4:6, that "the hearts of the parents will return to their children."

Remember never to crush the innocence of your child, who is born as the unique expression of the simple essence of the Divine.

Welcome to the fundamental parental paradox—that your children are both your children and not your children!

Your children are a sacred expression of life forever longing for itself.

Parents are the launching pad of the Divine, from which your children are set forth into the world; yet you are also, paradoxically, key companions on their life's journey.

May you appreciate this extraordinary gift that the Divine has provided through you, which is both yours and not yours.

May you understand that this gift is the opportunity to nurture, protect, and teach your child, so that each of your children becomes a good and holy human being.

May you understand and nurture the great potential your children have within themselves.

May you realize that how you raise your children will not only influence their lives but their children's lives, and their children's children's lives.

May you understand and appreciate your children for what they are rather than what you project onto them.

May you appreciate that your child is still shaped by the Divine because of their natural closeness to It.

May you know that the great secret to childhood is not that our children have much to learn from us, but that we have much to remember, through our experience of them, about who we are and what we will always be as the essence of the Divine.

May you understand that the most important component of shaping good behavior in your children is your own personal desire for living in the truth, which will then help you to guide your children in the perennial truths of right and wrong, the perennial ethics of what it means to walk as a full human being on the Earth.

May you remember the continual love nourishment that your own couple relationship needs while raising your family, so that you both walk as full human beings in complete intimate relationship on the Earth, for yourselves and as an example to your children.

May you be successful in helping your child learn clarity and conviction, so that they may clearly differentiate between the dark and the light.

May you always remember that your children do not belong to you, but belong to and are a gift from the Divine, entrusted to you to protect, nurture, and raise as full human beings who understand their purpose and ultimate mission in life.

May you understand that the Divine has asked you to raise your children with love, and to care for these precious souls with divine sensitivity.

May your children understand and honor you as parents—not because you are an authority but because you as parents are the ones chosen to bring them into this world, and because you are walking your talk.

As your children grow, may you succeed in helping them appreciate the subtle teaching of Maimonides that "A person should see the entire world as half-good and half-evil, so that with a single good deed they will tip the scales for themselves and the entire world toward the side of merit." In other words, our actions count, and make a difference.

May you remember that love is the first thing a child needs to feel as the foundation of leading a whole and healthy holistic life—a life that enables them to make the distinction between good and evil and right and wrong to clarify the direction of all their studies and life choices.

May the education you provide your children be one that sensitizes them to an entire world of moral, ethical, and spiritual awareness of absolute truth as a grounding anchor in the storming seas of relative egotistical truth, empowering them with the commitment to participate in a greater good than the desires of their limited ego.

May your children understand why the Ten Speakings begins with "I am your God"—because it establishes acceptance of a morality and ethics that is universal and perennial rather than relative and based on their own or society's egocentric needs of the moment.

May you have the strength to teach your children to stand strong in our current world, where the idea of perennial morality is often considered nostalgic fantasy.

May you thus teach them the "why" as well as the "how" of how to behave in alignment with the divine unfolding.

May you be blessed to understand—and teach—that true education is education for life in alignment with the Divine; and that this will sustain them individually and empower them to create a better world for their children and the whole world.

Before your children are taught the technology of reading and writing, may you always teach them to be good persons with good habits, and to know the distinction between life- and death-generating activities, and between light and dark, and to understand that these qualities are an increasingly rare commodity seldom respected in the world they are growing up in.

May you teach your children the extraordinary value of their souls as well as the value of learning mathematics and English.

May you empower them to maintain their inner strength to live in truth.

May you be so blessed in this process of parenting that you are more profoundly elevated than you ever expected.

—Rabbi Gabriel Cousens, MD

CHAPTER 1

The Alive Parent and Child

The Role of the Alive Parent is the Way of the Spiritual Warrior!

The choice to become a (parent) is the choice to become one of the greatest spiritual teachers there is. To create an environment that's stimulating and nurturing, to pass on a sense of responsibility to another human being, to raise a child who understands that he or she is created from good (and for good) and is capable of anything... (F)ew callings are more honorable. To play down (parenting) as small is to crack the very foundation on which greatness stands.

—Oprah Winfrey

The art and mystery of (parenting) is being the source of love, sweetness, and powerful, gentle discipline fused with the ability to bring, with holy, loving firmness, a fruitful order out of life's chaos, so that one's children are best empowered to reach the highest expression of their sacred design and holiness in the world.

—Rabbi Gabriel Cousens, MD

Parenting is a Living System.

—PCI (Parent Coaching Institute)

Whoever touches the life of a child touches the most sensitive point of a whole.

—Dr. Maria Montessori

———————

The question is often posed as to why, as a nation, we allocate so much of our resources to war while we continue to cut education funding for our children. Continuing this culture-of-death cycle when it has never worked for the health and spiritual well-being of society doesn't make any sense! And yet here we are still spinning and spinning on the same old merry-go-round, long after we've all gotten sick to our stomachs.

A starting point for getting out of this vicious cycle is to stop the ride long enough to clear the dizziness. When we find ourselves in stillness, we may begin to see that how our government prioritizes its budget is but one symptom of a materialistic and ego-driven culture of death. Big ego is the bully whose objective is to dominate rather than to serve and elevate all beings. With our heads settling and our vision less blurry, we may also begin to see how our ego-driven culture is bestowing on us a poignant reflection of ourselves.

As the mystic poetess St. Teresa of Ávila (1515–1582) once said, "Yes, overthrow any government that makes you weep inside. The child blames the external and focuses his energies there; the warrior conquers the realms within, and becomes gifted."[1] As we gaze into this mystical mirror of the self, we may receive key information, such as how *we* may be unintentionally contributing to the massive, whirling confusion.

All who share a relationship with children are invited to ask ourselves the central questions: How am I allocating my precious resources of attention, time, money, thought, and other energies? What is my true motivation for each of these expenditures? In any given moment, are my vital life forces directed toward egocentric pursuits, or are they directed toward the spiritual work of elevating the whole? Whether or not I spend a fair amount of time, money, and energy with children, what is the quality of these interactions? Am I bringing the aliveness of my Divine presence to the experience of breastfeeding, potty training, teaching literacy, or coaching ball?

When a child shares with me his drawing or his homework, am I in a hurry to say "good job" without even really looking, so that I can get on to something else? Are my affirmations sincere? Do I hastily make corrections for them, or do I take care to *see the child* in their work, appreciate their unique developmental journey, and explore how I might be of hidden assistance to them in their unique and holy process? The Huichol culture in Mexico does this consciously. When a child is born, the elders gather and attempt to attune the child's sacred design or unique gift to the world, and then help to create an early-life training plan to help the child manifest that sovereign life purpose.

We see a repeating pattern of governmental abuse of power interfering with our ability to authentically parent alive and conscious kids, through their unspoken agendas to program and use children for their own purposes, such as with the "Common Core" curriculum. We also see it in attempts to take away parents' rights to choose organic and non-genetically modified (GMO) foods and supplements, and even to choose whether or not to vaccinate our children. These attempts to undermine parents' responsibility and power of conscious evolutionary choice are about robbing the global community of its right to be alive, conscious, and to spiritually evolve.

Governments and bureaucrats have never been better parents than real parents, and they were never meant to be. Is there a valuable lesson for us parents here as well? Alive and conscious children call for alive and conscious parents who proactively take on full parenting power and responsibility. When we are willing to look deep within for this, we may discover that, as parents and grandparents, we sometimes forget that our role is one of enlightened, turned-on, "all-weather" mentors for our children. How often do we use the same societal tactics of fear, misinformation, legislation, and physical force in order to control our children?

As we come alive as parents, we start to see these unconscious trends of domination instead of dominion for what they are—enslavement to ego rather than conscious choices to love, support, and steward the unfolding of the new life with which we've been entrusted. This process leads us to courageously surrender the ineffective long-term fall back to power and control in exchange for the ever-increasing joy of awareness and being. As our parenting methods evolve, our children regain a sense of their unique divine expression, and are no longer taught to exist with a slavery mentality. This results in a profound support for the health and spiritual evolution of the global family.

Alive and conscious parenting is the ego's worst nightmare. Contrary to pseudo-parenting—analogous to politicians who like to have their pictures taken with kids in the classrooms yet continue to deplete government aid to education—it is understanding parenting as a golden opportunity for us to tap into our compassion, inner peace, and strength as part of our unique expression of the Divine. *Raising children is a way of the spiritual warrior.* We suddenly have a young and vulnerable human being who is relying on us to serve his or her development. For the biological mother, this means the sharing of a body for up to nine months, and perhaps years of breastfeeding. For the father, it means all forms of nurturing short of pregnancy, birthing, and breastfeeding. For the teacher or day care professional living in the U.S., this means accepting less pay and lower social status than what society deems to be more glamorous careers. Generally, the younger the child, the less we value this teaching work monetarily.

For all adults in childrearing roles, this means having our own childhood "ouchies" revisited. The inner-child buttons get a rigorous pushing like a dreaded electronic press-me toy, sounding over and over and over, demanding our attention until our tucked-away tender spots are noticed, cared for, and healed.

Holistic parenting and grandparenting is spiritual work! And when our egos want some kind of kickback—such as living vicariously, assuming bragging rights, having power over the weak, someone to look up to us, or someone to love us, or even to appear to be saintly—we also have a golden opportunity to find out that true aliveness and liberation require us to consistently discipline our own egos to serve the flow of Divine consciousness.

Not only does the path of parenting lead to service, self-discipline, and clues to our own healing, but thankfully this adventure also greets us with springs of spiritual joy. Yes—parenting is a gift for adults' spiritual growth spurts, and it's a challenge to think of anything else that fills a home with more laughter! Beyond description is the depth of love that we feel for our children. Beyond measure is the ecstasy of being the living vessel through which the Divine begets the spark of the Divine. And it is the teacher's pure, unadulterated pleasure to witness the Divine hand at work in his or her students' lives.

So we see that in the joyous role of alive parenting, we conscious choose an alternative to the culture of death and ego's domination-over-the-weak model. Alive parenting is a holistic alternative to what we might call "allopathic parenting." In the allopathic approach to health care, we use drugs to modify symptoms rather than treating the root cause of disease—often nutritional deficiency or imbalance—and forget that ADD, for example, is not a symptom of a Ritalin deficiency. With the allopathic approach, we devalue and deprive the innate intelligence and power of the body to heal itself.

Unfortunately, we see this allopathic strategy in our cultural approaches to childrearing as well. In parenting, for example, if we attempt to dominate and control children as we do our bodies, rather than going to the root of undesirable behaviors (which may require inner work on our part) we fail to recognize the innate brilliance of children who, under the right conditions, will correct themselves. In a culture where we drug and numb the body and mind in order to keep it quietly controlled, we also treat children in this way, with excessive television, video games, addictive and numbing foods, and an extraordinary recent increase in psychomedications given to children.

By contrast, the goal of alive parenting is to create a setting for the growth of alive and conscious children: We see our role as one of service to a new life that has an innate soul-intelligence and is worthy of our respectful support. This new vision guides our relationships with children and enhances our experiences of joy! Alive parenting is thus a powerful tool for fulfilling the overall purpose of *our* lives—to know God, Cosmic Source, or the Divine.

In this light, we can appreciate the uniqueness of our own part in the Divine play, knowing that these roles of dad, mom, grandpa, grandma, teacher, daycare provider and even spiritual warrior are not our identities. When we remember that we're all just playing dress-up, we are freer to relax, to forgive, to trust, and to keep going even after we've taken a few tumbles.

The Role of the Alive Child

> Every child comes with the message that God is not yet discouraged of man.
>
> —Rabindranath Tagore

Contrary to belief, in popular culture, the child does not exist to satisfy the egotistic needs of the parent, grandparent, teacher, corporation, government, or even clergy. The child is here for the same purpose as we are—to know God, Source, or the Divine. In other words, the child is here to develop their own potential to walk the Earth as a full human being. What is the child's role in *our* lives? The child's intention is not to be "naughty" or make our lives miserable (which is not always easy to remember when our cell phone is swimming in the toilet bowl). Nor is the child the enemy who is out to get us.

On the contrary, the child's innate intention is to thrive. A child who is not thriving is sending an unconscious message to the adult that they need our help with their specific life mission of unique soul expression and their general mission of spiritual liberation. In this way, the child serves us just as much as we serve the child. In so doing, we play the role of the vigilant prince whose enduring love breaks the evil spell cast upon Kingdom Earth, our symbolic Sleeping Beauty. In other words, we are all helping each other to wake up!

This is great news, because it means that there is no reason for resentment on either side. Adult and child alike, we are all playing the ultimate game of hide and seek: "Your turn to hide your Divine spark!" "Peek-a-boo!" "Now, it's your turn, and we'll try to find you!" And when the ghoulish night of the culture of death has passed, we'll all take off our array of costumes, able to delight in the treat of *I am that*. As the great traditions tell us, this is the sacred covenant between us and the Divine. So, may we all be blessed with the remembrance of the child's and our own true purpose, that we may all experience a deep appreciation for this role; and may this understanding guide us in our service to the child's unfolding and our own unfolding.

The Role of Grandparents

Grandparents are a gift to children from the Divine. In a magical, mystical way, grandparents are among a family's greatest treasures. They provide the lineage and generational support for a strong family foundation. This special love relationship enlivens the fun of growing up for children, and allows a family to maintain a close heart connection.

Grandparents are the carriers of life secrets that parents may not yet know. These secrets have come to them through direct experience over time, and from oral tradition. Children benefit greatly from the love and understanding of grandparents, who provide depth and comforting clarity in a rather confusing world.

Grandparents have the special advantage of being free to love and befriend their grandchildren without taking daily responsibility for them. They are able to gently, lovingly, magically, and spiritually bridge the gap between the generations. For this reason, grandparents have the opportunity to become unique educators.

In sum, grandparents have the potential to be subtle family heroes, as necessary for a child's growth as all levels of physical nutrition. Conscious grandparents naturally create a holistic body, mind, and soul setting for the fullest, optimal growth of their grandchildren.

A Grandfather's Prayer for the Newborn

You are my child. I have begotten you today.

—**Psalm 2:7**

Your birth is not an accident!

The moment of your birth is the beginning of your mission on Earth.

The Divine has chosen you to come into the world for a specific purpose.

This is the beginning of your personal mission. May you find, and thus be able to express, your sacred design.

You matter!

You are irreplaceable!

Every moment of your life gives meaning, and is precious.

The intention of the Divine is for you to reach your full potential and offer your sacred gift to the world.

May you may grow to deeply know your soul, which has incarnated with this birth, allowing you to become a full person.

May the entire world rejoice with the birth of a new world member.

May your parents feel the great joy of being blessed with a child.

May you, in time, also feel this joy.

May you be blessed with the joy of having entered this world.

You are blessed with the gift of a soul that is connected with the Divine.

May you always honor your soul connection to the Divine.

May you truly know in your life the greatness of your God-given soul, and may you truly live an alive life, attuned to the Divine.

Over your lifetime, may you consciously merge with the Divine in the inner and noncausal love, compassion, joy, peace, oneness, and ecstasy of liberation.

—Rabbi Gabriel Cousens, MD

A Grandfather's Blessing for the Youth

May the natural rebellious energies of your youth empower you to overturn the comfort zone of the status quo of materialistic futility into a sublime life of dancing in the Divine.

May you have the awareness that you have such a choice.

May you be blessed with the need to create for yourself a world and life of meaning.

May you find the soul and willpower to transition into a spiritually fruitful life as you enter adulthood.

As you move into adulthood, may you retain the awareness of the raw power and eternal light of your soul moving through you.

May you be blessed in your hunger for meaning so that you understand the spiritual nature of this hunger.

You are involved in a spiritual war between light and dark for your very soul; may you take on the spiritual "weapons" of love, peace, compassion, prayer, meditation, and spiritual endurance, in your quest to choose and maintain a higher purpose in your life.

May you use the raw power of youthful energy for good, moral, and ethical evolutionary needs, and create a revolution, returning to virtue and integrity in everyday life.

May you lead a successful revolution against your own hypocrisy and tendency toward ungrounded, idealistically driven acts of injustice and intolerance.

May you be blessed to take the full power and meaning of your youth into your blossoming into a full human being that walks the earth with consciousness and living experience of mitakuye oyasin—Lakota for "all my relations"—honoring the rock people, sprouting ones, walking, flying, and swimming ones, and the talking ones with written history.

In honoring all your relations, you naturally learn to honor yourself, your family, and all of humanity.

—Rabbi Gabriel Cousens, MD

CHAPTER 2

Creating an Alive Environment

The little child unconsciously imitates everything that streams toward him from his environment, and the impressions thus received work back upon his body functioning: breath, digestion, circulation, and the body building process itself.... A harsh, discordant, loveless, or even skeptical environment produces a slight freezing and congestion, prelude to physical or moral weakness in later life; a warm, gentle, loving and harmonious environment releases forces and quickens courage for life in years to come.

—Francis Edmunds, in Rudolf Steiner's
Gift of Education: The Waldorf Schools

You cannot teach a child any more than you can grow a plant.

—Swami Vivekananda, in his treatise on education

Just as the remarkable divine plan tucked within a tiny seed can be helped along with the right proportions of water, sunlight, soil pH, compost, etc., we can see that the luminous potential within each child is nourished with love, nutrient-dense food, opportunities for creative expression, and self-esteem-building parent-child interactions. And, as we all know yet often find challenging in practice, it is the environment surrounding the child that teaches the most, rather than what we say—no matter how loudly it is said.

A popular beginning-reader book for children called *Frog and Toad Together*, by Arnold Lobel, illustrates this point lightheartedly. It begins with the character Toad, who is planting his first garden. Shortly after the seeds are in the ground, Toad sees that the seedlings haven't yet come up, so he instructs the seeds to "Start growing." As this does not produce results, he tries raising his voice, commanding, "Now, seeds, start growing!"

Toad continues to yell at the seeds until his good friend Frog comes along and tells him, "You are shouting too much. These poor seeds are afraid to grow. Leave them alone for a few days, and let the sun shine on them. Soon your seeds will start to grow." So Toad alters his approach. He sings songs, reads poetry, and plays music to his seeds to help them stop being afraid to grow. In the end, the seedlings do grow according to their own timing, and Toad is pleased with the fruits of his rigorous labors of love (a.k.a. learning how to get out of the way).

Historically, we can see this same story played out in the evolution of education. Maria Montessori (1870–1952), for example, the first female Italian medical doctor, who also became a childhood-development scientist, is credited with making a profound discovery that turned the schooling system of her time on its head. Dr. Montessori reported that this discovery, which created a worldwide stir, took her too by surprise. What Montessori accidentally discovered was the normal characteristics of childhood, in contrast to deviant characteristics that the adults of her day mistook to be the inherent nature of the child.

Under optimal environmental conditions designed to support the holistic development of the child into a healthy human being—children exhibit healthy evolutionary characteristics such as deep concentration, self-discipline, spontaneous joy, social cohesion, a sense of dignity, and a love for order, silence, and work. In Montessori's day, describing schoolchildren with these attributes was completely unheard-of, and word spread quickly of the miraculous appearance of the "new child." By carefully observing children and thus seeing their healthy unfolding, Montessori sought to match the children's environment to the specific and general needs of human development, and saw that deviations from healthy childhood such as restlessness, inability to concentrate, aggression, and depression, as well as physical symptoms, began to naturally disappear.

Today we are seeing an alarming number of physical, mental, and behavioral childhood disorders. The spirituality of the child cannot help but be affected by this. We are now witnessing the ramifications of a society whose primary goal is to be industrially productive. This, at its worst, creates a culture of death, a culture that puts money, wealth, power, and materialism at the center of one's life rather than the Divine, spiritual evolution, and creative living as a full human being. If we are blessed with the discrimination to see this for what it is, we can choose to embrace an alternative experience, a culture of life and liberation strengthened by an alive environment for ourselves and our children.

What is an alive environment? It is a cultural atmosphere that supports the divine journey of human development—the unfoldment of our full potential for knowing and being the divine experience we are uniquely meant to be.

What does an alive environment look like? The specific form may vary from one family or education support team to another, because the culture of life and liberation is not limited to one specific religion, pedagogy, parenting approach, or educational method. At the same time, these tools or metaphors can lead us to our own aliveness; these are therefore likely to be a part of our supportive environment.

In this book we will be presenting Six Foundations for Spiritual Life (which are also foundations for an alive environment) and the Sevenfold Peace, all of which are universal to the human experience. We will present these foundations as optimal lifestyle support for the parent's unfolding aliveness, and the rest of the book will be devoted to the support of the alive child by using these same universal foundations to provide alive environmental conditions for our time.

Creating an Alive Environment for the Parent

> When we're on an airplane and flight attendants are instructing us on emergency procedures, we are always told that before you put your child's oxygen mask on, you put yours on first. It makes perfect sense. How can you look after your child if you can't breathe yourself? The same holds true for all the other things we do as a parent.
>
> —Barbara Desmarais, in *The Parenting Coach: Raise Your Child Without Raising Your Voice*

The first step in preparing an alive environment for the child is the building of an alive environment for the parents. For conscious childrearing, we need to first be open to receiving aliveness so that we can be equipped to give in this way. All of us have probably either experienced or witnessed parents burning out by denying their own needs for the sake of the children, which can more easily happen in child-centered parenting. Not only does this result in the depletion of what a parent has to give to the child, it may also inadvertently teach children that only their own needs matter.

Similarly, we run into problems if we attempt to meet the needs of the self through the child, or otherwise at the expense of the child, as can also easily happen with parent-centered parenting. Our children's lives do enhance our own spiritual development, but in order to maintain balance we need to go to our own Divine Source for replenishment and renewal.

As the adults, we are the ones who set the stage for vitality, love, or disharmony in the home. We set ourselves up for one or the other, and our children take their cues from us. If we live our lives with the Divine at the center rather than our ego (career, house and accessories, parties, entertainment, addictions, retirement, emotions, or even children), then our kids will receive what their souls cry out for most—a living example of how to stay connected with one's own divinity, and thus remain fully alive.

As we have all probably noticed, the path of human adventure is riddled with pitfalls. This is why an effective system of support is such a tremendous blessing! The following six foundations for spiritual life have been developed by one of this book's authors, Rabbi Gabriel Cousens, MD, MD(H), DD, Diplomate in Ayurveda, and Diplomate of the American Board of Holistic Medicine, psychiatrist, and family therapist, who has been acknowledged as having attained the highest goal of yoga by his two liberated teachers, Swami Muktananda and Swami Prakashananda. These foundations are practical ways to live out the ancient Kabbalistic teaching to *receive in order to share*. Or, as a kindergartener once emphatically put it while on the playground with her playmate, "Don't you see? It's all about sharing!"

Six Foundations for a Spiritual Life

1. SPIRITUAL NUTRITION

Spiritual nutrition includes: 1) A plant-sourced, organic, vegan, 80% live-food, highly mineralized, moderate- to low-sugar, high-hydration diet, individualized to one's unique constitution and prepared with love; and 2) spiritual fasting, primarily with a green vegetable juice rather than water or a dry fast. By live food, we mean organically grown plant-source-only food that is still alive because it has been prepared at a temperature below 118°.

Living-nutrition and spiritual-fasting workshops are available for adults at the Tree of Life Center U.S. While living foods provide optimal nutrition for childhood, which we will soon explore further, we do not recommend fasting for pre-pubescent children.

Living-food books, websites, films, recipes, coaching, chef services, classes, retreats, restaurants, potluck groups, and food products can be found in the "Resources" section (page 485) for additional live-food lifestyle support.

2. BUILDING LIFE-FORCE ENERGY

Yoga *asanas, pranayama* (breathing practices), the *ophanim* (the energetics of the Hebrew letters), t'ai chi, qigong, *vaastu* (sacred architecture), feng shui, sacred dance, and other energy practices enhance and expand the consciousness of the body-mind, filling it with increased life-force energy, also known as *prana, chi,* or *nefesh.*

3. SERVICE *(SHERUT)* AND CHARITY *(TZEDAKAH)*

In the process of service and charity, we are able to face our attachments to things and to feel our heart connection to the whole family of life (humanity, animals, and ecology) or, as the Native Americans say it, "to all my relations"—*mitakuye oyasin.* This helps to expand consciousness through direct experience.

As parents serving the vital needs of our children, service and charity are already somewhat built into our lives. Consider also the relationship-enhancing effect of a community-service project for the family. With younger children, this could be dog-walking together at the local animal shelter, weeding an elderly neighbor's garden, or cleaning up litter in a favorite natural habitat. Getting involved with bigger-scale local and global projects, such as joining up with a service group like Habitat for Humanity, can be meaningful experiences for families with teens. Service opportunities can provide positive role models for the child, strengthen self-confidence, and nurture a sense of purpose and fulfillment. According to The Search Institute, an organization dedicated to discovering what kids need to succeed, youth who volunteer just one hour a week are fifty percent less likely to abuse drugs, alcohol, or cigarettes, or engage in otherwise destructive behavior.[1] Reaching out to others beyond one's own family helps all members attain a broader perspective.

4. SPIRITUAL GUIDANCE AND INSPIRATION
FROM A SPIRITUAL TEACHER

People at every level benefit from teachers. Our parents are our first teachers. Being in the presence of an awakened teacher gives meaning, value, heart, and energy to spiritual wisdom teachings and spiritual life energetics. Spending time with spiritual people or community is part of expanding and refining the mind with teachings from great scriptures such as the Zohar, the Torah, the New Testament, the *Tao Te Ching,* the Vedas, or great mystery poetry such as that of Hafiz, Rumi, and Blake.

Wisdom literature helps formulate, focus, and expand our consciousness. Sacred music and spending time in nature are also part of this foundation. (See "Resources," page 485, for family-in-nature support.)

5. SACRED SILENCE

Meditation, prayer, repetition of a mantra *(hagia)* and chanting in the spiritual traditions elevate the awakening and nurturing power of family. In this context, children as young as three years old can be strengthened by sacred silence. According to Peggy Jenkins, PhD, in *The Joyful Child:*

> The stress of daily living can create a tremendous gap between what we know to do and what we actually do…. We often end up not modeling the best we know, and not showing the sensitivity and awareness that children need from us. The answer, we feel, lies in staying centered. Centering is an integration of mind and body that helps us develop a pool of inner stillness…. It is calming ourselves and turning inward. One way to get centered is through meditation.

Jenkins also quotes teacher Michael Nitai Deranja:

> It has been my experience that regular, deep periods of meditation provide the most direct means of effective teacher preparation, even taking precedence over time spent on lesson plans or background preparation.[2]

Family meditations can be powerful tools and experiences. We will discuss children and the role of silence and sacred music in "Supporting the Spirit of the Child with Silence" (page 354).

6. AWAKENING THE SACRED FEMININE

Kundalini is the energy of the sacred feminine that dwells within all of us. It is also known as *shekhinah, shakti,* the Holy Spirit, or the Divine Mother. The awakening of the sacred feminine is the awakening of the divine force that is resting in potential within us. This is known as "the descent of grace." It usually occurs through a living, enlightened, spiritual leader by touch, look, sound, or breath, but may occur spontaneously, such as during childbirth. Once the spiritual energy is activated, it begins to spontaneously move through our body, spiritualizing every cell, every aspect of the DNA, every subtle-energy vessel, every *chakra,* every *nadi* (channel of the subtle nervous system), every organ and every tissue, so that all consciousness becomes activated into the next evolutionary stage.

While it is fairly common to talk about holistic nutrition, yoga, spiritual teachers, and observation of silence, as well as service and charity, some readers may be less familiar with the awakening of the sacred feminine within all people. Teachings about this spiritually evolving energy are found in almost every culture or religion including Judaism, Christianity (such as on the day of Pentecost), Hinduism, Buddhism, and Native spirituality, and have been written about by Carl Jung. This awakening energy is a highly positive biological and spiritual process, marking a passage into the final stage of one's evolutionary development. More in-depth discussion is beyond the scope of this book, but this mystery is well explained in *Spiritual Nutrition* by Gabriel Cousens, MD.

The six foundations are not goals to be attained; rather, they are a way of life that creates *awakened normality* as a result of living in a natural way. When we plant, water, weed, and nourish seeds for Divine-merging and liberation throughout our daily lives, one happy day we see the sprouts of Divine awareness unfurling up from that fertile soil. In this way, we are like the wise gardener who, when complemented on the plants blossoming under his care, replies, "*I* didn't grow them." Spiritual growth cannot be forced, anymore than Toad could command his seeds to grow—but as on a fruitful plot of earth, it unfolds according to the plan of the seed, the potential within.

So it is with parenting. Try as we might, we cannot force our children to reach their full potential. Theirs is the life that they alone must live. The role of the parent is to prepare the most fertile soil and appropriately water the seedling so it can most fully blossom. When we construct our lives upon spiritual foundations, this naturally establishes greater balance in the home, creating an optimally supportive environment for the child's fullest Divine unfolding. The following passage expresses this beautifully:

There are many ways to get your children to behave as you wish. You can force, plead, and bribe. You can manipulate, trick, and persuade. You can use shame, guilt, and reason. These will all rebound upon you. You will be in constant conflict.

Attend instead to your own actions. Develop contentment within yourself. Find peace and love in all you do. This will keep you busy enough. There is no need to control others.

If you are able to release even some small part of your persistent need to control, you will discover an amazing paradox. The things you attempted to force now begin to occur naturally. People around you begin to change. Your children find appropriate behavior emerging from within themselves, and are delighted. Laughter returns to all.

—William Martin, in *The Parents'*
Tao Te Ching: Ancient Advice for Modern Parents

The Sevenfold Peace

1. PEACE WITH THE BODY

Peace with the body is experienced by creating an optimally functioning body, which allows us to manifest our optimal physical expression. It gives us the freedom to move in any direction, unburdened by self-made disease. It is part of the "alive" aspect of alive children.

2. PEACE WITH THE MIND

Peace with the mind is given major emphasis in this book because one cannot be alive and conscious mentally if one's brain and mind are malfunctioning due to physically, emotionally, and mentally toxic input. One of the most important roles of us parents is to both protect and optimize the functioning of our children's brains and minds.

3. PEACE WITH THE FAMILY

Peace in the family is the foundation of all interpersonal relations. It is where the capacity for intimacy is developed, which is the key to healthy, close, and loving relationships. Parents are children's primary role models for healthy intimacy. According to the Research of Dr. Innes Pearse in her pioneering ten-year study, the physical and mental health of the child is directly related to the physical and emotional health of the family. In this way, a healthy family is the foundation of healthy children and a healthy society.

4. PEACE WITH COMMUNITY

Peace with community means peace within and among all units of society. A sustainable, healthy society has worked out the optimal relationship between the individual's freedom to become the divine expression they are meant to be and government support of that expression for everyone.

Unfortunately, in most societies today, that optimal balance seems to have been lost; but it can be regained in time as we develop more and more conscious, alive children who can address this spiritual (not political) question. In other words, we seek our unique role in a world in which our souls and visions are equal, even though they appear unequal since everyone has a unique soul mission. Peace with community comes when politics is in service to the spiritual uplifting of society and the individual.

5. PEACE WITH CULTURE

This kind of peace acknowledges the validity and balance of all levels of culture—including the rock people (the living Earth), the sprouting ones (vegetation), the walking, flying, and swimming ones (animal kingdom), and the talking ones with recorded history (humans). It is creating respect for all levels, as the Native American teaching says—*mitakuye oyasin*—"to all my relations." On the human level, it means not only respect but designing a world society where all cultures and religions allow and support all others to flourish, as long as they respect the others' right to exist.

6. PEACE WITH THE ECOLOGY

Peace with ecology means seeing ourselves not as stewards but as one with the living planet. It is a relationship of dominion, not domination. Our role in a dominion relationship is to support the elevation of all creation, the harmonious uplifting of the whole network of life on the planet. It is in this context that veganism has a most potent holistic and evolutionary meaning.

7. PEACE WITH THE DIVINE

Peace with the Divine comes when we realize our oneness with the Divine on every level of creation.

For further explanation of the Sevenfold Peace, Rabbi Gabriel has written an in-depth description, now in its second edition, called *Creating Peace by Being Peace: The Essene Sevenfold Path.*

Sevenfold Peace Family Activities

Foundational for teaching our children is to be the living example of what we aim to teach. Then we invite the children to participate in the daily rhythms of a culture of life. The following exercises are a prototype for ways to invite children's involvement. These examples are merely a starting point to developing activities of your own.

Lifestyle changes take time and practice. Allow these new ways to enter your life gently, joyfully, and consistently, at a pace that feels balanced rather than overwhelming. These exercises are not to be forced upon children, but presented in a way that appeals to them. While we seek to inspire rather than to dominate, there may be times, such as in the case of an illness, where we need to thoughtfully inform children that "our situation is showing us that this is what we must do." Before inviting their participation, carefully observe their level of readiness for the task. This will help to boost confidence, foster enjoyment, and avoid frustration.

1. PEACE WITH THE BODY

Keep a journal of the seven healers

The "seven healers" are: 1) living nutrition, 2) fresh air, 3) pure water, 4) sunlight, 5) exercise, 6) rest, and 7) emotional, mental, and spiritual harmony. Keep a journal that records your family's lifestyle changes, logging meals served, bedtimes, exercise, time outside, etc. Also record how everyone felt that day, both physically and emotionally. Look over your log at the end of the week, and talk with each other about any cause-and-effect connections that you may notice.

Share your experiences

When you exercise, or eat foods that help your body to feel "happy" or "alive," as well as unhealthy foods that make you feel "sluggish" or "yucky," say aloud what you are feeling, for the child's benefit. Letting your child in on the experience gives them information that will help interpret what their own body is communicating.

2. PEACE WITH THE MIND

Making silence—daily prayer and/or meditation

Prayer and meditation are foundational to the experience of peace with the mind. When your child shows the ability to sit still (generally as early as age three and up), invite him or her to make silence with you. This should always be a voluntary activity rather than mandatory. Just before bedtime is often best, because the child has had opportunity for activity and is winding down to transition into restful sleep. Explain to your child that you will be meditating, or making silence to quiet your mind, and ask if they would like to join you. Dim the lights, and tell your child that when a candle is lit, silence has begun.

Especially with the very young child, start with short lengths of time (such as five to fifteen minutes) and increase the duration as their readiness permits. Mark your calendar to participate in the global Peace Meditations on each solstice and equinox. Books to help the child get used to the idea of silence include: *I Want to Hear the Quiet* by Aline D. Wolf,

When I Make Silence by Jennifer Howard, *Another Way to Listen* by Byrd Baylor, and *A Handful of Quiet* by Thich Nhat Hanh. These and other books are available at www.MontessoriServices.com. The parenting book *Seven Times the Sun* by Shea Darian has a collection of songs for children about quietness, including music notation as well.

Walking labyrinths

Labyrinths date back to 15,000 years ago and are recognized as paths to wisdom and peace. If you have access to a walking labyrinth, walk it with your child. This is a calming activity that helps balance the right and the left hemispheres of the brain and body. If you do not have regular access to a walking labyrinth, consider creating a simple one outside your home or classroom. Tabletop labyrinths can also be traced with one's finger.

3. PEACE WITH FAMILY

Forgiveness lightens our load

Forgiveness is key to the ongoing expression of love that is foundational for peace within the family. The following activity lends a physical experience that is analogous to being unnecessarily weighed down by carrying what is unforgiven: When you are working around the yard or house, carry a bucket of soil or a laundry basket full of clothes, setting it down only to complete other tasks. Invite the child to do the same. When the child asks why you are doing this, or complains about the weight, explain that he or she is right to question this practice, and that making the choice not to forgive is much the same.

Make—and use!—a talking stick

Collect a stick and decorate it with other natural items such as beads, feathers (found on the ground, not commercial byproducts), a special stone, etc. While you are decorating the stick, say a prayer or an intention of peace. Use the talking stick during family meetings, handing the stick to the person whose turn it is to speak. This sends a clear message that everyone's voice counts.

Blessings

Before bed each night, say a blessing over each child and your relationship together. Continue to affirm these blessings verbally, nonverbally, and with your actions throughout the day.

Seek support

If an unresolved issue is greatly impacting peace in the family, find the support that you need from extended family, friends, community, and/ or professional counseling.

4. PEACE WITH THE ECOLOGY

Quality time in nature

Observe the phases of the moon with your child each month, stop to smell the roses together, and place your hands upon the ground to feel the Earth's nurturing energy.

Magical connection

Show your child pictures of human lungs and how they resemble trees, and pictures of how our veins resemble rivers and streams. Talk about the resemblance between rocks or crystals and our bones, and explain that what the trees breathe out, we breathe in, and vice-versa. Show your child how both our bodies and atlases of the Earth are mapped with meridians like those on an acupuncture chart. We are not *stewards* of the Earth; we are *part* of the Earth.

Literature

Check out books from your local library on ways that children can care for the Earth—composting, recycling, making reusable shopping bags, conserving water and electricity—and incorporate these solutions into your home. If the books do not include eating low on the food chain, discuss this solution together as well.

5. PEACE WITH THE COMMUNITY

Host an alive tea with friends

Plan a tea party with your child in which your favorite healthy foods are served. Talk about compassion for all people no matter what they eat (sometimes a very young child can think a person is bad because they eat poorly), and about what it means to be a leader. Delight with your child in positive responses from their peers, and talk together about any negative reactions: How do they make you both feel, and do either of you have any ideas of how to handle it lovingly?

Find volunteer opportunities

Seek out ways to participate in volunteer activities with your child in your local community.

Life of service

When your child helps out around the house, point out how, thanks to them, the whole family has benefited. Talk about meaningful work outside the home (what they might want to do when they grow up) and how some roles uplift the whole while others may produce a paycheck but cause problems for the community, whether local or global.

Make a "caring can"

Recycle an old container and decorate it as a colorful bank. Invite your child to choose from a few nonprofit organizations and discuss their work and why they need contributions. Add money to this bank, and let your child know that they are free to give as well.

6. PEACE WITH CULTURE

In addition to sharing stories from your own culture and spiritual path, incorporate stories from wisdom traditions all around the world in your read-aloud time together (examples are the *Buddha at Bedtime* books, Native American legends, or Judeo-Christian teachings for children). This nurtures an awareness that differing cultural traditions point to many of the same teachings. The golden rule—"Do unto others as you would have them do unto you"—for example, can be found in most of the world's religions. Seek out music and other art forms from various cultures and historical time periods.

Make a point to interact with people, whether a neighbor or another family from the playground or school, with diverse ages, cultures, ethnicities, religions, and languages.

7. PEACE WITH THE DIVINE

Peace with the Divine is unique to each individual and each family. Whatever your tradition, invite your child to participate in your spiritual community through meaningful ceremony, inspirational songs, books, and other spiritually focused media. Look for opportunities to weave prayer and blessing into your daily family rhythm, such as your time of meal preparations, before eating, after eating, before bed, upon waking, before you drive your car, when you part for the day, or in notes or text messages. Offer blessings or set intentions during special occasions such as moving into a new home, welcoming a new family member, holidays, and birthdays. Post prayers, scripture verses, and/or spiritual quotes around the house. Live in such a way that your home is imbued with your commitment to peace with the Divine.

Supporting the Alive Child's Stages of Development

Now that we've looked at building a foundation of nourishment, renewal, core-strength, and inspiration for the parent, we'll delve deeper into the developmental needs of childhood. Although both parent and child share the same general soul-purpose, understanding that this unfolds according to different stages or rhythms in our lives is key. When we really "get" that children are not merely miniature adults but are in a continual maturation process, we can offer much greater support for their experience.

An obvious example of this is how an infant's digestive system develops over time. Their food sources need to match their younger physiology, rather than starting on grownup foods. A less obvious example is the two-year-old who may need to assert choices that oppose her parent's will—not because she doesn't want the bedtime story or dessert being offered, but because she is just starting to see herself as being separate from others and needs to have the experience of exercising her own will. After she has satisfied this age-appropriate, ego-development need of choice, she may then want the story or treat after all.

Similarly, the very young child who is beginning to grasp the relationship of cause and effect may benefit most from the adult stating simply, calmly, and clearly what is happening in this regard. "When we hit, there is no play" may be more effective than going into diplomatic negotiations that may be well-intentioned but require more advanced thinking skills than the child is ready for.

Education innovators such as Rudolf Steiner (founder of the Waldorf Schools and biodynamic farming) and Dr. Maria Montessori have metaphorically likened the child's stages of growth to the metamorphosis of a caterpillar into a butterfly. These sequential phases are very distinct, almost as if we are witnessing the unfolding of a new creature from one period of growth to the next. As Montessori noted, this is significantly different from the development of the oak tree, which grows by simply getting bigger.[3]

Montessori observed four specific stages marking a child's developmental journey, noted the qualities and needs of the growing child during each stage, and organized them by age accordingly. With the understanding that the unborn child is sharing the mother's experience, for example, we can aim to support all mothers in healthy thought and lifestyle choices. This is the first stage.

When we consider a baby's experience of childbirth, we can be sensitive to this major transition by welcoming him into a warm, natural, quiet, dimly lit, and otherwise tranquil environment, rather than treating an impressionable infant as if he has already experienced loud noises, bright lights, cool temperatures, restrictive clothing, invasive medical procedures, and unnatural settings.

With the understanding that the child age zero to three is unconsciously taking in his surroundings without the ability to filter out stimuli, we can also take greater care to provide natural, peaceful, and affirming stimuli. When we realize the highly significant role that movement plays in this second stage of development, as it is instrumental in moving from unconscious into conscious, we can minimize restrictions to the child's movements such as playpens, strollers, walkers, baby swings, etc., and set aside time to go for walks at the child's pace.

During the third stage of development (age three to six), we see children refining their movements and wanting to be helped to do things by themselves.

In the fourth stage, from age six to twelve, we see children entering into greater social collaboration and a place of greater developmental stability. This is a time when we can appreciate their emphasis on justice, as they are now really grappling with this concept. We are empowered to understand rather than judge when children may also be inclined to vocalize their own accomplishments at this stage of life.

In adolescence, which is the fifth stage (ages twelve to eighteen), we can appreciate that although children may take on the appearance of adults, because of the significant physical, emotional, mental, and spiritual changes they are undergoing, teenage years are a less stable time. During this stage they tend to be very sensitive to any form of criticism, yet may not yet be aware of their own negativities and judgments. This is also a time when heavy academic pressure may not be as beneficial to the child as hands-on character-building community service projects.

In the work of renowned psychologist Erik H. Erikson (1902–94), a student of Maria Montessori, we see a continuation of these stages into adulthood. In the Steiner model of human development, we see an observance of seven-year cycles. Steiner described cosmic energies that support the human journey with specific energetic themes in each cycle from age seven into adulthood. In the contemporary work of Pamela Levin, there are seven stages of growth accompanied by supportive affirmations specific to each of these times in the child's life, as well as for the adult years of integrating the experiences of childhood.

From birth to six months, for example, is a key time for adults to affirm, "We're glad you're here, because this is where you belong." From six to eighteen months, we want to send the consistent message: "When you explore and experiment, we will protect and support you." From eighteen months to three years, we affirm, "We are glad you're starting to think for yourself," and "You can say 'no' and push the limits as much as you need to, and we will keep you and others safe as you do so." From age three to six, the message is: "We delight in your discoveries." From age six to thirteen it is: "You can be responsible for your own needs, feelings, and behaviors, and still ask for our support," etc.

In Levin's work, we see what all of these human-development researchers have pointed to: The human journey is a spiraling cycle, coming back around to the same themes, each time with ever-greater expansion and understanding, in contrast to a linear timeline or stages through which we pass, never to visit again.

Understanding that there are "normal" stages of human development can guide us in how we support our children with living nutrition as well. With the understanding that the first five years of development are pivotal for laying the foundation for the rest of the child's life, we can see the tremendous value of the parents' personal healing on all levels prior to conception. With the understanding that our toddlers and pre-schoolers have a different and more impressionable and programmable mind than the adult mind, we can serve our children by protecting them from the commercial influences that seek to make a profit off of their vulnerability.

We can also create the foundation for healthy dietary and lifestyle patterns for the young child at this stage in order to protect them from cultural food addictions and patterns that have a high probability of creating chronic disease. Later in life, the child will be ready to make mature food decisions for themselves, guided by the foundation we have created. As Kelly Dorfman, MS, LND, points out in her book *What's Eating Your Child?: The Hidden Connections Between Food and Childhood Ailments,* brain research now indicates that the prefrontal cortex, which helps us to connect our actions with consequences, is not fully developed until the late teens or early twenties.[4] Dorfman confesses that if she were unable to connect the experience of ill health with the food that she eats, and therefore made dietary decisions based on taste alone, she would be eating ice cream for breakfast, lunch, and dinner!

As it stands today (in 2015), twenty percent of American children are obese. Because children are still developing food awareness, they need our positive help with welcoming new taste experiences and developing healthy eating habits, just as they need our help in learning to brush their teeth and to understand other safety issues. When children are raised on vegan, organic, living foods, their taste buds seem to be more trained to appreciate diverse and vibrant flavors and textures. Likewise, as we transition from processed foods to organic, whole and vegan, living foods, our taste preferences also begin to change. For example, we begin to experience white flour as lacking in flavor, and begin to receive great pleasure from eating fresh, ripe fruits and veggies.

As our children grow and begin to express an interest in justice, we can also support them with an education about how animals are enslaved in order to harvest their life-force energy. We can teach them about the hogging of global resources by animal-based eating habits. (See "Resources," page 485, for educational media on this subject.) For teens who might be dealing with concerns over weight gain, acne, or other body issues due to hormonal changes, we can sensitively offer an alternative to unhealthy food patterns and harmful pharmaceuticals that may support those patterns. As this age is emotionally more delicate, it may be helpful to be less direct with our guidance, and wait until we've been asked (directly or indirectly) before giving advice. As Steiner noted, this is also a time when the child delights in ideas and ideals. Adults who are a living example of the culture of life can thus be a profound inspiration to teens as they learn to make life-affirming choices.

In the human developmental journey, we arrive from that which is prior to consciousness. Through the experiences of physical life, which include ego development, we become more and more conscious of the Oneness from which we've come, and eventually cast off the chrysalis-like restrictions of the ego to enter into a love of the Divine and Divine-merged states of expression.

The metaphor of transformation deepens as we consider how a butterfly needs to struggle for its ability to fly. If the chrysalis is broken by someone in an attempt to help free the butterfly, its wings will be shriveled and immobile. This is because the effort that it takes to pass through the small opening is the very thing needed to force fluid from the body of the butterfly into the wings, preparing it for flight. So it is with our children's developmental journeys—we can offer a loving example, guidance, affirmation, and other forms of support, but setting themselves free like the butterfly is *their* evolutionary work, guided by the hand of grace.

CHAPTER 3

Supporting the Child's Physical Development

Blessed is the Child of Light who is strong in body,
For he shall have oneness with the Earth...
He who hath found peace with the body
Hath built a holy temple
Wherein may dwell forever
The spirit of God.

—Essene Gospel of Peace, Book 2

Living Foods for the Living Body

If there is one thing that will significantly change your child's enjoyment of food and the nutritional benefit that they get from the food—it is always fresh. There is no substitute for it. Any time that you can go fresh, do it.

—Tammy Algood, MS, Food Marketing Specialist, UT Extension, as featured on Nashville Public Television Report "Children's Health Crisis: Grocery-Store Shopping"

Why treat your child with drugs when you can cure your child with food?

—Kelly Dorfman, MS, LND,
in *What's Eating Your Child?*

Let food be thy medicine.

—Hippocrates, Father of Medicine

We live in a world where the health of children and adults is rapidly degenerating. According to a CDC and Health Resources Services Administration paper, one in six American children suffer from a developmental disability as of 2008; and the rate of parent-reported developmental disabilities in children increased 17% from 1997 to 2008, to 1 in 68 over a twelve-year period.[1] The first question is, "What is going on?" The bigger question is, "What can I, as a parent or grandparent, do about it?"

In 1990 the rate of autism was 1 in 10,000. Now, according to the CDC, the rate of autism is 1 in 68,[2] and for boys the rate is 1 in 42.[3] Autism reflects a problem that all children are facing. It seems to be a multi-factored problem related simultaneously to environmental pollution, poor nutrition, vaccinations, radiation exposure, and a variety of emotional and environmental stresses. Autism represents the extreme result of a synergy of toxic forces affecting our children and grandchildren.

As we look at the bigger picture, we begin to see a rather disturbing pattern of extraordinarily increased environmental toxicity, radiation exposure, and toxic emotional and physical forces, resulting in toxic health effects such as cancer rates. It is amazing that acute lymphoblastic leukemia (ALL) is the leading cause of death, aside from accidents, in children ages five to fourteen.[4] The leading nonaccidental cause of death amongst teenagers, aside from suicide—which has increased threefold—is, again, cancer. This is totally unnatural and counter to the order of life.

In looking at the whole picture, we see that each generation is given the medicine for that generation. The medicine for the current generation and for the future is holistic, live-food veganism. An organic, live-food, holistic vegan diet (comprising at least 80% live food) and lifestyle is best for helping curtail this progressive multigenerational disease disaster.

However, we have to ask another social-based question: "Is a live-food vegan diet safe?" In answering it, we need to get away from the extreme fear-mongering perpetuated by so-called experts who base their criticisms on extreme vegan/live-food diets that cause imbalances and have not been particularly successful except for a minority. These red-herring arguments are equivalent to citing omnivores living on an exclusive diet of junk food, white flour, white sugar, synthetic substances, and processed foods as exemplifying the health problems of an omnivore diet.

To consider these imbalanced diets to be the mainstream reality of a live-food vegan diet is a very cynical, biased perspective. The diet we are talking about is a science-based, holistic, live-food, organic, vegan diet organized according to one's constitution, age, and environment— nutritionally adequate, with sufficient water, and high in minerals. This science-based holistic diet works ninety-nine percent of the time when intelligently applied; it is a diet already successfully followed by many people.

We are not talking about an extreme diet advocated by an extreme minority. The world-famous pediatric authority Dr. Benjamin Spock, in the second edition of *Baby and Child Care* (May 1998), recommended a vegan diet. By 1998, Dr. Spock was scientifically concerned that a diet rich in animal products and dairy fat would lead to chronic adult diseases such as diabetes, heart disease, cancer, arthritis, Alzheimer's disease, and premature death—and his concerns were indeed well-founded. Dr. Spock's vegan position highlights a very important principle: We are talking about not simply a diet for children, but setting the foundation of a healthy diet for the rest of the child's and emerging adult's life.

Dietary patterns are set at a very early age—somewhere between four and eight years old. The research shows that children who have established a healthy diet are healthier in the longer range and less likely to develop cancer, heart disease, stroke, diabetes, and obesity. It's ironic that those who attack a vegan diet by cynically citing extreme dysfunctional examples of poor and ignorant application of the diet, which can create malnutrition by ignoring scientific principles, consistently miss the crucial larger picture of creating a wise, scientifically based, vegan (plant-source-only) diet that supports long-term good health.

Childhood and adult obesity, not malnutrition, are a real pandemic problem. Being overweight is defined as up to twenty pounds beyond a normal weight for one's height, and obesity as twenty to thirty or more. In 2011 and 2012, nearly 35% of U.S. adults (78.6 million) were obese.[5] The prevalence of childhood obesity in the U.S. also remains high. (However, among children two to five years old, obesity has declined, according to CDC's National Health and Nutrition Examination Survey [NHANES].) Obesity among young people age two to nineteen years has not changed significantly since 2003–2004, and still occurs in about 17% of the childhood population (12.7 million children).

The prevalence of obesity in children and adolescents shows significant racial and age disparities. In 2011–2012, obesity was far higher among Hispanics (22.4%) and non-Hispanic black youth (20.2%) than non-Hispanic white youth (14.1%). The prevalence of obesity was lower in non-Hispanic Asian youth (8.6%). In 2011–2012, 8.4% of two- to five-year-olds were obese, compared with 17.7% of six- to eleven-year-olds and 20.5% of twelve- to nineteen-year-olds.[6]

These so-called critics also miss "the cow in the living room" as evidenced by a skyrocketing increase in type 2 diabetes in children. During 2008–2009, an estimated 18,436 people per year under age twenty in the United States were newly diagnosed with type 1 diabetes, and 5,089 were newly diagnosed with type 2 diabetes.[7] The pandemic of obesity, type 2 diabetes, and cancer in childhood and teen years are all major chronic degenerative diseases that a science-based organic, vegan, live-food diet (with no components of dairy, eggs, fish, chicken, or meat) significantly prevents.

The Vegan, Live-Food Solution Is Safe

Research initiated by Gabriel Cousens, MD, MD(H), DD, and completed by Philip and Susan Madeley, MA, graduates of Cousens' School of Holistic Wellness, involving 119 vegan children, whose diets comprised an average of 80% live food and 20% vegan cooked food, suggests that a vegan, live-food diet is quite safe. Their vegan parents who ate approximately 80% live food had newborns with an average in the upper 58th percentile for weight. These newborns were in the upper 88th percentile for length, and their body mass index (BMI, comparing weight to height) was in the upper 71st percentile.

Although height, weight, and BMI do not entirely define health status, they are strong indicators of normal growth and development—indisputable, concrete correlations between a live-food vegan cuisine and general health. We have a most objective basis for discussion about how live-food and vegan children are doing compared to the U.S. and world population (per World Health Organization data). The upper-percentile birth weights, heights, and BMIs for newborns clearly indicate that women with an 80% live-food vegan diet bring forth very healthy, above-average babies in the overall upper third percentile of BMI.

It must also be noted that, based on Dr. Gabriel's forty years of clinical impressions, the occurrence of colds, flu, earaches, asthma, tonsillitis, allergies, and general immune weakness is also significantly less for children on an 80% or greater live-food vegan diet.

The study was continued to include babies from ages one to ten months on a spectrum from plant-source-only cooked food to up to 80% live vegan food. Again, these infants compared well to omnivorous infants both in the U.S. and worldwide. The babies who lived on an 80% live-food vegan diet ranked high compared to the general population. Their weight was in the 83rd percentile; their height was in the 86th percentile; and their BMI was in the 67th percentile. These basic growth data, again, strongly indicate that the 80% live-food vegan diet provided excellent support to the development and growth process from age one to ten months. Most of those mothers were breastfeeding, which also speaks to the nutritional quality of the breast milk. These high scores were obtained even though, in general, breastfed children temporarily have normal dips in their growth curves at this age. Fifty-two children were also followed from the ages of one to four years. Again, on a spectrum from a cooked vegan diet to an 80% live-food vegan diet, their weight increased to the 94th percentile (the top 6%).

This kind of study is far more meaningful than simply focusing on nonthriving children on nonsupplemented, imbalanced fruitarian or macrobiotic diets, and then generalizing that these exceptions represent all vegan and/or live-food children. We are not even talking about a science-based, holistic, supplemented, vegan, live-food diet, which provides another level-up in nutritional power.

At four years of age, these children's height was in the 65th percentile, and their BMI was in the 67th percentile. These are strong scores that indicate a better than normal growth and development. Based on this research, it is safe to conclude that these vegan and/or live-food children were at least in the top third of the U.S. child population in basic physical development. Although 119 children is a modestly small sample, it is the only evidence available on the topic. Many of the other opinions on this topic seemed to be based on fear, biases of the dominant omnivore culture, and social myth. We would love to do a much larger study, but it is hard to get parents to go public because of their concerns about the threatening biases of most public agencies against vegan and live-food children.

We can comfortably and scientifically say, with the only study available, that vegan, live-food babies, at least until the first four years (the limits of this study), stay in the top third of the general population in height, weight, and BMI. It's interesting that this population is heavier than the average population, where children are eating junk food, meat, etc.—an obesity-causing diet. This even more strongly indicates the efficacy of the diet in supporting children's growth.

Our data was compared to populations analyzed by the CDC and WHO. The American Dietetic Association has said that vegetarian children and adults obtain twice the amount of adequate protein for one's daily needs.[8] Harvard researchers have stated that it is difficult for a vegetarian to move into protein deficiency if they avoid an excess of fruit and sweets—which is also advised by an intelligent, science-based diet. *The Lancet,* a renowned British medical journal, stated that vegetarian protein is no longer considered second-class; vegetarian protein is actually safer and healthier than meat protein, and less likely to cause insulin resistance. If one tends to eat junk food, one will have an inadequate diet whether vegan, vegetarian, or omnivorous. But it is virtually impossible not to get enough protein if one eats enough healthy, natural, whole, unrefined foods.

When we look at all the data, the key is to eat a diet of healthy, organic, micronutrient-concentrated whole foods, high in vegetables and some fruits. In the twenty percent of the diet that is cooked, we include beans and legumes, which are a good source of protein. Additionally, vegans have concentrated protein available in spirulina, chlorella, and blue-green algae, and nuts and seeds and their concentrates. The proteins in meat, fish, and chicken are, respectively, 16%, 17%, and 18% assimilable, while protein in eggs is 44% assimilable. It is important to note that many children are allergic to eggs, and all blood types show some immune reaction to eggs.

Spirulina, chlorella, and blue-green algae are 95% assimilable, so vegans have no problem finding an adequate protein source. Their diet provides adequate protein, micronutrients, healthy carbohydrates, and healthy raw, plant-based fat. Cooked fats, trans fats (which are cooked, hydrogenated, and processed at high temperatures) and animal fats have been shown to be unhealthy, and are precursors for heart disease and cancer. In the big picture, a diet that supports thriving in utero through age four, successfully protected from chronic disease and safe in adulthood, will also be safe and supportive of thriving from the ages of four through teenage years, with age-appropriate adjustments.

The use of some superfoods commonly found in the live-food movement has a significant positive effect on both the mental and physical states. Between June and December, 1994, an interesting study was done in Nicaragua on first-, second-, and third-grade children in Nandiame,

Nicaragua, in conjunction with the Central American University.[9] In Nicaragua, as in two-thirds of the population of Central America, malnutrition is a serious health problem. It is associated with high rates of poor health, and mortality due to infectious disease. Malnutrition in children directly affects learning, school behavior, and academic achievement, as well as appropriate socialization.

In this exploration, children were given *Aphanizomenon flos-aquae* (AFA), a blue-green algae from Klamath Lake in Oregon. The sample group had 111 children, who were particularly selected for their deteriorated physical appearance, disheartened behavior, and origin in families of low socioeconomic background. They were given one gram of AFA five days per week, both at home and at school, for a period of six months. These children experienced significant changes in their nutritional status.

At the beginning of the six months, only 14% were found to have a normal nutritional status, but after six months of eating the algae, 79% were considered to have a normal nutritional status. At the beginning of the study, 86% of the children were found to be malnourished; after six months that had dropped to 21%—a fourfold improvement in nutrition amongst children who took AFA blue-green algae for six months.

It was clinically observed that the children's hair, skin, eyes, and mouth showed considerable improvement over the six months. Ninety-seven percent of the children in the AFA blue-green algae program were found to have normal hair, compared to 75% at the beginning of the study. Twenty-seven percent of the children had paleness and skin problems. After six months, there was a 100% improvement, after which no children had any skin problems. Twenty-nine percent of the children had conjunctiva in poor condition. This decreased over the course of six months to 3.6%, showing an 87% improvement. Eight-one percent of the children showed a normal overall rating at the beginning of the study, compared with 98% six months later.[10]

Change in behavior patterns and school attendance also reflected this shift in nutritional profile. Seventy-two percent of the children had "good" or "excellent" school attendance (zero to three absences per month) when the study began. This increased to ninety-five percent "excellent" school attendance by the end of the study. The percentage of children with "unsatisfactory" attendance (four or more monthly absences) dropped to a quarter of that number, from 28% to 7%.

There was considerable improvement in behavior as well. The number of children who initially showed hyperactive behavior and were not participating in class was 45%. This decreased to 13% after six months. The percentage of those who initially had been "passive" in class dropped to one-third of previous levels, from 36% to 12%. The percentage of children who were "active" in class was initially 11%, and this increased fivefold to 56% by the end of the study. Those who were initially described as "passive" and who increased their participation during this program more than doubled, from 10% to 21%.

Academic performance also significantly improved. At the outset of the study, 52% of the group was evaluated academically as "unsatisfactory" to "fair," with grades scored from 0–69. By the end of the study, the size of this poorly performing group had dropped from 52% to 20% of the total. At the beginning of the study, 48% of the group tested as "good" or "excellent," and by the end of the study, this group had grown to 80%, which includes children scoring 90–100. The number of students scoring 90–100 tripled in size throughout the course of the study, increasing from 7% to 21% of the total.[11]

There was also a control group of 111 children who were not taking the AFA blue-green algae. The percentage of these children who achieved "good" or "excellent" school performance rating dropped from 70% to 58% during the correlative six-month period. Those who initially showed an "unsatisfactory" school performance increased from 14% to 20%.[12]

The power of these high-quality vegan proteins appears to tremendously affect the physical, emotional, mental, and academic health of children. The blue-green algae *Aphanizomenon flos-aquae* improved the status of the Nicaraguan children by reducing malnutrition. This happened by taking one gram a day, which is close to half a teaspoon. School attendance, attitude, and participation changed dramatically in a positive way. Negative clinical signs and malnutrition were dramatically reduced.

Children were ill less frequently, became more interested in academic studies, and improved in school attendance.[13]

As demonstrated by the Nicaraguan study, vegan, live-food children have very high-quality protein available to them that can significantly improve, with small amounts, their physical, emotional, mental, and academic functioning. Those mothers who had taken blue-green algae during pregnancy reported feeling that their children's clarity of mind and IQ were positively impacted compared to other children, although this is anecdotal and not clinically documented. One gram of blue-green algae daily seems to be a good, simple, super-nutritional protein source.

There are clearly some potential deficiencies we need to consider in a live-food, vegan diet. One of these is, of course, vitamin B12. In the vegan, live-food books *Conscious Eating* and *Spiritual Nutrition* by Gabriel Cousens, MD, it is made clear that there are no viable vegan sources of B12 that actually increase B12 levels in the blood.[14] It is thus very important that all vegan and live-food infants and children take a B12 supplement. We strongly recommend a living B12 supplement, derived from living bacteria. Based on Dr. Gabriel's forty years of clinical experience, we also strongly recommend, if you are not actively monitoring B12 levels, taking a B12 supplement derived from a raw-food concentrate. At the Tree of Life Center U.S. in Arizona, we carry two different living B12 sources.

In Dr. Gabriel's clinical practice, he finds that not only vegan children and adults but most omnivorous children and adults as well tend to be deficient in B12. At least 30–50% of adult omnivores do not have the minimum recommended blood level of B12, and the percentage of adults below the optimal B12 serum range is closer to 80%. There are many reasons for this increased deficiency in the general population. There is a greater need for B12 in an environment where toxins, lack of healthy gut flora, chlorinated water (which kills B12-producing bacteria), and antibiotics all disrupt normal colon flora. Various environmental and emotional stressors also create a need for this supplementation. All of these considerations make regular B12 supplementation for everyone a good and necessary idea.

Recent research has shown that optimal (not minimum) B12 blood levels are needed to decrease homocysteine, a toxin to the nervous and cardiovascular systems. The optimal blood level of active B12 is 400–450 nanograms of B12 per cc, while the recommended minimum daily blood level of B12 is 200 nanograms. To obtain optimal, biologically healthy levels, it is safest for all children and all adults to supplement their diets with B12. Vitamin B12 deficiencies in childhood are linked to stunted growth and abnormal neurodevelopment, which may not be reversible, according to the limited research available.

Vitamin D is another nutrient in which all children are potentially deficient. People promoting an omnivorous diet talk about a vitamin-D deficiency in vegans, but in the reality of a science-based discussion, according to the CDC's recent findings published in the *Journal of Pediatrics,* research between 2005 and 2006 estimated the average daily vitamin-D intake of U.S. infants was such that only 20–37% of formula-fed infants were getting the recommended 400 IU of vitamin D.[15]

All children are born without vitamin D. Among breastfed infants, only 5–13% were getting the recommended 400 IU of vitamin D. This is important, as all children less than one year old are deficient in vitamin D unless they live in the sun, and most children less than one year do not get adequate sunlight. About 50–85% of omnivore adults have less than the minimum vitamin D measurement of 30 milligrams in their blood. Again, we would recommend at a minimum that both formula-fed and breastfed infants get a vitamin D supplement of as much as 400 IU daily. Vitamin D is essential, and affects the proper functioning of over 3,000 DNA programs. We need it for healthy brain, bone, and physiological and mental development, and also to protect against type 1 and type 2 diabetes, as well as all types of flu. More recent studies suggest that everyone—omnivore and vegan alike—needs a vitamin D supplement, even if they live in the tropics, to reach optimal levels.

A particularly spurious criticism of a vegan diet is that is causes iron-deficiency anemia. This is simply not true. Iron-deficiency anemia has been reported amongst some macrobiotic vegetarians following a limited diet low in leafy greens. However, a science-based, live-food, vegan diet does not normally cause iron deficiency, as leafy greens and beans contain more than adequate iron. Leafy greens, vegetables, and beans actually have more iron than chicken, turkey, and cow meat, and they are also higher in vitamin C, which helps iron absorption.

In comparing iron sources in food, we see that spinach is the highest, with 5.4 milligrams of iron per 100 calories—three times more than in 100 calories of steak. (Popeye had it right!) Collard greens, lentils, broccoli, chickpeas, and cashews all offer about 1.7 milligrams of iron per 100 calories. Steak contains 1.6 milligrams per 100 calories. Figs offer .8 milligrams of iron per 100 calories. Chicken contains .6 milligrams of iron per 100 calories, and turkey contains .4 milligrams of iron per 100 calories. Leafy greens, as previously stated, offer not only higher levels of iron but also vitamin C, which amplifies iron assimilation. Flesh food contains no vitamin C. However, it should be noted that a junk-food vegan diet lacking in legumes, nuts, seeds, and vegetables—just like a junk-food omnivorous diet—will not provide enough iron.

Another area of global deficiency that has been found in vegans, vegetarians, and omnivores is DHA and EPA (docosahexaenoic acid and eicosapentaenoic acid, which are essential long-chain omega-3 fatty acids). This deficiency will grow more prevalent because fish, particularly from the Pacific Ocean, are now filled with radiation, toxic pesticides, herbicides, and heavy metals, and thus are no longer a safe source for long-chain omega-3s, DHA, and EPA.

We strongly recommend, for a child's optimal brain and mental development once weaned off breast milk, 50–100 milligrams daily of DHA/EPA in the diet. The safest way to get these is from yellow algae (which is where the fish get them). At the Tree of Life Center U.S., we sell several different kinds of high-quality yellow algae concentrates. Omnivorous, vegetarian, and vegan children all need this supplemental support for optimal physical, emotion, mental, hormonal, cognitive, brain, and eye development.

There is general long-chain omega-3 deficiency amongst omnivores, vegetarians, vegans, and live-fooders alike, which includes approximately ninety-five percent of all pregnant women and about seventy-five percent of the general population. Hempseed, flaxseed, chia seed, and walnuts have short-chain omega-3s, which may convert to long-chain omegas at a rate of one to three percent. This conversion is more than doubled, up to six to ten percent, by adding coconut oil with these omega-3 nuts and seeds. In a recent pilot study by Dr. Gabriel, one tablespoon of chia oil and one tablespoon of coconut oil was the nutritional equivalent in the biological system of 200 IU of DHA and 100 IU of EPA—so we do have some non-supplemental ways to achieve adequate levels of DHA and EPA.

There is a dramatic countrywide and perhaps worldwide mental and physical degeneration happening in all our children. It is best described by Abram Hoffer, MD, PhD, one of the leading orthomolecular psychiatrists in the world, who comments on this unfolding degeneration:

> Recent intergenerational research on both animals and people shows that on a uniformly poor diet, the offspring of each generation deteriorates more and more, and in rats this continues up to eight generations. We don't know what the final stage will be in human deterioration, but I suspect that many of the people with psychiatric disorders today—the addicts, the high degree of violence, the tremendous number of depressions and tension states, and the great number of physical degenerations such as diabetes, arthritis, etc.—are the modern manifestations of this continued degeneration. I have seen no experiences, which show what happens when the diet continues to get worse with time. I shudder to think of the final outcome.[16]

A diet of junk food, fast food, GMOs (genetically modified organisms), and processed foods high in refined carbohydrates such as white flour and white sugar, full of pesticides and herbicides, and grown on depleted soil, creates an inadequate and degeneration-causing diet for Americans and most of the modern industrialized world. This can be corrected and reversed with diets that are high in concentrated, nutrient- and micronutrient-dense, whole, natural, organic, well-hydrated foods. This is the quality of nutrition we get from a science-based vegan, organic, 80% live-food diet.

Unfortunately, life and health are more complex than diet. Our children's brains and physical bodies are also facing documented challenges from environmental pollution, emotional stresses, poor or absent parenting, and vaccinations. For example, according to Dr. Robert Rower:

> Children born to women exposed to air pollution have a higher risk of reduced intelligence, behavior disorders, and anxiety.... (I)nfants of mothers so exposed had markers of DNA damage caused by hydrocarbons. This also suggests the placenta is not the perfect barrier (Journal of Environmental Health Perspective, July 14, 2014).

Data has also been published showing that children born to families living within 1,000 feet of major roadways in three different California cities had double the normal risk of autism.[17] In the Netherlands, one study found that breathing street level fumes for thirty minutes imbalanced electrical activity in brain regions responsible for behavior, personality, and decision-making.[18]

Separate research teams at Columbia and Harvard Universities found that breathing city air with high levels of traffic exhaust for ninety days can alter the way genes turn on and off in the elderly.[19] Other research teams on three continents found that children living in areas of high emissions had poorer scores on intelligence tests and were more prone to depression, anxiety and attention problems than children growing up in cleaner-air environments.[20] Dr. Gabriel, as mental health director for Head Start in Sonoma County, California from 1973–1976, found in a pilot study that in a 300-square-mile area, close to 90% of the children had excess lead, according to hair testing. A parent's vigilance can never be let down. Play in parks as far from exhaust fumes as possible, and if you live in a busy city, get air filters in your homes.

As stated earlier, diets learned in childhood set the pattern for diets that continue to evolve, if inadequate, into accelerated chronic degeneration and disease. For example, a high-protein, omnivorous diet has been shown to have a long-term negative impact on health. A 1983 article in the *Journal of Clinical Nutrition* showed that by the age of sixty-five, female omnivores had an average measurable bone loss of 35% compared to only a 7% bone loss in female vegetarians.[21] In other words, female vegetarians by the age of sixty-five had one-fifth of the bone loss suffered by those on an omnivorous diet.

Male vegetarians had a 3% bone loss, while males on an omnivorous diet had six times as much, at 18%. In 1984, the *Medical Tribune* reported that vegetarians had significantly stronger bones. A study in 1988 of 1,600 women, reported in the *American Journal of Clinical Nutrition,* showed that by the age of eighty those who had been vegetarians for at least twenty years had 18% bone loss, compared to a 35% bone loss in women on an omnivorous diet.[22] The reasons for this are well explained in *Conscious Eating.*[23] The Harvard School of Public Health released a study of 120,000 adults in 2012, showing that those who ate one palm-sized serving of meat per day had up to a 20% higher mortality rate from all causes.[24] In other words, a key to long-term prevention and healthy longevity is to set healthy, preventive diet patterns at an early age.

We will now look at some other nutrient deficiencies to dispel the myth that an omnivorous diet provides more nutrition than a vegan diet. One very important nutrient is vitamin C. According to German research, vitamin C is the most important vitamin for the heart and cardiovascular tissues.[25] Vitamin C is found in higher concentrations in a vegetarian diet, and is highest in a science-based, healthy, vegan, live-food diet.

Folic acid and vitamins B3 and B6 are also found in higher levels in a vegetarian diet. Silica, needed for collagen development, is found in mothers' milk and leafy greens, bell peppers, and horsetail grass. The primary sources for silica are vegan foods. Magnesium is extremely important for a healthy heart; it is responsible as a coenzyme for over 300 enzymatic neurotransmitter processes. Eighty percent of all Americans are deficient in magnesium, which is found in highest concentrations in leafy greens, some whole grains, legumes, seeds, almonds, alfalfa sprouts, avocados, black-eyed peas, mustard, bee pollen, beets, dates, dulse, figs, garlic, lentils, green vegetables, grapefruit, and kelp. Very little magnesium comes from meat, fish, and chicken.

Copper, potassium, strontium, and zinc are other minerals that are important for general health and wellness. The same plants that contain the highest concentrations of magnesium are also high in these minerals. Some soft findings suggest that vegans seem to need to put more emphasis on high-zinc foods like pumpkin seeds, which can be made into Nut/Seed Mylk (page 470) or purchased in the form of raw pumpkin-seed butter (which can be substituted for peanut butter in any recipe). Other sources of zinc are garbanzo beans, kidney beans, pinto beans, lentils, almonds, walnuts, pistachios, pecans, sunflower seeds, cashews, chia seeds, miso, and broccoli. Protein increases zinc absorption, so foods high in protein and zinc, such as legumes, nuts, and seeds, are good choices.[26]

Fulvic acid helps with all mineral absorption, so *shilajit* (a plant/rock-based exudate from the Himalayas) is another excellent addition to help maximize zinc absorption. Boron is important for bone development and the production of an active form of vitamin D. Three milligrams daily is very protective against loss of calcium, and helps to maintain levels of natural postmenopausal estrogen. Boron is primarily available from plant sources, especially kelp and alfalfa. Spinach, snap peas, lettuce, cabbage, apples, greens, and legumes are good sources of boron as well. This may be one of the reasons that vegetarians have less osteoporosis, as they consume many of these high-boron foods regularly.

Ninety-five percent of the U.S. population is deficient in iodine, which is essential for proper brain, thyroid, endocrine, heart, ovary, adrenal, lymph, and immune development. Natural sources of iodine are sea vegetables such as kelp, dulse, and agar-agar, and vegetables such as summer squash, mustard greens, Swiss chard, kale, asparagus, turnips, and spinach. Iodine deficiency is seen in children whose mothers were deficient during their gestation, and is the leading cause of developmental disability and cretinism in the world.

Children of mothers who were given iodine supplementation during gestation scored thirteen points higher on IQ tests than those not supplemented.[27] A randomized study was done in central Java, Indonesia of preschool children age twenty-five to twenty-nine months, in which 100 milligrams of iodine were added to their drinking water daily. After twelve weeks, the IQ scores of children who had been given the iodine showed an increase in 8.8 points compared to the controls.[28]

There are other long-term problems with an omnivorous diet. Vegetarians have an approximately 30–33% lower rate of heart disease[29] and approximately 3.6 times less breast cancer;[30] vegans have 35–50% less type 2 diabetes;[31] and two to three times less lymphatic cancer.[32] There is two to three times less colon cancer in vegans,[33] less obesity,[34] and fewer occurrences of almost all chronic diseases compared to people eating an omnivorous diet.[35]

As previously mentioned, Harvard School of Public Health data showed that people who ate a palm-sized piece of meat each day had a 20% increase in mortality rate compared to vegetarians. Omnivores had an 18–21% increased incidence of heart disease, and a 10–13% increased incidence of cancer.[36] Another study at Oxford showed a 32% increase in heart disease in people who ate meat regularly.[37]

There are, of course, variables in this data. Grass-fed beef is less destructive to health than factory-farmed meat, but there is a clear overall association between meat-eating and a higher rate of chronic disease. A high-protein diet in middle-aged men seems to accelerate the aging process, quadrupling the rate of cancer and doubling overall mortality. The general omnivorous diet has been associated with a far higher occurrence of high blood pressure—26% versus 2% in vegans.[38] A vegan diet is a clearly healthier diet, less likely to induce obesity and chronic diseases.

Other health and safety reasons for eating a vegan cuisine include eating lower on the food chain, which exposes us and our children to a smaller toxic load. Pesticides, herbicides, and other environmental toxins such as radiation are concentrated in meat—up to 15–30 times higher than in vegetation. In other words, if our children eat lower on the food chain, they consume significantly less radiation, pesticides, and herbicides. Vegetarian women have been found to have one-third to one-half the pesticides and herbicides in their tissues compared to omnivorous women, and only 1–2% of the pesticides and herbicides in their breast milk compared to omnivores.[39] There are approximately fourteen times more pesticides in flesh foods than in vegetarian produce.

Trace amounts of pesticides in an animal's environment lead to high dioxin levels within the animal's bodies, and also in eggs and dairy products. The Environmental Protective Agency (EPA) reports that 6.16 billion pounds of toxic chemicals were released into the environment in 2001, representing a 220-pound increase per person over the year before.

> These compounds persist in the environment and build up in the bodies of farm animals that eat contaminated feed or grass. While many of these toxic chemical compounds are resistant to degradation in the natural environment, they dissolve readily in oil and thus accumulate in the fatty tissues of fish, birds, and mammals....
>
> Every time an animal is exposed to a tiny bit of these toxic chemicals, it remains in the animal's body for life, only released when the animal (or animal product) is eaten by humans.[40]

This is one of the reasons we recommend eating lower on the food chain and avoiding all animal fat, which contains lethal and carcinogenic pesticide residues that build up over time.

Omnivores must also face the threat of toxoplasmosis and trichinosis in pigs, mad cow disease in cattle, and salmonella in chickens, as one-third of commercial chicken carring salmonella.

The overall data strongly suggests that a long-term, scientifically based, organic, vegan diet is the safest diet for ourselves and our children. As previously mentioned, dietary patterns established between the ages of four and eight are more likely to be maintained over a lifetime. The earlier we start our children on a scientifically organized, vegan, organic diet, the higher probability they will have of living longer and healthier, as well as uplifting the overall web of life on the planet.

A New Look at Transitioning from Eating Flesh Food

It is unusual for us as live-food vegans to recommend which flesh foods to eat as one transitions from an omnivorous to a plant-based cuisine. Realistically, however, the transition to a live-food, vegan diet may happen, if not immediately, over a few months or a few years. Dr. Gabriel used to recommend in this transition that people first give up red meat. But since that time, environmental pollution—in particular, since the Fukushima nuclear-plant catastrophe—has shifted the discussion.

The radiation from Fukushima contaminated many fish with toxic radioactive elements, and the oceans have become more plasticized and polluted. Unfortunately, the fish are eating the floating plastic waste in the ocean, and people who eat fish are consuming it as well. This can't be healthy. All flesh foods, in fact, because of increased environmental radiation, now contain approximately 15–30 times more radiation than plant-based foods.

Dr. Gabriel is now recommending that fish be the first flesh food eliminated by anyone transitioning into a vegan diet. The second flesh food he recommends eliminating is pig flesh, followed by poultry. This takes us to a new consideration, which is that organically raised, grass-fed, finished beef may be the last flesh food to give up. Of course, beef too has the same problems with contamination by radiation, transmutable diseases, high pollution levels, and also ecological and cruelty issues, as do all fish, chicken, poultry, and pig meats.

Unfortunately, eating higher on the food chain exposes one to potentially serious radiation contamination. For example, following the Chernobyl nuclear disaster in 1986, the perinatal mortality rate in Boston jumped 900% because the radioactive I-131 (an iodine isotope) from Chernobyl had traveled around the globe and was recognized as falling on the grass in the Boston area, where free-range cows were eating it. Consequently, the cow milk became high in radioactive iodine, and was consumed by pregnant and nursing mothers in the Boston area— and their embryos and infants began to die from I-131 poisoning. This concentration of I-131 from the grass through the cows yielded a higher risk of radiation exposure, as the concentration of radiation in animal flesh is approximately 15–30 times greater than in vegetables, especially greenhouse-grown vegetables. Chernobyl, Fukushima, and myriads of unpublicized radiation-spill contaminations have dramatically and negatively impacted the safety of flesh foods.

In addition, the infectious protein prion called TDP-43 found in beef seems to be associated with mad cow disease, Creutzfeldt-Jakob disease, chronic wasting disease, amyotrophic lateral sclerosis (ALS), and also Alzheimer's. Thirteen percent of people dying from Alzheimer's are found to have mad cow disease,[41] so we can't assume mad cow disease does not exist in the American public; it may exist concurrently (perhaps even causally) with Alzheimer's. The only difference may be one of time-dependent physical change, as mad cow disease is more pathogenically active and thus acts more rapidly. The prion TDP-43, commonly found in Alzheimer's disease, is also attributed with shrinkage of the hippocampus associated with memory loss.

It also appears that mad cow disease may be more closely linked with concentrated animal feeding operations (CAFOs), in which animal parts are fed back to the same species, thus amplifying the transmission of the TDP-43 prion disease. There appears to be a spreading of TDP-43 via CAFO feeding of factory-farmed animals. Research strongly suggests that Alzheimer's, Creutzfeldt-Jakob, and mad cow diseases may be more easily contracted from eating food from CAFO-fed animals, especially cows. The statistics suggest that beef-eaters have a three times higher risk of developing Alzheimer's than vegetarians.[42]

As we follow this down the rabbit hole, research is also suggesting that connected with Alzheimer's/Creutzfeldt-Jakob/mad cow diseases is an age-related reemergence of food-borne, antibiotic-resistant bovine tuberculosis, which incidentally is on the rise throughout the world. Although organic, grass-fed meat is the safest meat compared to CAFO-reused animals, fish, pig, and poultry, for these reasons one may consider being cautious about jeopardizing brain function for a hamburger. The chronic wasting disease in deer and elk also appears to be related to these human diseases, so wild game should also be reconsidered as a potential carrier of the mad-cow prion.

If one is still having trouble with flesh-food addiction—often caused by meat's dopamine-spiking effect—your best choice at this point is grass-fed beef, while avoiding fish, poultry, and highly *tamasic* (an Ayurvedic term for "sloth-energy") foods such as pig flesh. It is best, of course, to just stop eating flesh foods altogether.

Additionally, meat is far more ecologically polluting than fish or poultry. Of all meats, beef production creates the highest level of global-warming climate emissions. Researchers at Bard College found that the production of beef releases over five times the greenhouse gasses released by the production of other meats.[43] The tons of carbon-dioxide generated per year per red meat-eater is 3.6 tons. A person who avoids red meat and focuses only on chicken and fish has a carbon input of 2.5 tons yearly. A lacto-ovo-vegetarian generates two tons yearly. A vegan has a carbon footprint of 1.5 tons yearly.

Ultimately, in trying to decide whether we should choose grass-fed beef versus poultry or fish, given all the factors, it is safest and simplest to go vegan; that is the easy way to resolve the dilemma.

Don't Eat the Fish

Fish consumption, especially if the fish is from the Pacific Ocean, may be the most dangerous flesh-food choice today. The FDA has quietly and repeatedly increased its "allowed-radiation doses" in flesh for human consumption to further obfuscate the radiation issue. Seafood is also the number-one cause of food poisoning in the U.S. More than 80% of the farmed fish consumed in the U.S. comes from Asia, where pig and chicken feces are commonly fed to fish as a primary food source.

Fish are commonly contaminated with toxins such as mercury. They also eat plastic and other manmade materials, which poison them and the people who eat them. According to University of Illinois research, fish-eaters with high levels of PCBs in their blood have difficulty recalling information they learned just thirty minutes earlier.[44] Farmed fish are also fed high levels of antibiotics and genetically modified (GMO) soy. And the more that people use factory-farmed fish, the more they support GMOs.

Unless the current situation improves, stocks of all wild fish species currently fished for food are predicted to collapse by 2048. The world's oceans are in a state of silent collapse, threatening our food supply, marine economics, recreation, and the natural legacy we are leaving our children and grandchildren. With the ever-increasing toxicity of the oceans, plus the ongoing Fukushima radiation disaster, fish from every ocean will eventually be contaminated.

Aside from radiation, the biggest water contaminants are PCBs and mercury. PCBs, along with dioxin, DDT, and dieldrin, are among the most toxic chemicals on the planet. The Tenth Annual Report of the Council on Environmental Quality, sponsored by the U.S. government, found PCBs in 100% of all sperm samples.

According to a *Washington Post* article in 1979, PCBs are considered one of the main reasons that the average sperm count of the American male is approximately 70% of what it was thirty years ago. This same article also points out that 25% of college students were sterile at the time, compared to one-half of one percent thirty-five years earlier. The Environmental Protection Agency estimates that fish flesh can concentrate up to nine million times the level of PCBs in the water in which they live.[45]

In a month, an oyster will accumulate toxins at concentrations 70,000 times greater than the toxin concentration of the water they live in.[46] Generally speaking, larger fish contain higher levels of toxins because they eat smaller fish, and assimilating and concentrating the toxins in their own tissues. Mercury toxicity from ingesting fish is a well-known source of illness. Mercury exposure can negatively impact the brain, heart, lungs, kidneys, and immune system. Methylmercury in the bloodstream of unborn babies and children harms their developing nervous systems, making them less able to think and learn.

Fish and shellfish may also carry their own toxins. The most common of these toxins is ciguatera poisoning. Ciguatoxin is both a neurotoxin and a gastrointestinal toxin, and may cause nausea, abdominal cramps, numbness and tingling of the lips, paralysis, convulsions, and even death.

Because there do not seem to be any fish available that are not potentially filled with toxins, one should consider carefully whether it's worth the risk of eating fish. The *Tufts University Health and Nutrition Letter* reports that the more fish pregnant mothers ate from Lake Michigan, the more their babies showed abnormal reflexes, general weakness, slower responses to external stimuli, and various signs of depression.[47] They found that mothers eating fish only two or three times a month produced babies weighing seven to nine ounces less at birth, and with smaller heads. Jacobsen, in a follow-up study that was reported in Child Development,[48] found a definite correlation between the amount of fish the mothers ate and the child's brain development, even if fish were eaten only once per month. He found that the more fish the pregnant mothers ate, the lower the children's verbal IQ. Children are usually the most sensitive to toxins, and they are prime indicators of what may be happening to adults on a more subtle level.

With the March 2011 Fukushima disaster, a new danger of eating fish has arisen—radioactivity. Presently the danger is mostly in Pacific fish, but it is predicted to spread to all fish throughout the world. Approximately 60% of fish have shown to have detectable levels of radionuclides.[49] Japanese data from November 2011 shows that 18% of cod, along with 21% of eel, 22% of sole and 33% of seaweed, exceeded the new food-radiation ceiling implemented in Japan earlier that year.[50] Overall, one in five of the 1,100 catches tested that month exceeded the new ceiling of 100 becquerels per kilogram. (Canada's ceiling for radiation in food is much higher, at 1,000 becquerels per kilogram.)

Scientists have detected radioactive cesium from the Fukushima Unit 1 nuclear plant in plankton at all ten gathering points in the Pacific, with the highest levels at around 25° north latitude and 150° west longitude.[51] In July of 2013, a sea bass caught in Japan had 1,000 becquerels per kilogram of radioactive cesium—ten times Japan's ceiling level. It was the second-highest amount found in a sea bass since the disaster occurred.

February 2013, a greenling in the Fukushima plant's harbor had a record 740,000 becquerels per kilo of cesium—7,400 times Japan's ceiling. Two in five fish tested in July 2013 had detectable levels of cesium-134 or -137, radioactive isotopes released from Fukushima. Radioactive cesium has been found in 73% of mackerel, 91% of halibut, 92% of sardines, 93% of tuna and eel, 94% of cod and anchovies, and 100% of carp, seaweed, shark, and monkfish tested.[52] Fish from the waters around the Fukushima nuclear plant in Japan could be too radioactive to eat for a decade or more, as samples show that radioactivity levels remain elevated and, a marine scientist has warned, show little sign of subsiding.

According to a paper published in the journal *Science,* large and bottom-dwelling species carry most risk of radiation contamination. This means that cod, flounder, halibut, pollock, skate, and sole from the waters in question could be off-limits for years. "These fish could have to be banned for a long time. The most surprising thing was that the levels [of radioactivity] in the fish were not going down. There should have been much lower numbers," said Ken Buesseler, senior scientist at the Woods Hole Oceanographic Institution in the U.S., who wrote a paper entitled "Fishing for Answers off Fukushima." Scientists tagged a bluefin tuna and found that it crossed between Japan and the West Coast of the U.S. three times in 600 days. *The Wall Street Journal* quotes the studies' authors:

> "The tuna packaged it up and brought it across the world's largest ocean," said marine ecologist Daniel Madigan at Stanford University, who led the study team.
>
> "We were definitely surprised to see it at all, and even more surprised to see it in every one we measured. We found that absolutely every one of them had comparable concentrations of cesium-134 and cesium-137," said marine biologist Nicholas Fisher at Stony Brook University in New York State, another member of the study group.[53]

I have presented many reasons why one would want to give up eating fish. There are no nutrients found exclusively in fish, including long-chain omega-3s, that cannot be found in safer, healthier, vegetarian sources. Although once considered safer to eat than mammals, fish is now the most dangerous flesh food to eat because environmental toxicity has shifted. The bad news is that it is only going to get worse, as Fukushima continues to spew radioactivity across the planet.

Don't Pig Out

Pork is one of the most-consumed meats in the world. China is the largest producer of pigs, which were first domesticated around 7,500 BCE.

Today it is estimated that 38% of the world's meat production is pork. The Centers for Disease Control and Prevention (CDC) states that more than 100 viruses come to the United States each year from China through pigs.[54] The infamous H1N1 virus, better known as "swine flu" is a virus that has made the leap from pig to human.

It is possible that trichinosis, a parasite infection primarily contracted from pork consumption, was the cause of Mozart's rather sudden death at age thirty-five. An American researcher theorized this after studying all the documents recording the days before, during, and after Mozart's death. He found that Mozart suffered many of the symptoms of trichinosis, and had in fact recorded in his journal the consumption of pork just forty-four days before his death.

Pigs are also the primary carriers of the *Taenia soleum* tapeworm, hepatitis E virus (HEV), PRRS (porcine reproductive and respiratory syndrome), Nipah virus, and Menangle virus. Each of these parasites and viruses can lead to serious health problems in humans that can last for years.

The flesh of swine is said by many authorities to be the prime cause of much ill health in Americans, causing blood disease, weakness of the stomach, liver troubles, eczema, tuberculosis, tumors, cancer, and trichinosis. Cattle are often infected with an incurable disease of the hog called the "mad itch." It is transmitted by the hogs' saliva left on corn, which cattle then eat. The itching in the cattle becomes so intense that they will run from stump to stump until they rub the skin from their mouths, and they will die shortly afterward.

Professor Hans-Heinrich Reckeweg's article entitled "The Adverse Influence of Pork Consumption on Health"[55] provides powerful insight into why there was a prohibition in the Bible against eating pig flesh, at least 3,300 years ago.[56] His points of concern were:

- Consumption of all forms of pork, including fresh, smoked, and cured, cause many acute inflammatory responses including inflammations of the appendix and gall bladder, biliary colics, acute intestinal catarrh, gastroenteritis with typhoid and paratyphoid symptoms, acute eczema, carbuncles, sudoriparous abscesses, and more.

- We are what we eat—and pigs eat anything, including urine, excrement, dirt, decaying animal flesh, maggots, and decaying vegetables. They will even eat the cancerous growths off of other animals. These toxic qualities are carried in the pig flesh, and amplified because pig meat and fat absorb toxins like a sponge. This is part of the reason pig flesh can be thirty times more toxic than beef or venison; and it is exacerbated by the fact that pigs don't sweat, so more toxins are retained in their flesh.

  It takes eight to nine hours to digest beef or venison, so the toxins filter through the liver and into the body at a slower rate. Pork takes only four hours to digest, which means more toxins are absorbed into the system in a shorter time, and are therefore more concentrated and more likely to be stored in the body.

- Pigs and swine are so toxically contaminated that they are practically immune to strychnine and other poisons. Pigs have acclimated to such a high level of internal toxicity that if a pig is bitten by a rattlesnake, it won't be harmed by the venom.

- A myriad of baffling and sinister parasites lurk in the pork that Americans eat. Swine carry about thirty diseases that may be passed to humans, and over a dozen kinds of parasites—tapeworms, flukes, worms, and trichinae. There is no safe cooking temperature to ensure that all of these are killed. *Trichinella* worms (trichinae), among the most serious parasites, are microscopically small, and once ingested can lodge themselves in our intestines, muscles, spinal cord, or brain. A single serving of infected pork—even a single mouthful—can kill, cripple, or condemn the victim to a lifetime of aches and pains.

  The trichina is just one parasitic worm found in the swine. There are also a large roundworm, a gullet worm, three kinds of stomach worms, a tiny hairworm, a hookworm, and the thornheaded worm, found in the small intestine. There are several species of nodular worms and one species of whipworm in the large intestine, as well as the kidney worm. The large roundworm can be eighteen inches long. A special report given to medical personnel in 1962 at a Doctors and Nurses Conference on Communicable Disease at the Wesley Medical Center in Wichita, Kansas estimated that one out of every three Americans is infected with trichinosis.[57]

- Cows have four stomachs and will digest their food in twenty-four hours. Pigs take only four hours to digest their food and turn their foul diet into flesh. This rapidity of digestion further increases the toxicity of their flesh, since toxins are not as thoroughly broken down, so pork is more toxic than beef.

- On a more subtle level, people are influenced by the astral bodies of the mammals they eat; thus, one who eats pig flesh will take on pig qualities. Pigs, although intelligent, are not considered a spiritually evolving food in most religious traditions; eating their flesh is associated with toxicity and degeneration. In Ayurveda it is considered a *tamasic* (sloth-producing) food. Pork is forbidden in both the Jewish and Islamic traditions.

  People have twisted scriptural passages to rationalize the eating of forbidden foods, but the scriptural directive[58]—has not changed, nor has the biological structure of animals. Jesus never ate unclean food, nor declared all food clean. The verse, "Jesus made all foods clean" was added later; it is not in any of the original manuscripts, which is why it is usually published in parentheses. Neither Paul nor the disciples ate forbidden foods, even after Jesus was resurrected.

  And the pig, because it parts the hoof and is cloven-footed but does not chew the cud, is unclean to you. You shall not eat any of their flesh, and you shall not touch their carcasses; they are unclean to you (Leviticus 11:7–8).

Poultry Problems

Many people switch to poultry when they stop eating red meat. Unfortunately, poultry, which has a profile of dangers similar to that of red meat—such as fifteen to thirty times as much pesticides, herbicides, and radioactivity—has outstanding problems of its own, including high incidences of salmonella and *Campylobacter* infections. According to research published in the series Advances in Meat Research by Pearson and Dutson, over 80% of chickens and 90% of turkeys are infected with *Campylobacter*.[59] These bacteria cause an intestinal infection similar to salmonella, and have become antibiotic-resistant because of the near-universal use of antibiotics in poultry. This means that when they cause an infection, antibiotics will not work effectively to kill the pathogenic bacteria.

According to the Project Censored ratings, a news report in the June 8, 1990 *Pacific Sun,* the "fowl" play in the chicken industry was voted one of the ten most underreported stories of 1989. This article points out that the incidence of bacterial salmonella infection is now 2.5 million cases per year, including an estimated half-million hospitalizations and nine thousand deaths. Apparently the epidemic is caused by a huge leap in consumer demand for "healthier food"—which people mistakenly consider chicken to be.

The dangers are made worse by a massive failure of the U.S. Department of Agriculture to inspect the chicken. The article states: "The USDA has placed gag orders on inspectors and destroyed documents disclosing that the agency has approved massive amounts of contaminated food."

In the *Pacific Sun* article, Dr. Carl Telleen, a retired USDA veterinarian, revealed how "… (C)hicken carcasses contaminated with feces, once routinely condemned or trimmed, are now simply rinsed with chlorinated water to remove stains." According to Telleen, "Thousands of dirty chickens are bathed together in a chill tank, creating a mixture known as 'fecal soup' that spreads contamination from bird to bird." This creates what Telleen calls "instant sewage." Articles like this encourage many readers to transition away from consumption of poultry.

A 2009 USDA study found that more than 87% of broiler-chicken carcasses sold in American stores had detectable levels of *E. coli*, indicating fecal contamination. In other words, if you're eating chicken flesh, you're almost certainly eating chicken poop.[60] Consumer Reports states there are "1.1 million or more Americans sickened each year by undercooked, tainted chicken."

Both the Centers for Disease Control and the World Health Organization say that if the avian flu virus spreads to the United States, people could be infected simply by eating undercooked chicken flesh or eggs, eating food prepared on the same cutting board as infected meat or eggs, or even by touching contaminated eggshells.

Nine billion chickens a year in factory farms produce enormous amounts of excrement, and fecal pollution from chicken farms is especially disastrous for the environment. In West Virginia and Maryland, for example, scientists have recently discovered that male fish are growing ovaries, and they suspect that this freakish deformity is caused by runoff from estrogen- and drug-laden chicken feces at factory farms.

Men's Health magazine recently ranked supermarket chicken number one in their list of the "10 Dirtiest Foods" because of its high rate of bacterial contamination.[61]

Grilled chicken—a popular alternative to fried chicken—commonly contains PhIP (2-Amino-1-methyl-6-phenylimidazo[4,5-b]pyridine), which may contribute to the development of certain types of cancers including breast and prostate.

A common industry practice involves feeding chickens arsenic in order to make them grow faster. Chicken flesh is loaded with dangerous levels of arsenic, highly toxic to humans, which can cause cancer, dementia, neurological problems, and other ailments.

HCAs (heterocyclic amines) are found even in meats cooked at high temperatures, including chicken, and have also been linked to an increased risk of cancer. A *Consumer Reports* analysis found that 83% of fresh, whole broiler chickens purchased across the U.S. had high levels of *Campylobacter* or salmonella, the leading cause of food poisoning in the U.S. Avian flu may have dropped out of the mainstream media's attention, but it's still a very serious illness that is transmitted through poultry.

In addition to bacterial contamination, there may be a virus-like organism in chicken tumors that is transmittable to humans. This organism is thought to be identical to the microbe found by Dr. Peyton Rous in chicken tumors, which he demonstrated to be transmittable to other chickens and humans. For this pioneering work, he received a Nobel Prize in 1966. Dr. Rous, a longtime researcher at the Rockefeller Institute for Medical Research, stated that 95% of the chickens for sale in New York City are cancerous. The extent to which the Rous virus might be associated with human cancer is still debatable, and its transmissibility to humans has not been conclusively proven; but as consumer advocate Ralph Nader points out on this issue, there is no proof that the cancer is *not* transmitted.

The work of Virginia Livingston-Wheeler, MD also strongly suggests that most chickens are at least microscopically infected with cancer. This chicken cancer, like the Rous virus, may be transmittable to humans.

Several recent studies have shown that chickens are bright animals, able to solve complex problems and demonstrate self-control, and that they worry about the future. Dr. John Webster of Bristol University found that chickens are capable of understanding cause and effect; and that when chickens learn something new, they pass on that knowledge—which means that chickens have what social scientists call "culture."

Chickens are the most abused animals on the planet. Chickens raised for their flesh are packed by the thousands into massive sheds. They are fed large amounts of antibiotics and drugs to keep them alive in conditions that would otherwise kill them. There are more than fifty-five times as many chickens slaughtered each year as pigs and cows combined.

To eat animals and fish in today's world is to incorporate into our bodies the psychology of victim consciousness, as these living beings are made into victims by the way they are treated. Once we are informed of the dangers, it is hard to separate the eating of flesh food from a passive kind of death wish. For those who are concerned about getting enough protein, it is important to understand that, as was mentioned previously, meat, fish, and chicken yield, respectively, 16%, 17%, and 18% assimilable protein. The protein in eggs—the so-called "perfect food," to which all blood types react negatively—is 44% assimilable. In comparison to the so-called "perfect protein" in eggs, chlorella, spirulina, and blue-green algae are far more (95%) assimilable, in addition to being great raw protein sources. At the Tree of Life Center U.S., because of Fukushima pollution, we've made deliberate efforts to carry chlorella and spirulina that is sourced away from these contaminated waters. There are also many vegan-source protein concentrates in powder form. For a vegan there is no problem getting adequate protein.

It should be noted that there is a danger of ingesting excess protein. Research indicates that optimal protein intake is thirty-five to seventy grams of protein daily, which optimizes the mTOR genetic pathway that turns on the anti-cancer and longevity genetic programs.[62] A long-term excess of protein (above seventy-five grams daily) is an enhanced precursor of chronic disease.

Another and lesser-known advantage of vegan nutrition is that it creates a later menarche (onset of menstruation) because plant-sourced nutrition is lower in hormone additives than animal food. However, because soy is so high in phytoestrogen, we do recommend that children minimize soy in their diets. The good news is that late menarche is associated with lower rates of breast cancer. Women whose menarche occurred at twelve years old or younger have over five times the incidence of breast cancer in their adult lives.[63]

Don't Do Dairy

I would call milk perhaps the most unhealthful vehicle for calcium that one could possibly imagine, which is the only thing people really drink it for, but whenever you challenge existing dogma ... people are resistant.

—Neal Barnard, MD, President,
Physician's Committee For Responsible Medicine

> For everyone who lives on milk is unskilled in the word
> of righteousness, since he is a child. But solid food is for
> the mature, for those who have their powers of discern-
> ment trained by constant practice to distinguish good
> from evil.
>
> —Hebrews 5:13–14

There was a time when dairy was considered *rasa*—the subtle energy of richness, sweetness, and delight. In India, the general population would regularly consume a small amount of dairy, which was a way of supplying vitamin B12. The cows were treated with a great deal of love and respect, and milked by human hands. Even so, Swami Muktananda, a world-acknowledged master in *kundalini* and *shaktipat* energy transmission, taught that consumption of any dairy product clogs the *nadis* (subtle energy channels).

The message from research indicates that dairy may be a less-than-appropriate food for our time. Dairy clogs the *nadis* (channels of the subtle spiritual nervous system), and brings the energy of death, misery, and suffering into our spiritual bodies. At this time in history, the choice to be vegan and not use dairy returns us to the original Garden of Eden diet, which is one precondition for a massive upgrade of human consciousness.

The focus of this section is to clear some of the confusion about the purity, safety, and so-called "harmlessness" of consuming dairy products, including those that are organic and raw (unpasteurized). Dairy products include milk, cheese, cream, butter, yogurt, and whey from lactating animals.

Stopping dairy intake is not just about our personal health, but is also associated with the prevention of cruelty to cows, and the protection of the planetary ecology and energy. In this context, the choice to eat a vegan diet is putting our own self-serving needs aside and moving toward elevating planetary healing. We can do this if we choose a diet that serves both the healing of the planet and ourselves.

The time for considering dairy *rasa* is gone. This is clear from looking at how the industry has changed the historically acceptable practice of dairy farming. It is interesting today that many yogis from India refuse to drink milk in the U.S. The famous nutritionist Paavo Airola, PhD would never eat or drink dairy products in the U.S. because of the intolerable cruelty to dairy cows, as well as the other problems associated with commercial or even raw dairy.

For spiritual and environmental reasons, dairy has become *ama,* or toxic. For eye-opening, heart-stopping details about the treatment of cows, watch the film *Earthlings,* which illustrates the cruelty and mistreatment of cows and other animals. You will quickly understand how cruelly cows are treated before they are killed. The changed relationship in India with what was once the "sacred cow" and now is the "suffering cow" has sadly changed the animal's milk from *rasa* to *ama,* or pure toxins.

Today, although you can get "organic raw milk" it is very difficult to get non-commercial, truly grass-fed, free-range, organic milk. Even with the best grass-fed cow milk, there are no guarantees of purity and, of course, the cows are still milked artificially. Whether raw or pasteurized, opioids called casomorphins are produced by the digestion of dairy products, making it easier for humans to become addicted to milk. According to Dr. Neal Barnard in his book *Breaking the Food Seduction,* the morphinogenic compound we get from dairy is actually one-tenth as powerful as pure morphine.

Following are some of the reasons we do not recommend consumption of dairy products:

Dairy production causes cruelty and suffering: Ongoing cruelty in the dairy industry is widespread. If you are a lactovegetarian (a vegetarian who eats dairy) because you think that dairy animals are not killed for food and therefore do not experience suffering, think again! Not only does the dairy cow end up on the plates of your carnivorous friends, she also experiences tremendous amount of cruelty in the production cycle, making death a final horrific release from suffering. And the male cows are use for clothes, fertilizer, animal feed, and pet food, among other things. This is, of course, after their sperm has been used to produce more females.

To keep the dairy animal's milk flowing, she is artificially inseminated two to three months after giving birth. The result is a crushing, life-depleting double burden of pregnancy and lactation for seven months out of every twelve. The dairy cow is the hardest-worked of all farmed animals, nurturing a growing calf inside her while simultaneously producing thirty to fifty liters (about ten gallons) of milk a day. No other farmed animal carries this dual load of pregnancy and lactation. Professor John Webster has likened the workload of the high-yielding dairy cow to that of "a jogger who goes running for six to eight hours every day." He believes that "the only humans who work harder than the dairy cow are cyclists in the Tour de France."

Today, dairy cows are usually confined in very limited spaces, and milked by machines. Reproduction happens through artificial insemination. The cycle of cruelty begins at the time the calf is born, ready to nurse from its mother. These bonded animals both suffer greatly when the female baby calves are taken away after only three days. The mothers are left to be suckled by automated machines. The male calves are taken away in the first few hours to enter the cruel death-cycle of the veal industry. Before being slaughtered, male calves are kept caged and immobilized without sunlight or nutrition for six weeks. The mother cow certainly senses that her calf is being taken away from her to be harmed or killed. Her distress, which can last for days, causes toxins to be secreted into her milk.

In historical times, dairy practices in India recognized that the milk belonged first to the calf. The mother cow fed her calf first, and only after the calf had taken its fill was the remaining milk taken for human consumption. In this way, the abundance of the cow's milk was shared with the family who owned her.

Overproduction and genetic alteration: Cows today are genetically bred to produce up to twenty-five times more milk than previously. Fifty years ago, the average cow created 2,000 pounds of milk per year. Now the top dairy producers give 50,000 pounds each per year. This results in a shortened lifespan for the cow.

Shortened lifespan of cows: Before the industrial age, cows lived a more natural lifestyle. The normal average lifespan of a cow was eighteen to thirty-five years. Today, their artificial lifestyle creates an array of diseases in both the animals and those who eat or use their products. What is happening to the cows being used for such an unnatural over-production of milk?

Increased milking, combined with being constantly pregnant and lac-tating, milks away the cow's life-force. The average milk-producing cow lives an average of three years—a sixth to a twelfth of a normal lifespan. In human terms, we can say that rather than living to a ripe old age of eighty, one's life as a cow would end before reaching puberty. Cruelty and exploitation take a toll!

Factory-production techniques: To produce such astounding pro-duction quotas, the cow has become part of an elaborate industrial pro-cess. Milking machines have been used since the 1870s. Today, the cow is attached to these machines for hours on end. This overproduction is achieved by the use of recombinant bovine growth hormone (rBGH, genetically engineered by Monsanto), which creates a fifty- to seventy-percent increase in mastitis, a painful mammary infection. The mastitis is treated with even more antibiotics than the cow is "normally" given. These herbivorous cows are also fed an unnatural diet that includes sheep, fish parts, and other animal parts ground into meal. It is difficult to believe what goes on in the life of the cow!

Wasted resources and ecological damage: Our dairy system also creates a massive wasting of resources. It involves a tremendous loss of energy, materials, labor, and caloric value. Better use of these resources could help solve the food crisis on the planet and prevent the deaths of an estimated 21,000–40,000 starving children per day, according to United Nation statistics, and approximately 40 million total humans who starve to death each year.

A tremendous amount of energy and grain is required to feed cows. The food required to feed 100 cows could potentially feed 2,000 people. Cows worldwide consume twice the total calories as world's entire human population. In the United States, cows consume five times the amount of grain as humans do. Cattle farming, including dairy cows, causes a major loss of the topsoil each year. Furthermore, the water used to produce dairy and its byproducts is *extremely* high. A vegan lifestyle, in a lifetime, can potentially save 1,500,000 gallons of water and an acre of trees per person per year, and feed the human population seven times over with resources conserved by avoiding meat and dairy.

Genetically modified dairy: Why is American milk banned in Europe? Dairy from the United States is considered to be genetically modified (GM) unless it is labeled "no rBGH." It is believed that the genetically modified bovine growth hormone (rBGH) in milk increases cancer risks. While American dairy farmers routinely inject rBGH into cows to increase milk production, European nations and Canada have banned rBGH in order to protect citizens from the hazards of a hormone called IGF-1 (insulin-like growth factor 1), which is elevated in the bloodstream of milk drinkers. IFG-1 has been associated with increased incidence of cancer in several specific tissues.[64]

Not only is the use of rBGH legal in the U.S., but due to corporate influence by Monsanto Company, which manufactures rBGH, the sale of _unlabeled_ rBGH milk is also permitted. While IGF-1 is a normal growth factor in the human body, excessive levels are linked to human cancer development and growth. According to Eli Lilly and Company, another manufacturer of rBGH, the milk of cows receiving the hormone showed a tenfold increase in IGF-1 levels.

Cow milk is not for humans: Another aspect confounding the intent of nature is that human mother's milk is designed for the nervous system of infants, while cow's milk is designed to grow a calf. Cow's milk is four times higher in protein than human milk. It is designed for the massive skeletal and muscle growth that a 400-pound cow needs.

Human milk has six to ten times as much essential fatty acids as cow milk—especially linoleic acid and DHA, needed for human brain and overall nervous-system development. Research shows that breastfed children have 5.32 points higher IQ than children not given mother's milk.[65]

Osteoporosis: Drinking a lot of milk (three or more glasses a day) increases the risk of osteoporosis, according to research, because of milk's high protein content. The U.S. and Scandinavian countries consume more dairy products than anywhere else in the world; these are the same countries that have the highest rates of osteoporosis. In another study involving ten countries, higher dairy consumption correlated with an increased risk of bone fracture. The United States and New Zealand, which have the highest intakes of milk products, also had the highest rates of hip fracture.[66] [67]

Chernobyl reaches Boston: The Chernobyl nuclear disaster made it very clear that the world is one interconnected global village. Cows are relatively high on the food chain, and concentrated toxins from the Chernobyl event with unexpected and disastrous results. For example, there was a 900% increase in perinatal mortality in the six weeks to three months after Chernobyl in the Boston area.

It was found that the cows as far away as Boston were consuming radioactive iodine from Chernobyl that had landed in the water and on the grass. Human mothers consuming the cow milk ingested the radioactive iodine, which poisoned their babies. Now we are facing depleted uranium in the atmosphere as well as iodine-131 and other radioactive nucleotides from Fukushima contamination—which the cows are also concentrating, especially if they are range-fed cows with access to grass.

Creutzfeldt-Jakob disease: The result of all the cruelty and industrialization of livestock, especially of cows, is that cows have become carriers of a significant disease. The 2004 edition of *Friends of the Earth* cites several autopsy studies in the United States suggesting that between three and thirteen percent of people diagnosed with Alzheimer's actually had "mad cow disease," or Creutzfeldt-Jakob disease. These studies suggested that the disease can be transmitted to a person who consumes less than one gram of the diseased tissue from any part of the cow, including the milk. It also suggests that there may be at least 120,000 unreported cases of Creutzfeldt-Jakob disease in the United States.

Pus cells, blood, and mucus: According to www.notmilk.com, the average liter of milk in Florida contains 633 million pus cells, which is the highest in the nation. Montana is the lowest, with 236 million pus cells per liter. This is not a healthy situation, whether it is 236 or 633 million. Besides pus cells and blood cells—which are now normal in milk produced during machine suckling—the milk is also high in pesticides, herbicides, antibiotics, hormones, radioactive iodine, and disease factors such as mad cow prions and bovine leukemia virus.

Research cited by Robert Cohen of www.notmilk.com has made the point that up to a gallon of extra mucus in the human body is created as a result of drinking dairy. The mucus problem is associated with the fact that eighty percent of milk protein is casein, the main ingredient of Elmer's glue.

Disease organisms in milk—*Mycobacterium paratuberculosis:* Milk is a carrier for very significant disease vectors. One of these is *Mycobacterium paratuberculosis,* which causes not tuberculosis—although TB may also be present in some raw milk—but chronic diarrhea and colitis. In babies, this diarrhea is often seen as irritation that can cause significant blood loss and anemia.

This bacteria causes Johne's disease, which manifests as chronic diarrhea and colitis in cows. It seems to be transmitted to humans as well, particularly through unpasteurized milk. Studies performed in the United States, the UK, and the Czech Republic have found that live, viable *M. paratuberculosis* organisms are even present in pasteurized milk sold in stores. These studies show either that the organism is capable of surviving conventional pasteurization (the more likely explanation), or that there is a significant source of post-pasteurization contamination in the milk supply.

While it has not been definitively proven that *M. paratuberculosis* causes disease in humans, there are a number of researchers who believe that the organism is a primary cause of Crohn's disease. They cite clinical similarities between Johne's disease in ruminants and Crohn's disease in humans, as well as studies showing that a significant number of Crohn's patients also have the *M. paratuberculosis* organism in their gut. However, there is no consensus yet about the pathological effects on humans of *M. paratuberculosis*. What is clear is that all known mycobacteria can cause disease, that these bacteria cause disease in ruminants, and that they are present in retail milk.

Disease organisms in milk—Salmonella, *E. coli, Yersinia enterocolitica,* and *Staphylococcus.* Those are some of the main disease vectors found in milk. In 1984, the *Journal of the American Medical Association* reported a multistate series of infections of Yersinia enterocolitica (which causes a disease in cows related to bubonic plague). In a study in UCLA, over one third of all cases of salmonella infection in California from 1980 to 1983 were traced to raw milk.

Disease organisms in milk—bovine immunodeficiency disease: This is another disease caused by a virus that is similar to HIV, and is often found in cow's milk. In Russia it was found that this disease can be transmitted to humans. The *Canadian Journal of Veterinary Research*, as well as the Russian literature, reports the presence of an antibody to the bovine immunodeficiency virus protein in human serum.

The Diabetes Epidemic: Children who drink cow's milk before the age of three to six months have eleven times the rate of type 1 (formerly known as "juvenile") diabetes than breastfed children. Type 1 diabetes is an autoimmune disease, different from type 2 diabetes, which is primarily diet-driven. Although few are aware of it, milk consumption is directly associated with type 1 diabetes. Over 100 antigens are found in milk, which tends to increase type 1 diabetes because the children's bodies create antibodies in response to the cow's-milk antigens. Researchers found up to eight times as many antibodies against milk proteins in dairy-product consuming children who also developed type 1 diabetes.[68]

Finland, which has the world's highest milk consumption, also has the world's highest rate of insulin-dependent type 1 diabetes. The antibodies the child's body produces to the milk antigens cross-react with the Beta cells, or B-cells, that produce insulin in the pancreas. This reaction creates inflammation, scarring, and destruction of the B-cells and the outlets where insulin is released from them. This blocks or inhibits the production of insulin.

Autism and schizophrenia: There is a strong link between milk protein and autism and schizophrenia. When there is a digestive problem, the milk protein, particularly the casein element, is not broken down, and exorphins are created. These morphine-like compounds affect different areas of the brain that can be involved in activating autism and schizophrenia.

One study cited by Dr. Joseph Mercola showed that 95% of a group of 81 autistic and schizophrenic children had 100 times the normal levels of milk protein in their blood and urine. When researchers injected rats with a compound from milk called beta-casomorphine-7, which has been found in the bloodstreams of those with autism and schizophrenia, the rats developed schizophrenia- and autism-like symptoms.

A human study on thirty-six autistic children was published in *Panminerva Medica* (the journal of the Italian Medical Association) in 1995.[69] The children showed a marked improvement in behavioral symptoms after eight weeks on a dairy-free diet. They found high levels of IgA antigens, specific antibodies for casein, lactalbumin, beta-lactoglobulin, and IgG and IgM for casein, in higher quantities in the blood of the children studied than that of a control group. There was a significant improvement when dairy was removed from their diet.

Another study, published in Frontiers in Human Neuroscience, found a major reduction in autistic behavior in children put on a casein-free diet.[70] A study from the University of Rome[71] showed a marked improvement in the behavior of autistic children who were taken off dairy products. Research suggests that certain children may be triggered into autism and schizophrenia. Other research suggests that after a dairy-free diet for one year, there is a significant reduction in schizophrenic symptoms in children. This all points to the possibility that certain subsets of schizophrenia and autism are allergic reactions to casein or other milk components, including approximately 100 antigens, or from exorphins that are created when milk protein is incompletely digested.

Cancer—bovine leukemia virus: This virus, which causes cancer of the blood cells in cows, is found in about sixty to eighty percent of the dairy herds in the U.S. It is mostly destroyed by pasteurization—which means that in raw (unpasteurized) milk it is not killed. *In raw milk, the bovine leukemia virus is found in two-thirds of samples.*

The bovine leukemia virus is associated with an increased rate of leukemia or lymphomas in humans. To support these statements, we would expect that the states highest in dairy use—such as Iowa, Nebraska, South Dakota, Minnesota, and Wisconsin, as well as countries like Sweden and

Russia—would have a statistically higher incidence of leukemia than the national average. That is indeed the case. Dairy farmers themselves also have a significantly high leukemia rate.

Cancer—lymphoma: Researchers in Norway followed 422 individuals for 11.5 years. Those drinking two or more glasses of milk per day had 3.5 times the incidence of cancer in their lymphatic organs compared to the normal population.[72]

There seems to be a high correlation, found in fifteen countries, between increased death from lymphomas and beef and dairy ingestion. In England there was also found a strong positive correlation between lymphoma and milk drinking. The reason for this is that dairy intake creates chronic immunological stress, which tends to cause lymphomas in laboratory animals and possibly also in humans. We know that ingestion of cow's milk can produce generalized lymphadenopathy, swollen liver, swollen spleen, and significant adenoid hypertrophy.

Cancer—lung: Persons who drank three or more glasses of milk a day were found to have twice the incidence of lung cancer.[73]

Cancer—prostate: Men who drank three or more glasses a day of whole milk were found to have 2.49 times the incidence of prostate cancer.[74]

Veganism is a choice for the benefit of health and spiritual life, for the prevention of cruelty to animals, for the benefits of a way of life that furthers the healing of the planet, and for the benefit of being fully in the natural cycle. By holding a vegan position—which gives joy because we are conscious and socially responsible for what we consume—we give a spiritual and health message about the importance of addressing the issues of dairy consumption.

Eliminate Eggs

There are a number of reasons why we do not recommend regular (or even supplemental) chicken-egg consumption, whether the laying hens were fed organically, allowed free range, or horrifically battery-caged.

From an immune-health perspective, eggs are not readily tolerated by most people. According to researcher Laura Power, PhD, eggs elicit an increase in negative immunoglobulin G (IgG) in all blood types. Immunoglobulin G (IgG) is an antibody. Simply put, this means that all blood types respond to eggs as a foreign invader, and fight against them to some extent; this creates an inflammatory response in the egg-eater.

In her research published in the *Journal of Nutritional and Environmental Medicine* as "Biotype Diets System: Blood types and food allergies,"[75] Dr. Laura Powers found that people with blood type A1 had "severe" IgG antibody responses to eggs, in specific quantifiable measurements. Blood type A2 had the most "severe" IgG antibody response to eggs of any blood type, and blood type B had the second-highest. Blood type O also had a "severe" reaction, and blood type AB had a "strong" (the second most pathogenic after "severe") reaction.

Blood types that were Rh-negative also had a "severe" antibody reaction to eggs. While the various blood types reacted to many different foods in different ways, the IgG defensive responses against eggs were consistently high in all blood types. This is significant, as egg protein is also contained in many vaccines, and has been noted to cause severe allergic reactions in egg-sensitive children and adults.

As we've seen with dairy and will also see with vaccinations, when we take in animal products such as milk and the various animal tissues and viruses present in vaccines, we are opening ourselves up to receiving transmittable diseases from the animal kingdom. In addition to the production of antibodies that egg consumption elicits in all blood types, eggs also pose risks of salmonella poisoning and other illnesses. Salmonella enters the eggs through the insides of contaminated hens. The hens contract salmonella bacteria from rodents, birds, and flies in their environment—which deliver the bacteria to all farms—conventional, organic, or free-range. So this is an issue for all chickens, from all sources.

Most cases of food poisoning reported yearly in the U.S. are from salmonella. Salmonella bacteria thrive once they get inside a chicken, as conditions are ideal for them at internal temperatures of about 102° F. Unfortunately, chickens harbor salmonella without exhibiting any signs of illness, making it nearly impossible to know which animals are infected. The few contaminated eggs that come out of a hen usually contain between two and five microorganisms. While it takes a level of at least 100 bacteria to make a person sick with salmonella, they multiply fast if the eggs are not quickly cooled. If there is a lapse in cleaning practices, or an undetected outbreak among the chickens, the percentage of infected animals—and tainted eggs—can also increase rapidly since salmonella bacteria double every twenty minutes under ideal conditions.

Even if chickens remain salmonella-free, their eggs can become contaminated externally. Each egg contains about 9,000 pores that can admit salmonella from contaminated environmental sources. While salmonella is becoming less frequent due to strict FDA sanitation regulations, chickens in Europe are already being vaccinated against it, which creates another unknown potentially dangerous variable.

While the body can generally fight salmonella infection on its own, in rarer cases salmonella has led to complications of bacteremia, enterocolitis, and severe local infections such as meningitis and osteomyelitis. As in the case of the young Australian girl Monika Samaan, whose family was awarded 8.3 million dollars in compensation from KFC (formerly Kentucky Fried Chicken) due to severe disability from food poisoning, salmonella poisoning can even lead to severe brain damage. After emerging from a six-month-long coma, Monika is now paralyzed, in a wheelchair and unable to speak.[76]

Although rare, there have been documented cases of death from salmonella infection, most of these being among elderly persons with compromised immunity. While a small percentage of people following a raw-food lifestyle have experimented with eating raw eggs for vitamin B12, this strategy puts the child at a very high risk of salmonella poisoning, whereas appropriate dosage of a quality vegan B12 supplement is not associated with any risk to a child's health.

Recently, in one year, an estimated 2,400 Americans were sickened from salmonella specifically from eggs, and more than 550 million eggs were recalled. It is the young child who runs a particular risk of sickness from salmonella infection. About a third of the salmonella cases in the United States are in children four years and younger.

In humans, *Campylobacter* causes intestinal infections similar to salmonella. It is possible that these bacteria are transmitted through the eggs as well. *Campylobacter* infection is found in eighty percent of chickens and ninety percent of turkeys.

Cross-species infection is another serious problem; in one study of monkeys fed milk from leukemic cows, one hundred percent of the monkeys developed leukemia after one year. This may explain why in Denmark, where there is a high rate of leukemia in cows, there is also a high rate of leukemia in children. In other words, transmission of animal disease to humans is not unusual.

As previously mentioned, the work of Dr. Peyton Rous, Dr. Virginia Livingston-Wheeler and others indicates that cancers are highly prevalent in chickens, and they may be transmittable to humans. While this issue specifically relates to the health of chickens, the primordial question remains: "Which came first, the chicken or the egg?" In other words, is there a cancer virus, such as the Rous virus, that may be transmitted through the eggs, and which can cause cancer in humans? As of now, it is not completely clear. But, as we consistently are teaching, "If there is doubt, leave it out!" It also helps to remember that no one suffers from a deficiency of eggs.

Eggs, since they are higher on the food chain, like meat and dairy, have a higher concentration of chemical toxins, including radioactive pollution, than plant-based foods. Periodic testing in the United States, for example, has revealed eggs and chickens to be highly contaminated with PCBs (polychlorinated biphenyls) after being fed fish that were contaminated with PCBs. Fish is the food that is highest in PCBs, and eggs come in second. We now have the issue of not only pesticides and herbicides but also the toxins that accumulate and concentrate in the bodies of animals higher on the food chain. Eating animal products higher on the food chain, such as eggs, exposes one to higher levels of toxins of all kinds.

Highly toxic industrial compounds such as PCBs pose serious health risks to fetuses, babies, and children, including developmental and neuro-logical problems resulting from prolonged or repeated exposure to small amounts. In an article addressing the content of dioxin (a form of PCB) in eggs, *Poultry Science* states, "Dioxins are considered to belong to the most toxic substances known, and present a serious threat to the food chain."[77]

The Institute of Medicine, which advises the federal government, has stated that "the most direct way for an individual or a population to reduce dietary intake of dioxins is to reduce their consumption of dietary fat, especially from animal sources that are known to contain higher levels of these compounds."[78] It is important to note that PCB is even of concern for "organic," free-range, and locally produced eggs, which commonly come from chickens fed oyster shells as a calcium supplement. While testing of both soil and worms do not show exceptionally high levels of dioxins, eggs from foraging chickens have been found to actually have a higher dioxin content than caged hens. (Please note that this in no way supports the horrific practice of factory farming, nor does it suggest that commercial eggs are healthy.)

Energetically speaking, eggs present a number of problems for any-one seeking to balance their constitution and support their spiritual life. From an Ayurvedic perspective, eggs tend to aggravate the emotional and physical heat and aggressiveness of *pitta* types. Yoga also considers eggs the most *tamasic* food. *Tamas* is a subtle energetic state that creates a veil of spiritual darkness and death, and thus impedes spiritual development. Therefore, in traditional yoga paths, eating eggs is strongly discouraged because it dulls spiritual consciousness.

In addition to medical considerations, the present-day egg industry is mistreating the sacred feminine through cruelty to chickens, possibly the most mistreated animals of all. It is also associated with sexual exploita-tion of the sacred feminine as expressed in the chicken's reproduction. From a macrobiotic perspective, eggs are considered an extremely *yang* food (causing heat and stimulation). Because of this, they are indicated only in cases of extreme *yin* conditions. By macrobiotic standards, they are certainly well outside of the margins considered for balanced food.

Clearly, based on the above evaluation—especially for those who base their food choices on more than just protein and calorie content—eggs are a poor choice. The risks and negative effects on consciousness associated with egg consumption outweigh their nutritional benefit as a high-quality protein, unless there are no other choices—which is definitely not the case in America and other first-world countries, where plenty of high-quality vegan proteins are available.

People who eat meat are also at a higher risk of various viral, bacterial, fungal, and parasitical infections such as toxoplasmosis and trichinosis. Given the level of various kinds of contamination in meat products, and the toxicity that is concentrated in animals as we go up the food chain—and the fact that there is nothing in flesh food that we cannot get with a vegan diet and supplementation—there is no biological reason to eat any type of flesh food.

Other Factors that Support Health and Wellness

STAYING IN TOUCH: MOVE TO PHYSICAL SUPPORT

Through numerous studies in hospitals and orphanages, where babies are most at risk for touch deficiency, we now know the importance of life-affirming touch to a child's physical development. Premature babies who are touched and held regularly, for example, put on weight more quickly than babies who are not. We also see that nurturing touch affects infant mortality. In 1938, for example, Bellevue Hospital in New York set a new standard that all infants should be picked up and "mothered" on the pediatric ward. That year, the infant death-rate dropped from thirty-five percent to under ten percent.[79]

In addition to statistics, we've all likely heard anecdotal stories of babies whose lives have been saved by another's loving touch. In 1995, for example, there was the heart-warming story of Brielle and Kyrie Jackson of Westminster, Massachusetts, twin sisters who were born prematurely and hospitalized in intensive care. Brielle, being smaller and weaker than her sister, was struggling to survive. Luckily, however, her wee twin Kyrie was placed next to her in the incubator and instinctively initiated physical contact with Brielle, even putting her arm around her as in embrace. From that point, Brielle began to gain strength and weight, and to show fewer signs of distress, resulting in both babies going home alive and well.[80]

Another inspiring story of therapeutic touch is of Kate and David Ogg, an Australian mother and father who were told just after their son's birth that, although the hospital staff had tried everything they could, sadly, he hadn't made it. The doctors pronounced baby Jamie dead, and the mother held her son's lifeless body next to hers, skin-to-skin, as she began to say a long, heartfelt goodbye. The father was also saying his goodbyes when little Jamie suddenly gasped for breath. Hospital staff thought this was only a reflex, but the mother followed her intuition and offered her baby a bit of breast milk, at which point Jamie received the milk and opened his eyes! The medical staff was astounded by the inexplicable life-giving power of parental love, colostrum, and life-affirming touch.

The receptors in human skin, when stimulated, release beneficial hormones that help a baby's digestion and healthy physical growth. Learned midwives and hospital staff also tell us that skin-to-skin contact between baby and mother directly after birth not only lends physical benefits to the baby, but also supports the child's emotional health and neurodevelopment.

Nurturing touch has an effect on the child's social life as well. Unfortunately, children who have not received supportive physical contact from others are more likely to seek out negative touch such as physical aggression. Survival instincts direct a child to find whatever form of touch may be available, and negative touch is better than no touch at all.

Studies conducted by American developmental psychologist James W. Prescott indicate that cultures that lavish more affection on infants and young children, and that show tolerance of sexual affection expressed by teens (illustrative of a lack of repression rather than promotion of promiscuity), tend to have less violence than cultures that do not.

A look at the animal kingdom reveals the need for touch among other mammals as well. Primates, for example, have been observed to show antisocial behavior when the vital need for physical contact has not been fully met.

How does life-affirming touch support the spirit of the child? Not surprisingly, it is through touch that children have so often been blessed in spiritual ceremony, as in Judaism, Christianity, and Buddhism, for example. We also see the ancient traditions of laying-on of hands in prayer, and of therapeutic massage for the healing of mind, body, and spirit.

In a fast-paced, competition-driven culture that has disconnected itself from the slower-moving organic processes of life, our babies spend a great deal of time held by inanimate objects such as car seats, baby swings, cribs, playpens, baby walkers, and strollers. How then do we provide our children with the uplifting gift of our life-affirming touch? If our lifestyles do not foster a hands-on relationship with our children, what can be done to modify this? Fortunately, ancient wisdom is still available to guide us. Parents are rediscovering what caregivers have practiced worldwide for thousands of years—postnatal bonding, breastfeeding, baby-wearing, and caressing. Thankfully, the longstanding custom of infant-massage has also traveled from India to the West.

Is touch just for babies? Not at all! Our children need physical nurturance too, as do adults of all ages—seniors being at highest risk for touch deficiency. If we parents didn't receive it in childhood, offering nurturing touch to our children may feel foreign. Yet if the child is willing, we can begin with one hug at a time, one hand extended to hold, one hand placed on our child's shoulder as we speak face-to-face, or one gentle stroke of our child's head when in need of comfort. As we keep offering this, while respecting the child's preference, both parent and child can begin to feel more at home with the giving and receiving of life-affirming touch.

Inappropriate touch from others can be a delicate yet important subject to discuss with our children. A good opportunity to bring this up is in the context of social experiences such as getting pushed in line or hit by another child. In a classroom or a family setting, it can be in a community discussion or family circle. Listening to each other's thoughts and feelings about touch is instructive. Based on the discussion, everyone can come to an agreement that hitting and pushing are against the rules.

The key in a variety of social settings, whether family, school, or elsewhere, is that everyone has the right to say whether or not their own body is touched; and if a child says, "No, don't touch me," and the other person doesn't listen, they need to go to a trusted adult for help.

THE IMPORTANCE OF SLEEP

While the introduction of a new child affects every family member's sleep cycles, the sleep cycles in turn have a profound effect on family life! For starters, the amount of sleep that we get affects the serotonin levels of the brain, which, in turn, affects our mood. Sleep deprivation is a real factor in many mothers' experiences of postpartum depression, as well as exaggerating any existing family tension. When we grownups are sleep-deprived, we tend to have less energy, alertness, and patience, while our children can experience the effects of moodiness, hyperactivity, and even extreme behaviors contributing to ADD/ADHD.

Lack of sleep also contributes to aggression and anxiety. It is estimated that over 100 million Americans are sleep-deprived. Working as much as possible with our natural desire to sleep at night and be awake during the daytime also links us in to the supportive cosmic energies of day and of night. Our eyes, for example, are designed to receive sunlight, not just artificial lighting. As we see in cases of seasonal affective disorder (SAD), as well as vitamin-D deficiency, receiving the blessing of sunlight each day plays a key role in our quality of life.

How much sleep is enough? Individual needs vary but, as a rule of thumb, if you're tired upon waking, you need more sleep. If you need coffee, caffeinated tea, or cocoa to get you going in the morning, you likely need more sleep. The experience of tiredness when adequate hours of sleep are received may be an indication of stressed adrenals or other health concerns.

Sleep requirements do vary at different developmental stages. The following are general sleep recommendations for supporting health and wellness. The hours below are cumulative for the younger years, with waking periods in between nighttime sleep and naps.

- Newborns (1–3 months): 10.5–18 hours
- Infants (3–12 months): 10–14 hours
- Toddlers (1–3 years): 12–14 hours
- Preschoolers (3–5 years): 11–13 hours
- School-aged children (5–12 years): 10–11 hours
- Adolescents (12–18 years): 8.5–9.5 hours
- Adults (18 years to the end of life): 7.0–8.0 hours

SLEEP FOR BABY

While some families find cosleeping to be a helpful way to bond with baby, if this interferes with the overall family sleep cycle—including the baby's—there are other healthy options. For the first two to three months of life, a baby's biological need is to wake at night for feedings, but around the age of three months many babies sleep six to eight hours through the night. Sometimes babies are actually asleep when they appear to be awake, and we inadvertently wake them.

When learning infant elimination communication with her son, Leah also discovered that infants will wake at night to urinate; but if the baby is taught to nurse during this time because the mother thinks hunger is waking them, it makes for numerous unnecessary nighttime wakings! With careful observation, sometimes a mother can learn to distinguish between her infant's cry for hunger and the need to eliminate.

If consistently frequent nighttime wakings continue far beyond three months, it may be in the best interest of the family to check in with an infant-sleep specialist. Coaching services and literature are available online for exploring gentle ways to help the baby develop nighttime sleeping skills while continuing to be attentive to baby's needs. To serve the baby in this way may very well serve the health of the whole family.

Information on infant sleeping that is also supportive of breastfeeding is available through La Leche League International (see "Resources," page 485).

Disrupted sleep may also be due to teething, overtiredness, or health-related issues such as ear infections/ear fluid, allergies, stuffiness, headaches, rashes/itching, reflux, gas/bloating, constipation, tummyaches, low calcium or magnesium intake, or illness. It may also be helpful to note that extended nighttime feeding has been linked to dental cavities because the breast milk or formula tends to pool in the mouth while the child is asleep. However, we strongly encourage full-term daytime nursing for however many years that may last.

The main idea about sleep for baby—and in parenting in general—is that there is not just one acceptable way of doing things. Each family must find its own balanced and loving approach. These early months can also be a critical time to ask for and accept help from friends and family, in order to get the sleep that is so important for being able to care for oneself, the baby, and the rest of the family.

SLEEP FOR PRESCHOOLERS AND OLDER CHILDREN

Some preschool children require daily naps, and others do not. Having afternoon quiet time provides a helpful break in daily life for both parent and child, without any unnecessary pressure. Having a daily winding-down time before bed is also very helpful to a child's consistent and restful sleep. Peace-promoting prebedtime interactions such as prayer, meditation, song, storytelling, footbaths, or therapeutic massage can be enhancements to family life in and of themselves. Older children may also express the need to talk about their day one-on-one with a parent. Weaving an opportunity for this into the evening rhythms can also become a treasured experience for both parent and child. Television time before bed, conversely, is found to be disruptive to healthy nighttime sleeping. We do not recommended allowing TV before bedtime.

SLEEP FOR TEENS

Teens need to receive adequate sleep during this time of rapid physical and emotional change. While our teens may look like adults, they still need our support in making life-affirming sleep choices. Sleep-deprivation in teens interferes with appetite satiation function, and is linked to obesity, depression, anxiety, diminished problem-solving and decision-making capabilities, and stimulant use. Tragically, over fifty percent of asleep-at-the-wheel car accidents are caused by sleep-deprived teens.

The American Academy of Sleep Medicine and the National Sleep Foundation have posted the following general recommendations to get teens into healthy sleep cycles:

- Consistency—go to bed and rise at the same time each day, including weekends and holidays.
- Create a relaxing evening routine and setting to aid the transition into sleep.
- Allow the bedroom to be quiet, dark, and a little bit cool. Nature generally provides us with this kind of sleep-supportive nighttime environment; in doing this we are harmonizing with natural law.
- Avoid caffeine and other stimulants, especially before bed.
- Avoid going to bed hungry.
- Avoid rigorous exercise three to six hours before going to bed.
- Avoid late-night cramming for tests or other homework assignments.
- Keep computers and TV out of the bedroom, or at least turn these off before getting into bed.
- Get a full night's sleep every night.

CHAPTER 4

Why Authentic, Vegan, Organic Food?

"Authentic food" is a concept that helps us optimize our idea of what quality food should be. The goal of authentic farming is to produce the most nutritious, high-energy food possible while protecting and building the soil for future generations. The farmers that are involved in this noble adventure probe deeper each year into the soil-plant-animal nutrition cycle and how to optimize it.

The life-optimizing power of authentic foods stands in contrast to the approach of agribusiness giants, who are beginning to undermine the word "organic" and who do not understand the traditional small organic farmer's commitment to producing the highest-quality food and regenerating the soil. The authentic approach is a pushback and a healthy response to the degenerate transition of organic-food production from small farms to large-scale agriculture.

Authentic farming does not discount organic farming; it is just one step more refined and advanced in the modern evolutionary process of returning to the natural, "old" (but progressive) ways. Organic food production plays a very important role in healing our world. A major focus of the Organic Consumers Association is getting toxic chemicals out of agriculture. Authentic-food production further focuses on enhancing the biological quality and energy of the food. So we are talking about a new set of concepts that do not simply dictate what to avoid in order to be considered "organic." They tell us how to maintain and add energy to food and soil through love and devotion in its production. This allows us to derive the highest possible energy from our food, which is the main way that we derive energy from the planet. Authentic food lifts food to a new level of quality and meaning.

The term "authentic" refers to farmers who are more concerned with quality than with mass production, even organic mass production. There is emerging evidence that organic food production is not only safer but also more productive than commercial or GMO farming. "Authentic" refers to fresh, organic food produced by local growers who focus on what they are doing instead of not doing. The concept of authentic food goes right down to the fundamentals of food production and distribution in the past. These principles are:

- All food is produced by growers who sell it directly to local consumers or local CSAs ("community-supported agriculture" entities providing food baskets or similar arrangements).
- Fresh fruits and vegetables are produced within a 50–150-mile radius of the location of their final sale.
- Seed and storage crops are produced within a 300-mile radius of their final sale.
- The growers' fields and greenhouses are open for inspection at any reasonable scheduled time on request, so that customers themselves can be the certifiers of their own food.
- All of the agricultural practices used on the farm selling "authentic" food are chosen with the aim of producing food with the highest possible nutritional and vibrational qualities.
- Soils are nourished, as they are in the natural world, with farm-derived organic matter, minerals, and particles from ground rot.
- Green manures and cover crops are included in broadly varied crop rotations to maintain biodiversity.
- Pest-positive rather than pest-negative philosophy is involved—recognizing that pests appear in imbalanced numbers when there is an imbalance in nature in the immediate soil and other factors. Authentic farming focuses on how to correct the cause

of the problem rather than treating the symptoms. This is a holistic approach to farming. The goal, of course, is vigorous, high-energy, healthy crops that are endowed with inherent power to resist pests.

- Any authentic farm or garden land would be a zone free of genetically modified organisms (GMOs). Authentic farming by definition emphasizes local, seller-grown, fresh, organic food—advantages that are not easy for agribusiness to co-opt. Authentic food production supports the health of the ecosystem, our bodies, and the local economy. And the food is fresh, meaning that it is three days or less from soil to salad.

Organic Foods

Organic foods are produced without using genetically modified organisms or toxic chemicals. Organic production methods, whether or not they are employed in conjunction with authentic farming, are vastly superior to commercial, chemical-based agriculture in producing foods with optimum nutrition. Foods produced by organic-farming practices exhibit improved vitamin and mineral nutrition, as well as superior taste and shelf life, and significantly higher phytochemical and antioxidant content.

Investigations show that wildcrafted foods—foods harvested from the wild—have the highest nutritional content and life-force, as measured by Kirlian photography; organically grown foods are next, and conventionally grown foods are lowest.

The USDA periodically publishes data on the nutritional content of food. Historically, since the 1940s, each of these publications shows a decline in the average nutritional content of food. Wheat, for example, used to average a protein content of 19% in the 1940s, but today it averages about 12%. The same trend exists for fresh fruits and vegetables and other foods. So the nutritional content—even of whole, fresh foods—is declining, even before additional losses from cooking and processing.

There appears to be a strong correlation between the declining nutritional content of foods and the introduction of a heavy reliance on chemical fertilizers, pesticides, deep tillage, gene manipulation, and other practices of conventional agriculture. These practices have been well documented as leading to loss of topsoil and a decline in soil quality and fertility. Further evidence of this relationship between conventional practices and the decline in nutritional content of foods is the fact that, on a fresh-weight basis—which is the critical way to look at nutrition for consumers of raw food—organic foods have about twice the vitamin and mineral content as conventional foods.

On a dry-weight basis, this difference in nutritional quality is less obvious, so scientists like to use the dry-weight comparison if they want to claim that foods produced by chemical-based farming are not nutritionally different from organic foods. Organic, authentic foods are better hydrated with biologically active water. However, this obscures the fact that food includes life-force energy, whereas food ash does not. Biologically, humans are genetically designed to consume authentic, organic food!

Organic farmers are performing an incredibly valuable service to society through their efforts to reform food production methods to better conform to nature, and to protect against environmental degradation and the degradation of human health.

Organic Veganic Farming

In Rabbi Dr. Gabriel's previous books *Spiritual Nutrition* and *Conscious Eating*, several key themes emerged regarding using diet as a tool to advance human consciousness and evolution. His book *Rainbow Green Live-Food Cuisine* details how a raw-food, moderately low-glycemic, organic, vegan diet is the best form of nutrition for humans, to optimize health and longevity and to expand consciousness.

Research shows that what works and is healthy for adults also works well for children, if adjusted to be age-appropriate. Children, like adults, do not suffer from a deficiency of white sugar, white flour, junk food, or processed foods. A growing child as well as an adult is hurt by junk foods and benefited by healthy foods.

At the Tree of Life Center U.S., we have gone one step further on the continuum of organic farming and authentic farming by developing our Tree of Life Foundation-sponsored Organic Veganic Farming Program. In this vegan farming method, we employ effective microorganisms (EM) to energize the soil so that it delivers the highest amount of energy into our fruits and vegetables.

There are at least five organic veganic farms in the U.S. at this time. The Tree of Life Foundation's own farm has a variety of veganic organic teaching programs to spread the practice both in the U.S. and for international students.

Background of Organic Veganic Farming

Vegan "Nature Farming" originated in 1935 when Mokichi Okada, a Japanese philosopher and spiritual teacher, began to develop a new method of organic food production. At the time, chemicals were being introduced into agriculture in Japan. Okada recognized that these methods were contrary to the patterns of nature, and created more problems than they solved. In particular, Okada believed that the use of toxic chemicals contaminated food, and that chemical methods of farming produced foods nutritionally inferior to those produced by nature farming methods. He demonstrated the principles of Nature Farming to his followers, who took up the method and continued to spread it after he left his body in 1955.

Nature Farming is based on keenly observing natural ecosystems such as forests and prairies, and then imitating and adapting the pattern of nature to human food production. Okada observed that in nature, "living soil" is the key to the health and stability of forests and prairies. He advocated that his followers imitate nature by seeking to create living soil on their farms. Natural compost, composed principally or exclusively of plant materials, were the key inputs in Nature Farming. Mulching the soil with plant debris and designing the farm layout based on natural forests and prairies further enhanced soil quality.

The Nature Farming method received a great boost in the late 1980s when Professor Teruo Higa, PhD, of the University of the Ryukyus in

Okinawa, Japan, shared his amazing discovery of "effective microorganisms" (EM) with the proponents of nature farming. Dr. Higa began his research on microorganisms in the early 1960s, discovering that certain combinations were beneficial and "effective" in their ability to change the microbial characteristics of soil.

"Effective" means that these microorganisms were able to alter the dynamics of the microbial ecosystems of soil, water, plant surfaces, and other environments, and to enhance the growth and activities of the beneficial components in the soil, which led to a decline in the activity of the detrimental components. Dr. Higa realized that this was a great tool that could have many uses in agriculture and the environment, where destructive practices had created microbial imbalances. In the context of Nature Farming, EM proved to be the key to creating "living soil" in a reliable and predictable manner. EM also helped to solve many practical problems in transitioning farms to sustainable organic methods.

In 1998, Nature Farming and EM were introduced to the Tree of Life Center U.S. by John Phillips, who had been working with Nature Farming since 1988 and with Dr. Higa since 1990. In December 2001, John joined the staff of the Tree of Life Center U.S. to work more closely with us in developing a model for Organic Veganic Farming using EM and other subtle techniques. We now offer one-week intensives and apprenticeships on this system of organic veganic farming.

As mentioned above, Nature Farming is modeled after nature itself. Natural ecosystems can have a very high productivity of plant and animal life, even though they are self-sustaining. Indeed, one characteristic of such systems is that they are always naturally accumulating fertility. Also, they are naturally resistant to pests and diseases, and can recover easily from fires, earth movements, windstorms, and other damaging events. This is in stark contrast to most commercial farming systems, where productivity is continually threatened by loss of fertility, insects, diseases, weeds, and other pests, and where fire, wind damage, and other catastrophes can cause the system to fail entirely.

The basis of Nature Farming is an appreciation for the power of "living soil," the key factor that makes the system sustainable and resilient.

Living soil is created through the interaction of plants and the life of the soil, especially the microorganisms, earthworms, mites, and countless other creatures. In the forests and prairies, living soil is created by the accumulation of plant debris from season to season. Plants provide the primary food for these ecosystems, thereby supporting the extended food chains that develop there.

Next to the plants, the microorganisms and other soil life are the most critical to the stability and productivity of the system. Microorganisms recycle the plant material, releasing nutrients to further promote plant growth. Microorganisms form symbiotic relationships with plant root systems and help provide nutrients such as phosphorus to plants in exchange for exudates from the plant roots. Animals, from earthworms and mites on up, dwell and feed upon the soil-plant complex. This is the natural scheme of things, and humans evolved from this ecological base.

In stark contrast, the newest, deadliest version of Roundup®, the glyphosate-based pesticide, has a combination of toxins that will destroy normal soil ecology. E. B. Szekely, one of the earliest holistic physicians of the twentieth century, who reactivated the ancient Essene movement, proposed that humans originally evolved from a subspecies he called *Homo sapiens sylvanus,* because the forest (*silva,* in Latin) was our natural home. Szekely also proposed that the raw foods of the forests—fruits, herbs, and vegetables—were our natural diet; he believed that when humans existed in harmony with the forest on their natural diet, life spans were much longer, and humans lived free of debilitating diseases.

Szekely suggested that we could return to this paradise by creating interdependent agrarian communities producing an abundance of plants for a raw-food, vegan diet to promote health, longevity, and conscious evolution. This is what we are creating at the Tree of Life by developing Organic Veganic Farming and the Rainbow Green Live-Food Cuisine.

To create an Organic Veganic Farming system, we eliminated all use of fertilizers that contain animal byproducts from the slaughter industry, such as bone meal, blood meal, feather meal, fish emulsion, and similar products. This has essentially been the approach since the beginning of our Tree of Life Foundation Gardens, but we have learned that many blended organic fertilizers also contain some form of animal product as a source of nitrogen. So it is important to look closely at the ingredients in fertilizers. Organic food can be produced without using animal wastes and byproducts, and for some vegans this is distinctly preferred. Vegan farming is the only farming system in the world that has virtually no GMO contamination. Vegan farming also provides protection from the possibility of mad cow disease and other potential contamination from animal products.

Many plant materials used for composting are now suspect because of GMOs, so cottonseed meal, alfalfa meal, and soybean meal, for example, are less desirable sources of nutrients for organic production than they used to be, and must be sourced from organic producers who avoid GMOs. Even hay—so commonly used as mulch in organic farming— now must be sourced from organic producers not only because of GMOs but because the latest herbicides being used in conventional farming are more resistant to natural breakdown in the environment and are causing herbicide damage to crops, even where the hay is only used as an ingredient for making compost.

Composting kitchen waste from an organic, vegan kitchen recycles nutrients that can be used for vegan food production. At the Tree of Life Center U.S., we employ EM—Dr. Higa's special blend of eighty-two beneficial microorganisms—to inoculate and energize compost and to make compost teas and vegan organic sprays for crops and soils.

Vegan farming does not necessarily exclude animals as companions and coworkers to help balance the agro-ecosystem. Ducks and geese may be used for weed control, and chickens and turkeys may be used to control harmful insects such as grasshoppers. Earthworms also can be used to recycle wastes, and their castings make a fine compost and organic fertilizer. Since these coworkers are willing to work for chicken feed and garden scraps, are kept compassionately in a natural environment, and are not used for human food, we see a mutual benefit in this arrangement. With the exception of worms, however, we do not use these coworkers at the Tree of Life Foundation Gardens.

We are especially interested in Nature Farming and the use of effective microorganisms in developing our vegan organic gardens because a masters student of the Cousens' School of Holistic Wellness has produced evidence with Kirlian photography that foods produced by these methods significantly exceed regular organic foods, and equal wildcrafted foods, in terms of energetic and nutritional content. This is likely because the synergy of Nature Farming with EM approximates nature's own system of growing.

Evaluation of this new system of Nature Farming using EM and a vegan ethic to produce authentic live foods is a work in progress at the Tree of Life Foundation Gardens, where we continue to explore the growing and utilization of authentic live foods in this way.

What Does "Organic" Really Mean?

There is no shortcut to health and happiness except by following the natural and spiritual laws of life to the best of one's ability and present knowledge. Humanity and all sentient beings are sustained by the same radiating light of the universe within and around us. If we are to be in harmony with this light as we receive it through the natural interplay of earth, water, air, and fire via the vegetable kingdom, then it is essential to choose to eat authentic, organic agricultural products that are grown in the fullness of this light. We should be very cautious when we attempt to tamper with nature.

In an evolution of multiple recent studies, organic produce was found to have an average of 25% more nutrients, significantly more antioxidants, about one-fourth of the pesticides and herbicides, and significantly less cadmium than conventional produce. The nutrient-density of organic foods varies, but on average they are more nutrient-dense than conventional produce. In a new study entitled "New Evidence Confirms the Nutritional Superiority of Organic Foods," a compilation of a variety of studies, the organic foods were found to have 20% more phenols, 80% more antioxidant capacity, 60% more quercetin, 50% more vitamin C, and 30% more vitamin D.[1]

A study in the western suburbs of Chicago also showed, on a per-weight basis, that organic produce contained many more nutrients than conventionally grown produce. Organics averaged 63% more calcium, 78% more chromium, 73% more iron, 118% magnesium, 91% more phosphorous, 125% more potassium, and 60% more zinc. Besides having less of the toxic heavy metal cadmium, organic produce also averaged 29% less mercury.

We would like to make it clear that the words "natural" and "locally grown" can be misleading to the public. They do not necessarily mean the food was organically grown. "Organic" means that the food was grown without pesticides, herbicides, or genetically modified seeds. "Certified organic" is the only label we can trust at this point.

Unfortunately, even the word "organic" is tricky. Under certified-organic regulations, foods must be at least 95% organic, which allows plenty of room for flavorings and additives that are not necessarily organic. For example, castoreum is a natural substance secreted into sacs in the anal areas of beavers, which is used in the food-flavoring industry, particularly in raspberry-flavored foods, ice creams, fruity drinks, and candy. (It is often listed as "natural flavoring.") Organic products can carry this anal-area secretion in their 5% margin, and still be considered organic. This is a problem we face if we buy processed "organic" foods.

The only final solution to this obfuscation is to not purchase any products in any store unless they are, or are made from, certified organic produce.

Organic food does not mean that it is 100% free from pesticides, as our entire environment is so polluted; but it does mean that organic farmers are not using pesticides directly. Federal rules do not require organic produce, or the soil it is grown in, to be tested for synthetic fertilizers or pesticides. The USDA allows 245 nonorganic ingredients in the production of organic produce and livestock.

In 2005, a federal court ruled that organic food couldn't be made with synthetic ingredients, but agribusiness lobbyists complained, and Congress rewrote the law to permit synthetics. It is even legal to use bisphenol A, a component of epoxy resins, which has been clearly linked to developmental problems in children. Bisphenol A may be used in canned organic food. We end up, to solve this issue, only buying organic produce. If we want to guarantee that we have no GMOs in our organic produce, we must transition into organic, veganic farming, which does not use any animal products such as blood meal, bone meal, or manure in its production. It is the only way we can guarantee that we are getting only organic food with no GMOs.

Organic farming is part of a general regeneration of the planet. Organic farming not only rebuilds the soil but pulls about 3,700 pounds of carbon dioxide out of the air each year per acre—and an acre of organic avocado trees pulls as much as 5,200 pounds. One study revealed that the area of certified organic farmland around the world has increased 3,300% since modern organic methods and standards of certification have been developed. There are now 91 million acres of certified organic farmland worldwide.[2] This is, however, still less than 1% of all agricultural land, and interestingly enough about the same as GMO acreage.

When we buy organic, veganic produce, we are actually creating support for all forms of organic farming. Holistic veganism, including buying organic produce, is a way of life, of loving ourselves, loving our children and loving the planet.

AN ORGANIC EXERCISE FOR CHILDREN OF READING AGE

(This exercise could be also be engaging for a child who is not yet reading, if the places where you shop have color-coded labels distinguishing organic and commercial produce.)

When you are at the grocery store or farmer's market, show your child how to look for the word "organic" on signs and labels, explaining that this is what you are looking for. It can be like a treasure hunt. When you are in the produce department, explain that the word "conventional" or the absence of the magic O-word generally means that "harmful chemicals were sprayed onto the plants. People do this to kill pesky insects, but they don't understand that this also kills the soil, and harms animals and people. We want clean food from clean soil to help us grow strong, healthy, and happy. When we buy organic foods, we are helping the soil, the animals, and the people. Yay!"

If you come upon a produce stand at farmer's market that is not certified as organic, make a point to ask the farmer (in front of your child) if the foods were grown with the use of pesticides, herbicides, fungicides, or chemical fertilizers, and politely choose not to purchase from them if the answer is "yes." (Your child may be interested in knowing that the suffix "-icide" means "kill.") At some point, you will want to also explain that some labels trick people by saying "natural"—but unless they are organic, they are not truly natural.

Further Exercises: As your child quickly catches on to label reading, explain other ingredients that you want to include (such as non-GMO, raw, vegan, veganic, sprouted, live, fair-trade, etc.) or to avoid (such as animal products, anything "artificial," MSG, hydrogenated oils, high-fructose corn syrup, etc.).

AN ORGANIC EXERCISE FOR TEACHERS

As a part of your environmental science curriculum, an adapted version of this exercise can be done in the classroom with organic and nonorganic food packaging. It is better not to ask students to bring in the packaging from home, because some children may feel badly that theirs was not organic. Encourage your students to ask their parents if there is an organic choice to replace foods that do not have "organic" on their labels.

An online curriculum resource for teaching about organics in schools is www.lessonplanet.com.

The reader may be wondering why we have spent a lot of time explaining organic, veganic farming and the growing of authentic foods. As parents whose interest is helping to foster the growth of alive, conscious children in this world, the deep philosophical teaching here reaches back to part of our purpose in life, which is to repair our world and create optimally healthy children who will thrive in that world.

The modern human world has damaged its connection to nature, as evidenced by the destruction of our ecology on many levels. At the root of this is both unconscious and conscious distortion of the directive that we should have dominion over creation, and should bring the Garden of Eden to its highest function. As pointed out previously, "dominion" does not mean "domination" and the right to destroy, desecrate, and exploit the living planet. "Dominion" means to be in right and harmonious relationship to the living planet. It is to go beyond stewardship, to the *dharma* (natural law) of elevating all life on the planet to its highest octave, including human life. The challenge is for us and our children to reestablish, by our own lives and diet, the proper dominion in which all of creation is elevated. By understanding the teaching and practice of organic veganic farming, we begin to reestablish this proper dominion.

Pesticide Pestilence

Although we see authentic food at the cutting edge, beyond organic, we want to make it very clear that the organic movement is playing an incredibly important role in the healing of the planet. We strongly urge everyone to go 100% organic regardless of their overall diet.

Presently, more than twenty percent of pesticides currently registered in the U.S. are linked to cancer, birth defects, developmental harm, or central nervous damage. We cannot even imagine how much this is involved with the current epidemic of hyperactivity and adult attention deficit disorder. Some research has shown that when children are simply put on an organic diet, without doing anything else, there is a 50% cure rate for ADHD. This is not surprising, since most pesticides and herbicides are neurotoxins, and the developing nervous systems of children are more vulnerable to these toxins.

This means that approximately half of the eight to ten million children who are presently on Ritalin may no longer have to take the drug. The other half, given the natural ways of healing of the brain that are available, would require a more extensive approach for healing. Although the Tree of Life Center U.S. is more about preventing ADHD, Dr. Gabriel and other physicians have reported up to a 90% cure rate for ADHD and ADD as part of a more comprehensive approach of healing and rebuilding the brain, which will be discussed later.

More than 12,000 children in the U.S. are diagnosed with cancer every year. Cancer is now the main cause of death, after suicide, for children under the age of fifteen. These high cancer rates in children were unheard-of before the age of pesticides, herbicides, and genetically engineered food. At least half the food on our grocery shelves contains genetically modified ingredients, and these GMO ingredients have not been adequately tested for their impact on human health. One of the most significant effects of an organic vegetarian diet is the tremendous health benefit of eliminating chronic poisoning from pesticide intake and exposure to GMOs.

We need to understand clearly that pesticides are designed to kill living creatures and, in case we forget, human beings are living creatures too. The organic movement is one of our most important ways to begin to rectify the destruction of our soils, the rampant rate of cancer and brain dysfunction in children and adults, and the literal poisoning of the planet. The only people who benefit from this pollution are corporations that profit directly from the sale of these poisonous chemicals.

Once again, farmers using the "Green Revolution" production-boosting techniques, GMO-production techniques, and heavy pesticide and herbicide use are simply less able to produce high-quality foods. And their total agricultural output seems to be subtly dropping, contrary to the promise of the Green Revolution and GMO companies. One of their problems is that the pests are smarter than the corporations.

The poisoning of our global environment is a threat that has to be faced directly. If we are to stand up to corporate practices that threaten the health of farmers, rural communities, consumers, bees, and other sectors of our ecosystems, we must vote with our mouths. By refusing to eat irradiated, commercial pesticide- and herbicide-laden, and genetically engineered foods, we and our children are making a very clear statement to the corporations and to the governments that are so influenced by corporate donations. We are saying that we, the public, will not buy your story or your food; we will not support the poisoning of the plants, all living creatures, ourselves, and our children on this Earth. For this reason, we cannot stress strongly enough the importance of going 100% or close to 100% organic in our food choices. At the Tree of Life Café, we have guaranteed to sell only 100%-organic, veganic live food since 1994.

The tide has begun to turn. In May of 2001, ninety-one countries and the European community signed a treaty to phase out persistent organic pollutants (POPs), including notorious pesticides such as DDT, PCBs, and dioxins that are wreaking havoc around the globe. More and more people are waking up to the fact that pesticides have been proven not only unsafe and counterproductive in the long run of agricultural practices, but that the pesticide treadmill forces farmers to continually increase their use of poisonous substances to combat worsening, chemical-resistant pest outbreaks.

An additional problem is that, at the same time as these pests develop resistance to poisons, their natural predators are being wiped out by them. Some of the corporations have gotten more clever about this; not only have they created pesticide-dependent farmers, they are now promoting genetically engineered crops as "essential to feed a hungry world." This technology, which is being more seriously combated and rejected in Europe and other places than in the U.S., raises very serious concerns about biodiversity in the environment, about who controls the food supply, and about the lie that GMO foods are essential to food productivity. The scientific reality is that their productivity is about the same as, or 1%–10% less than, organic farms.[3]

Unfortunately, pesticides do not recognize borders once they are released into the environment. Pesticides can travel thousands of miles through the atmosphere, waterways, and ocean currents, as well as in imported foods and fibers. What we are seeing, even in supposedly pristine polar habitats, is high levels of toxic pesticides, especially POPs. They are showing up in the tissues of native peoples, whales, penguins, and other animals. The same is true with genetically altered foods; once they are released into the environment, they have the serious potential to disrupt delicate ecosystems in devastating ways. By going organic, we make a strong vote with our mouths to break this cycle of poison and ecological destruction.

Unless we eat organic fruits and vegetables, we are continually exposed to pesticides. Research shows that children who eat primarily organic foods have one-quarter to one-sixth the pesticide levels in their blood as those eating commercially grown foods.[4] One of the most important pathological effects of these toxins, besides initiating cancer, is the neurotoxicity to the brain and the rest of the nervous system. These produce more subtle symptoms in our children, such as reduced mental functioning, poor concentration, hyperactivity, and ADD.

We have some very suggestive evidence that the use of pesticides and herbicides affects our mental function and brain physiology, including increasing the incidence of Parkinson's disease up to seven times in those most heavily exposed to them. This is not exactly a surprise when we realize that pesticides are designed to be neurotoxic to the pests. Does it surprise us to realize that we are biologically similar to the insects we are poisoning? Our nervous systems are more sophisticated and may take longer to poison, but we are still vulnerable; we still get poisoned, over time.

The following excerpts are from a study titled "An Anthropological Approach to the Evaluation of Preschool Children Exposed to Pesticides in Mexico" by Elizabeth A. Guillette, María Mercedes Meza, María Guadalupe Aquilar, Alma Delia Soto, and Idalia Enedina García, published in *Environmental Health Perspectives.*[5] The following study is the most stunning we have seen illustrating the powerful neurotoxic effects of pesticides and herbicides on our children. It represents more evidence that an organic diet is important at any age, but probably most important for children whose brains are still developing.

The children of the agrarian region were compared to children living in the foothills, where pesticide use is avoided. The RATPC [a physical, psychological, and mental assessment] measured varied aspects of physical growth and abilities to perform, or function in, normal childhood activities. No differences were found in growth patterns. Functionally, the exposed children demonstrated decreases in stamina, gross and fine eye-hand coordination, 30-minute memory, and the ability to draw a person. The RATPC also pointed out areas in which more in-depth research on the toxicology of pesticides would be valuable....

The 33 children exposed to elevated levels of pesticides, hereafter referred to as valley children, came from three towns and corresponding rural areas within the Yaqui Valley. The towns were Quetchehueca (n=10), Bacum (n=12), and Pueblo Yaqui (n=11), all 10–30 feet above sea level. All of the towns, regardless of location, were similar in infrastructure and the interfacing of tradition with modernization....

Pesticide use is widespread and continues throughout the year, with little governmental control.... An initial site visit revealed that household bug sprays were usually applied each day throughout the year in the lowland homes. In contrast, the foothill residents maintained traditional intercropping for pest control in gardens and swatting of bugs in the home. These people cited their only exposure to pesticides as the governmental DDT spraying each spring for the control of malaria. (Identical DDT spraying also occurs in the agricultural areas and is repeated if a case of malaria occurs.) ...

Group play was observed more frequently in the foothills, with pretend parties for dolls and street games. Valley children appeared less creative in their play; they roamed the area aimlessly or swam in irrigation canals with minimal group interaction. Some valley children were observed hitting their siblings when they passed by, and they became easily upset or angry with a minor corrective comment by a parent. These aggressive behaviors were not noted in the foothills. Such clues indicated that additional aspects of development may be affected by environmental change, as opportunities and toys for play were available at both sites. In both areas, mothers were generally home on a full-time basis and showed interest in their children....

The rapid assessment tool did show that psychological and physiological differences in functional abilities exist between the valley and foothill children at 4 and 5 years of age.... Of increased concern were the differences found with activities involving mental/neurological functioning. The inability to remember a meaningful statement after 30 minutes has implications for school performance and performance in social activity. The drawing of a person, often used as a nonverbal screening measure of cognitive ability, could also indicate a breakdown between visual sensory input and neuromuscular output, as found with brain dysfunction. The decreases in eye-hand coordination, as with catching the ball and dropping raisins into a circumscribed area, could also correlate with this type of brain dysfunction. This concept of breakdown between incoming sensory signals and neuromuscular output certainly deserves greater attention in future research....

Valley children had a significant decrease in their ability to catch a large ball ($p=0.034$) at the distance of 3 meters. This inability to catch a ball increased as the ball size decreased. Foothill children outperformed the valley children in catching the tennis ball at 1, 2, and 3 m ($p=0.05$, 0.01, and 0.003, respectively). A stronger difference was found between the two groups in regard to fine eye-hand coordination; foothill children were better able to drop a raisin into a bottle cap ($f=7.3$; $df=1.44$; $p=0.009$). Interestingly, the location of the child's home (valley versus foothills) had a significant effect on these measurements, but the child's sex had no relationship to any of these outcomes.

Children in both locations performed equally well in the immediate recall of numbers up to four digits. The valley children had more difficulty grasping the concept of repeating the numbers, although marked differences were found between towns. Children with such difficulty were encouraged to repeat one and then two vowel sounds made by the interviewer. Thus, the movement into repeating numbers became more comprehensible. Marked differences in recall were seen with 30-minute memory (X2=14.3; P=0.027). In recalling their gift, 59% of the 17 foothill children remembered both the object

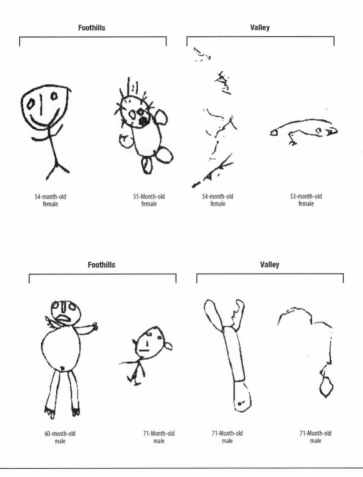

Figure 1. Representative drawings of a person by four-year-old Yaqui children from the foothills (lower pesticide exposure) and valley (higher pesticide exposure) in Sonora, Mexico. Studies like these graphically make the case for going organic to protect the health and brains of our children. No money saved by buying commercial food is worth risking damage to a child's developing brain.

From *Environmental Health Perspectives,* Volume 106, Number 6, June 1998.

and its color, with all but one of the remaining children remembering just the balloon. In contrast, 27% of the 33 valley children recalled the balloon and color, 55% recalled the balloon only, and 18% could recall neither the object nor the color.

An article in the *San Francisco Chronicle* ("Polluted Bodies," February 3, 2003) is also quite revealing. It tells us that Michael Lerner, a twenty-year resident of seaside Bolinas, California, and the president and director of Commonweal, a health and environmental research group in Marin County, thought he was eating a healthy diet and avoiding exposure to industrial chemicals. Yet he found that his body was polluted with 101 industrial toxins as well as elevated levels of arsenic and mercury.

Lerner was one of nine people in a collaborative study by the Mount Sinai School of Medicine in New York City, the Environmental Working Group of Oakland, and Commonwealth, of the body burden of monotoxic chemicals in the body. On the average, each person studied was found to have fifty or more chemicals in their bodies that have been linked to cancer in lab animals, are considered toxic to the brain and nervous system, or interfere with hormones and reproductive systems.

Andrea Martin, founder and former executive director of the San Francisco Breast Cancer Fund, was found to have ninety-five toxins, fifty-five of which were carcinogens. Further information on this research can be found at www.ewg.org. The point is that no matter who we are—whether we are living on the ocean in Bolinas or in a large urban area—we are all in the same toxic world neighborhood. To minimize the damage, we need to eat an all-organic diet, have a regular detoxification program, and begin to clean up our planetary neighborhood.

One of the most significant effects of an organic vegetarian diet is the tremendous health benefit of decreasing chronic poisoning from pesticide intake. In 1987, the National Academy of Sciences concluded that in our lifetime, pesticides in American food may cause more than one million cases of cancer in the United States.

The pesticide 2,4-D comprises half the content of Agent Orange, which was used to devastate forests and people in Vietnam. There are estimates that there will be a 500–1,400% increase in the use of 2,4-D in corn and soy over the next nine years. The use of Enlist Duo (Dow Chemical's newest herbicide, a combination of 2,4-D and glyphosate) will particularly affect fruits and vegetables. It is horrifying to see pictures of the increasing number of third-generation Vietnamese children who are born with severe congenital defects caused by the use of Agent Orange in the Vietnam War in the late 1960s and early '70s. The residual effects of Agent Orange have created a hell on Earth for these people for at least three generations. Its use represents the darkest of dark human actions.

According to pesticide-industry authority Lewis Regenstein, those who eat beef get a dose of dioxin that is concentrated as it moves up the food chain. The EPA has officially recognized that cattle grazing on land sprayed with dioxin accumulate it in their fat. Dioxin has been shown to produce cancer, non-Hodgkin's lymphoma, birth defects, miscarriages, reproductive and immune system problems, and death in lab animals in concentrations as low as one part per trillion. It has also been linked to an increase in human cancer, a variety of reproductive problems, and increased incidence of type 2 diabetes.

It is no wonder, according to David Steinman in *Diet for a Poisoned Planet,* that deaths from cancer in this country have risen from less than one percent in the beginning of the nineteenth century to one in four American men and one in five American women today. Although other factors, such as nuclear radiation and cigarette smoking, do play a role in increasing the incidence of cancer, we wonder how much the cancer rate would drop if we stopped all pesticides from entering our food chain. Even if their toxicity is acknowledged and they are banned, once pesticides have been introduced into the environment, their chlorinated hydrocarbons are extremely stable compounds that do not break down for decades or longer.

We do not think scientists have discovered the full extent of the damage pesticides have already done to the nation's health. The types of cancers that are emerging statistically suggest that they originate from the effects of specific pesticides. According to *Diet for a Poisoned Planet,*[6] urinary-bladder cancer increased by 51% between 1950 and 1985; kidney and pelvic cancer increased by 82%. These cancers are directly associated with toxins in the drinking water.

Testicular cancer, which occurs in significant proportions among farm workers and manufacturers of pesticides, has increased 81%. In 1985, non-Hodgkin's lymphoma, which is linked with pesticide exposure, increased by 123%. The 1988 *Surgeon General's Report on Nutrition and Health* estimated that as many as 10,000 cancer deaths annually may be caused from the chemical additives in food; this does not even include cancer from pesticides. It is extremely difficult to know the exact percentage of cancer increases due to pesticides, additives, and other environmental factors in our food, water, and air, but it is most likely significant.

In addition to the single-pesticide effect, which can be directly tested in the laboratory, there is often a more powerful synergistic effect from the use of multiple toxins that react together. This synergistic effect is difficult to assess. The cumulative effect of widespread, chronic, low-level exposure to multiple pesticides is only partially understood. One National Cancer Institute study found that farmers exposed to herbicides and pesticides had a six times greater risk than nonfarmers of getting one specific type of cancer.

Research at the University of Southern California discovered in 1987 that children living in homes where household and garden pesticides were used had a sevenfold chance of developing childhood leukemia.

The foods most likely to contain high levels of toxic pesticides are peaches, apples, nectarines, popcorn, and pears. The baby foods most likely to have unsafe levels are pears, peaches, and apple juice. This study found that approximately one in four peaches and one in eight apples had levels of organophosphates that are unsafe for children. Can we afford *not* to protect our children by buying nonorganic produce?

If you think this increase in pesticides and herbicides is just a bunch of statistics and has no effect, think again. According to the EPA, the incidence of childhood cancer increased 10.8% from 1973 through 1990, and cancer now kills more children under the age of fifteen than any other disease. A child born today has a one in 600 chance of developing cancer by the age of ten, according to the EPA. By a child's first birthday, the combined cancer risk of just eight pesticides on twenty foods they may have eaten exceeds the EPA's lifetime level of acceptable risk.

Children eat more food and take in more water relative to their size than adults do, and thus they suffer increased exposure to pesticides and other contaminants. Industrial pollution is a form of national domestic violence. With these kinds of statistics, it's clear why we so strongly stress the importance of feeding ourselves, pregnant mothers, and our children as close to 100% organic foods as possible because, although no one can avoid all exposure, it is important to minimize exposure.

Because children's bodies receive proportionally higher doses of toxins for their body weight than adults, and their organs are not fully developed, the organs are more vulnerable to toxin damage. Furthermore, many of the most frequently used pesticides affect the nervous system, and children are more susceptible to neurotoxins than adults.

Evidence has accumulated that many industrial chemicals (including many common plastics and pesticides) mimic estrogen hormones, thereby disrupting reproduction and development in humans, mammals, birds, and fish, just as diethylstilbesterol (DES) did to mothers and fetuses who received the drug in the 1960s. These estrogenic industrial chemicals may be causing or contributing to the increasing incidence of cancer of the breast, testicles, and prostate. They have affected us in a variety of ways:

- Average sperm counts in men worldwide are now 50% of the average fifty years ago.
- The incidence of testicular cancer has tripled, and prostate cancer has doubled, in the past fifty years.
- In 1960 the incidence of breast cancer was one in twenty, but by 1998 it was one in nine.
- Young male alligators in pesticide-contaminated lakes in Florida have such small penises that they are unable to function sexually. Estrogen-mediated hormonal imbalances can create all these changes and more.

One study showed that the mothers' milk of vegetarians contained only 1% of the amount of pesticides as that of meat-eating mothers. Many of these estrogen mimics will cross the placenta barrier and pass into the developing fetus. The resulting high estrogen exposure is one reason we recommend minimizing the use of soy, which is high in natural phytoestrogens. Soymilk is especially important to avoid for infants (as discussed later in this book).

Even the conservative *Journal of the American Medical Association* has reported that estrogenic chemicals have an effect. Ana Soto, a researcher at Tufts University, combined ten estrogenic mimics, each at one-tenth the dose necessary to produce a minimal response. She found that when all ten were combined, they were strong enough to produce an estrogenic response. This is significant, because the U.S. government has been regulating based on its testing of individual chemical effects. They have almost no data on the amplified synergistic effects of the many pesticides, herbicides, fungicides, plastics, PCBs, etc., interacting together, which is a far more likely scenario in actual exposed humans.

Since the 1960s, most researchers in the U.S. have expressed the opinion that the findings connecting the estrogenic pesticides with breast and other cancers are only preliminary, but the Israeli government has already acted on the evidence with exciting results. From 1976 to 1986, Israel was the only country among twenty-eight countries studied where the breast cancer death rate dropped. One explanation was that in 1978, Israel banned three estrogenic pesticides. Within two years after the ban, lindane levels in the tissues dropped by 90%, DDT by 43%, and BHC by 98%. By 1986, the death rate for breast cancer among Israeli women below the age of 44 had dropped by 30%. Conscious action to protect citizens from pesticides actually works.

Scientists can pretend to discern "safe" levels for an individual chemical, but they have no idea of any safe level for the synergistic use of chemicals. In fact, there are no "safe" levels. Political decision-makers need to understand that we have to abandon the chemical-by-chemical regulation approach, and regulate whole classes of chemicals. Furthermore, instead of setting standards according to pesticide effects on healthy adults, their effects on children should be used to set maximum exposure limits. Certain categories of dangerous chemicals, such as those that cause cancer and disrupt nervous system and hormone function, need to be immediately discontinued if we are to survive as a species.

In the *Journal of Food Science,* one of the few studies on the synergistic effect of pesticides reported that when three chemicals were each tested separately on rats, there was no obvious ill effect. When two of the three chemicals were added together, the health of the rats diminished. When all three were used synergistically, the rats all died within two weeks. This synergistic pesticide-porridge of our food and water is probably creating the most overall amplified damage to the health of all living forms in our environment. People who do not use purified water or organic food are exposing themselves significantly to these dangers.

Dr. David Pimentel of Cornell University, one of the world's leading agricultural experts, estimates that more than 500 species of insects are now resistant to pesticides. It is no accident that crops destroyed by insects have nearly doubled during the last forty years in spite of an almost tenfold increase in the amount and toxicity of insecticides. One study showed that recent pesticide usage by Filipino rice farmers costs the individual farmer more in medical bills than it generates in increased rice production. The amazing conclusion is that pesticides do not even achieve their stated purpose—yet we still are willing to risk our lives to use them.

In 1986, the Indonesian government sponsored a plan to decrease the use of pesticides. The rice production since then has increased by 10%, and there is far less capital outlay for pesticides and their concomitant medical problems. In Bangladesh, farmers using integrated pest management spent 75% less money on pesticides and increased their crop harvest by 14% over those using high levels of pesticides.

In summary, pesticides can negatively affect every living organism. Human beings are no exception. The more detrimental effects of pesticides, herbicides, and fungicides include cancer, brain dysfunction, ADD, nervous system disorders, birth defects, alterations of DNA; liver, kidney, lung, and reproductive problems; and an overall disruption of ecological cycles on the planet. According to Dr. David Pimentel, an entomologist and agricultural expert at Cornell University, pesticides cost the nation $8 billion annually in public health expenditures, groundwater decontamination, fish kills, bird kills, and domestic animal deaths. Pesticide usage is a major public health problem worldwide. It reflects a consciousness that is completely out of touch with the laws of nature and the laws of soil and human health.

Most genetically engineered plants are bred to act as pesticides themselves, or to withstand increasingly heavier applications of herbicides such as Monsanto's Roundup® weedkiller. The result has been a threefold increase in pesticide use in some places, because the plants can withstand them—which of course creates three times more toxic pollution. In the process of using genetically designed plants, corporations have taken control over seed supplies and the pesticides that they have designed to control them. The result is that this technology works powerfully against farmer-controlled, ecologically sensitive, sustainable, and organic methods that obviously reduce the amount of pesticides and help to protect agricultural biodiversity.

The good news is that many people and parents are listening to the basic facts. The total of organic products sold has grown about 20% per year in recent years, and many major supermarkets now stock organic products. In 2011, 91 million acres of farmland were certified organic.[7] Please support this positive shift in the supermarkets, and buy organic foods. Yet, in the midst of consumers waking up, the large corporate use of pesticides continues. For example, in the year 2000, Monsanto sold more than 2.6 billion dollars' worth of Roundup® around the world. Monsanto's genetically engineered seeds are grown on more than 100 million acres. In 2015, the World Health Organization (WHO) identified glyphosates as "possibly carcinogenic (cancer-causing) to humans."[8]

What sort of intelligence and consciousness does it take to continue to deliberately poison yourself and your family—in order to get less effective crop outputs? What sort of consciousness does it take to manufacture these poisons and sell them—especially to sell poisonous chemicals banned in the U.S. to developing countries, where the people may not understand how to even minimally protect themselves, due to ignorance and poverty? This is what is meant by the culture of death. Pesticides not only lead to human disease, but directly destroy the life-force of the soil. In our commitment to raise healthy, conscious children and create a healthy world, it is hard to understand how people can choose to spend money for something that not only does not work, but poisons humans and the environment. The energy of domination gets so out of control that it is consuming and destroying even the unethical dominators and their families.

Protect Yourself Against Food Chemicalization

According to the *Pesticide Monitoring Journal,* published by the Environmental Protection Agency (EPA), the major source of U.S. pesticide exposure comes from foods of animal origin. *Diet for a New America* points out that 95–99% of all toxic chemical residues in our diet comes from meat, fish, dairy, and eggs. One can substantially avoid this high toxic exposure by choosing vegan foods such as fruits, vegetables, nuts, seeds, and grains, which are lower on the food chain and thus have less accumulation of these poisons.

As mentioned earlier, *The New England Journal of Medicine* published a finding that the breastmilk of vegetarian women has only 1–2% of the pesticide contamination of the national average for breastfeeding women on a flesh-centered diet. This is a significant indication of how much you can decrease your pesticide exposure by becoming vegetarian or vegan. It is possible to further decrease exposure by only eating organically grown vegetarian foods. In some places it is not possible to obtain organic, vegetarian foods; it is still a safer choice to eat commercially grown fruits, vegetables, grains, nuts, and seeds rather than flesh foods. The body can adequately detox minor and occasional pesticide exposures, but becomes overwhelmed if the exposure is chronic or too high.

David Steinman, in *Diet for a Poisoned Planet,* has done an enormous amount of work in studying exactly which fruits, vegetables, nuts, seeds, and grains have the lowest toxic residues. He analyzed foods for more than one hundred different industrial chemicals and pesticides, using laboratory detection limits that were five to ten times more sensitive than the normal FDA detection standards. This work has been continued by the Environmental Working Group (EWG)'s *Annual Shopper's Guide to Pesticides in Produce.*[9]

The fruits and vegetables with the highest pesticide load in 2013 included: apples, celery, cherry tomatoes, cucumbers, grapes, hot peppers, nectarines, peaches, potatoes, spinach, strawberries, sweet bell peppers, kale, collard greens, and summer squash. These are therefore the most important to buy from organic sources only. Those with the lowest pesticide load included: asparagus, avocado, cabbage, cantaloupe, eggplant, grapefruit, kiwi, mango, mushrooms, onions, pineapple, sweet peas, and sweet potatoes.

The best way to be safe, of course, is to avoid commercial foods altogether. If enough people care about themselves and their children to buy only organic foods, the law of consumer demand on the market will force a shift that will increase the amount of organic farming that will occur, which will make more organic foods available at lower prices. Fortunately, a subtle shift toward organic farming and produce is already happening in many parts of the U.S. and throughout Europe. Prince Charles in England is one of the outspoken leaders of this movement.

Genetically Engineered Foods

Genetically engineered foods provide a more significant threat to our delicate worldwide ecosystems than even pesticides and herbicides. John Hagelin, an award-winning quantum physicist and presidential candidate on the Natural Law Party ticket, says,

> When genetic engineers disregard the genetic boundaries set in place by natural law, they run the risk of destroying our genetic encyclopedia, compromising the richness of our biodiversity, and creating a genetic soup. What this means for the future of our ecosystem, no one knows.[10]

Dr. John Fagan, internationally recognized molecular biologist and former genetic engineer, says,

> We are living today in a very delicate time, one that is reminiscent of the birth of the nuclear era, when mankind stood on the threshold of a new technology. No one knew that nuclear power would bring us to the brink of annihilation, or fill our planet with highly toxic radioactive waste. We were so excited by the power of a new discovery that we leaped ahead blindly, and without caution. Today the situation with genetic engineering is perhaps even more grave because this technology acts on the very blueprint of life itself.[11]

When you do not know what you are doing, and you insist on meddling, you have the potential to create a great deal of damage. There is an old saying: "If it's not broken, don't fix it."

The dangers of genetically engineered foods (GE foods, also known as GMOs, or genetically modified organisms) are multiple:

- Once a gene is inserted into an organism, it can cause unanticipated side effects. Mutations can cause genetically engineered food to contain toxins and allergens, and also to be reduced in nutritional value.
- GE foods have the potential to damage the ecosystem, harm wildlife, and alter the natural habitat. Our plant and animal species have evolved over millions of years, and introducing genetically engineered species upsets the delicate balance of the ecology.
- Gene pollution can never be cleaned up.
- The use of GE crops increases pesticide pollution of our food and water supplies. Approximately 57% of the research done by biotechnology companies is focused on genetically engineering plants that can tolerate larger amounts of herbicides.
- GE foods may cause unpredictable, permanent changes in the nature of our food because they can potentially disrupt the genetic structures of plants and animals that have been

nourishing the human race for thousands of years. Because genetic engineering is a new and far from exact science, the new genetic structure of a plant could give rise to unusual proteins that could easily cause unforeseen problems for humans and our health.

Examples of "leaky genes"—genetically engineered plants cross-pollinating with traditional varieties and passing on the genetically engineered traits—have been reported in several places. In 2000, the National Institute of Agricultural Botany reported the first genetically modified superweed in Britain. Pollen from a genetically engineered canola crossed with wild turnips, and the turnips inherited the herbicide-resistant genes. In Mexico, cross-pollinating from genetically engineered corn has spread as far as sixty miles away. Reports have come from Canada since 2000 that weeds are now able to tolerate herbicides originally designed for herbicide-resistant GMO crops.

- GE foods may be missing important elements, or have changes in the nutrient ratios. Genetic engineering may accidentally or intentionally remove or inactivate substances in food that the engineers consider undesirable, but the new food or the missing substance may have qualities that we do not quite understand. For example, the nutrient chemistry in genetically engineered soy reveals that it has 29% less choline (needed for nervous system development), 27% more trypsin inhibitor (which inhibits protein digestion), and 200% more lectins (associated with greater food sensitivity).
- The use of GE foods may result in decreased effectiveness of antibiotics. It is now commonplace in genetic engineering to introduce antibiotics in genes as a marker to indicate that the organism has been successfully engineered. GMOs may be foods with the potential to neutralize antibiotics.
- GE foods can cause allergic reactions. One of the problems of these newly identified proteins is that the human body is simply not equipped to deal with them. One of the body's responses to

unnatural and toxic food is to create an allergic reaction. Reports of increased allergies to GE soy products are already coming out. Soy, 92% of which is now genetically engineered in the U.S., has moved into the top ten allergenic foods. It is now associated with significantly more severe allergies.

- Harmful effects of GMOs may not be discovered for years, in the sense that we do not have an idea of what could potentially happen as we introduce these new foods into our diet. As pointed out in *Conscious Eating,* in the chapter on the biologically altered brain, there have been significant changes in the quality of our health since we introduced refined, fried, fast, and junk food into our Western diet in the 1930s. What makes us think that, by further interfering with natural foods through genetic engineering, we are not going to cause more and more serious problems, and further alter the already biologically altered brain? There are no long-term studies to prove the safety of genetically altered foods. We do not even want to wait to see these studies, because results will not be available until decades after the fact, and by that time it may be too late for us and our children—and their children.

- GE organisms may have unanticipated negative ecological impacts. Some genetically engineered bacteria looked useful in some limited way, and then researchers discovered that they are capable of making the land infertile. One case of this is a soil bacterium called *Klebsiella planticola.* This bacterium has been genetically engineered to dispose of wood chips, corn stalks, and waste from the lumber business and agriculture.

- As it turns out, *K. planticola* also produces ethanol in this process. When seeds were planted in soil that contained its waste products, they sprouted and then died. Independent researchers found that the genetically engineered *Klebsiella* is highly competitive with native soil microorganisms, and strongly suppresses their activities. We need the more than 1,600 species of microorganisms found in a teaspoon of soil, in order to maintain the vital force of the soil. If it is not obvious, it should be: We cannot predict the effect of a new microorganism on the ecology and the environment, and the unforeseen consequences could be dire.

• GE foods have been shown to create newer and higher levels of toxins in the environment. Many plants produce a variety of compounds that are toxic to humans or alter the food quality. Generally speaking, as pointed out in *Conscious Eating*, these toxic elements do not cause problems in the levels normally found in plants, unless we consume those plants in large quantities. The practice of combining plant and animal species in engineered foods, however, has the potential to create new and unpredictable levels of toxins.

Even the FDA and the EPA now classify as insecticides certain corn and potato strains that were engineered to produce toxins that kill insects. These plants are no longer even classified as vegetables! Insect-resistant crops make up about one-quarter of the acreage of transgenic plants. One of the most serious ecological threats is crops carrying a gene from a soil bacterium called *Bacillus thuringiensis* (Bt). The Bt gene, when transferred into corn and cotton plants, kills leaf-eating caterpillars. Every cell of these plants contains the Bt gene, and produces Bt toxin, which is one of the world's most important biological pesticides.

This is a direct threat to organic farmers. In 1999, the International Federation of Organic Agricultural Movements joined with Greenpeace and the Center for Food Safety in a lawsuit against the EPA, which had approved genetically engineered Bt cotton, corn, and potatoes. Monsanto's Bt cotton harms a wide range of insects, including lacewings and ladybugs, and confuses bees' ability to distinguish the different smells of flowers. Monarch butterfly caterpillars, according to the journal *Nature*, were being killed by pollen from Bt corn. What potential damage might toxic Bt crops have on the flora that live in our own intestines?

- How much proof do we need before we realize that genetic engineering can potentially create biological chaos? Genetic engineering companies try to claim that genetically engineered foods are natural and equivalent to the original genetic strains. But that simply and scientifically is not the case.

  For example, although the industry has presented more than 1,400 analyses to demonstrate that Roundup Ready® soy is the "substantial" equivalent of natural soy, the manufacturer's own studies suggest that when the herbicide Roundup® is sprayed on Roundup Ready® soy, the defensive response of the plant leads to increased plant estrogen levels. Therefore, it is possible that the sprayed soybeans contain a higher level of plant estrogen than the natural beans, which is already high. The implications of this for the sexual development of our male and female children are obvious, yet beyond our full understanding. We also know that a significant amount of people have become allergic to soy protein with stronger allergies than ever before, when exposed to genetically engineered soy.

- Using bacteria to make genetically engineered tryptophan is another example of how toxins are created that are beyond our current understanding. In 1989, there was an outbreak of a flu-like, sometimes fatal, disease called eosinophilia–myalgia syndrome (EMS). A company selling the supplement L-tryptophan that was produced by genetically engineered bacteria was found to be the source of the problem. The tryptophan itself did not seem to be causing the EMS, but rather the contaminants, which made up only .01% of the product by weight.

  When the bacteria were genetically altered to produce larger quantities of tryptophan, the increased concentration of tryptophan reached such high levels that unexpected chemical reactions produced new kinds of toxins, which led in turn to the EMS. The result of this genetically engineered tryptophan disaster was that thirty-seven people died, 1,500 people were partially paralyzed, and 5,000 were temporarily disabled.

That toxic tryptophan would have passed as a "substantial" equivalent of trypophan, and would also have passed the test for known toxins. We cannot test for toxins we do not yet know about—and there is much we do not yet know about the consequences of GMOs on our health and our children's health.

- One of the biggest problems with genetically engineered plants is their presumed ability to tolerate almost unlimited quantities of pesticide, which means that the public, including our children, will be exposed to an ever-increasing pesticide load unless they eat an entirely organic diet.

- GMO crops, because of the way they are commercially grown, are less nutritious. Some studies have found a reduction in IQ of up to ten points in the generation of children brought up on these "green revolution" foods. Genetically engineered crops— because they are so strongly tied to the monoculture approach, chemical fertilizers, herbicides, and pesticides, will probably cause an increase in all of the health and mental health problems associated with the "green revolution"—and possibly on a grander and more serious scale, because the gene pool will have been disrupted. One clear example is the significantly increased use of Roundup®. According to the U.S. Fish and Wildlife Service, at least seventy-four plant species are endangered by Roundup®, and it kills fish at concentrations of 10 parts per million, impedes the growth of earthworms, and is toxic to soil microbes that help plants take up nutrients from the soil.

The active ingredient in Roundup® is glyphosate. In the 1990s, glyphosate was listed as the third most common cause of all forms of pesticide-related illness in California. Studies have also linked exposure to glyphosates with an increased risk of developing non-Hodgkin's lymphoma, the third-fastest-growing cancer in the U.S. Already, the Roundup Ready® crops (engineered to survive Roundup®) need to survive higher doses of glyphosates than ever as superweeds too become more pesticide-resistant. This story of increasing resistance in weeds is all too familiar. As previously mentioned, Round Up Ready has been identified by the WHO as potentially causing cancer.

Genetically engineered soy is in soy flour, soy oil, lecithin, soy protein isolates, concentrates, vitamin E supplements, tofu dogs, cereals, veggie burgers, sausages, tamari, soy sauce, chips, ice cream, frozen yogurt, infant formula, sauces, margarine, soy cheeses, cookies, chocolates, cakes, fried foods, shampoos, bubble bath, cosmetics, and enriched flours and pastas. It is hard work, but it pays off to keep our children away from all those foods.

Genetically engineered corn is in cornflour, cornstarch, corn sweeteners, corn oil, and many syrups. Products that may contain GE corn derivatives include vitamin C, tofu dogs, chips, candies, ice cream, infant formula, salad dressing, tomato sauce, breads, cookies, cereals, baking powder, alcohol, vanilla, margarine, soy sauce, tamari, sodas, fried foods, powdered sugar, and enriched flours and pastas.

Because genetically engineered canola is so prevalent, it is found in most products that contain canola oil derivatives. These include chips, salad dressings, cookies, margarines, soaps, detergents, soy cheese, and fried foods. Genetically engineered cotton is found in many fabrics and in cottonseed oil, as well as in products that contain fabrics or cottonseed oil, such as clothing, linens, chips, peanut butter, crackers, and cookies. With GE potatoes we are obviously looking at not only fresh potatoes, but potato chips, fries, mashed potatoes, baked potatoes, mixes, Passover products, vegetable products, and soups.

We find GE tomatoes in sauces, purees, pizza, and lasagna. It appears that no plum or Roma tomatoes have been genetically engineered, and only one cherry tomato has been, but this may not even be true by the time this book is published. Most nonorganic papayas grown in Hawaii are genetically engineered. Some crookneck squash and zucchini are genetically engineered. Since 95% of the soymeal and approximately 90% of the corn grown in the U.S. are used as livestock feed, almost all nonorganic meat, poultry, dairy, or egg products sold in the U.S. contain genetically engineered substances.

The potential dangers of eating genetically engineered foods and/or foods that contain genetically modified substances were highlighted by the research of Dr. Árpád Pusztai, a senior scientist at the Rowett Research Institute in Aberdeen, Scotland. He fed genetically engineered potatoes to rats. The rats developed smaller hearts, livers, and brains, and had weaker immune systems. Some rats showed significant brain shrinkage after only ten days of eating genetically modified potatoes. We consider this a most significant piece of data on the health dangers of GMOs and an ominous warning.

Public relations for GE foods talk about how important these are for "feeding the world's hungry." This is a cruel joke. The GE companies' products are primarily intended as feed for livestock, not to provide nutrition to people. However, their GE/GMO corn and soy is also in a high percentage—some estimate 67%—of packaged and processed foods at organic-food chains such as Whole Foods. Fortunately, thanks to consumer pressure, Whole Foods may be phasing out these GE/GMO foods by 2018.

Contrary to GE food corporations' public relations claims about producing more per acre, genetically modified soybeans actually produce 4% less than conventional varieties, according to the research of agronomy professor Ed Oplinger at the University of Wisconsin. His study covered soybean yields in twelve U.S. states. Other studies on Monsanto's transgenic soybeans showed 10% less productivity compared to traditional varieties.

Part of the argument against genetically engineered food and for going organic is the importance of preserving heirloom seeds, which contain the original seed genetics. Heirloom seeds work on a deeper energetic soul level as well. Heirloom seeds contain the entire history of a people and of a land. These seeds nourish our souls, and strengthen our connection to the land. They were bred for nourishing people, not for making money.

This shamanistic, Earth-based understanding is in sharp contrast to the intent of the genetic engineering corporations. This contrast is becoming clearer to many people throughout the world. For example, the Indian scientist Vandana Shiva determined after an international meeting in 1987 that the corporate chemical and food companies were attempting to control agriculture through patents, genetic engineering, and mergers. She believes that what the global-economy corporations call "growth" is really a form of theft from nature and from people. These are ecological teaching points for our older children.

In summary, we have made an extensive effort to make information available to the reader on the potential dangers of GMOs. Based on the data we have seen, GMOs are a significant threat to the health and well-being of our offspring. But we can choose not to involve ourselves and our children in this culture-of-death experiment. We can choose to eat only organic certified produce—especially since many efforts to mandate labeling of GMO foods have not yet succeeded, as of the writing of this book. That is the only way to escape this culture-of-death misuse of power. One step further, because even manure from GMO-fed animals can contain GMOs, is to practice organic, veganic farming, or eat produce from these farms, which also sustains their work.

A key scriptural teaching is, "Don't eat what may be harmful to you." One should act to protect one's physical, mental, and spiritual health by not eating anything that may be dangerous to human existence. As the old saying goes, "Better safe than sorry."

What can we do to protect ourselves and our children from GMO exposure?

- Vote for labeling GMO foods. As interest gathers, there will be a time when the U.S. will label or outlaw GMOs. At the time of this writing, sixty-four (and counting) other countries require GMO labeling. Fifty-one countries currently place strong restrictions or outright bans on GMOs. Currently a crucial legal battle is raging between the people of the U.S. and Monsanto and its lobbyists, who are working to restrict our food choices by not labeling GMOs.
- Buy fruits and vegetables that are rarely genetically modified. These include onions, avocados, pineapples, peas, asparagus, mangos, eggplant, kiwi, cantaloupe, cabbage, sweet potatoes,

grapefruit, watermelon, and mushrooms. Avoid produce that is most likely to be genetically modified, including apples, celery, bell peppers, peaches, strawberries, nectarines, grapes, spinach, lettuce, cucumbers, blueberries, potatoes, green beans, kale, collard greens, sweet corn, yellow squash, zucchini, cherries, and hot peppers.

- If you choose to eat meat, stay away from all factory-farmed animal products, CAFO-raised meat, and conventionally raised dairy, as they are almost certainly using GMO products. Simply purchase and consume only certified organic products from your local farmers.
- There is a 60% chance that any processed foods, even from a health food store, contain GMO-contaminated food. The safest approach for you and your children is to only use non-processed, organically certified foods.

Irradiated Foods—Another Hazard

Irradiated food is a health hazard. Irradiating food completely disorganizes its energetic field. This is also true of microwaved food. It is believed that irradiation kills all bacteria infecting food, but even *E. coli,* the bacterium most often cited by proponents of food irradiation, has evolved new forms that are radiation-resistant.

Irradiating food significantly decreases the quality and energy of food. A substantial number of studies show that irradiated food, when given to certain animals, caused increased incidence of tumors. In one study in India, researchers fed irradiated wheat to children, and after about a month, the children began to develop leukemoid reactions (increased white blood cells, as in leukemia, in response to infection or other stresses). When researchers stopped giving the children the irradiated wheat, their blood tests went back to normal. The implication is to go back to basics and respect the natural laws by avoiding irradiated food. With this approach, we can have a healthy diet that will sustain our lives and the quality of our DNA.

By eating authentic, organic, whole foods as nature has given them to us, we have a sound, delicious, and healthy way of eating that begins to bring us back to health as a nation and a planet. This is not about being deprived! Not eating genetically engineered and junk foods, irradiated foods, white flour, and sugar is a blessing, and not a deprivation. Unfortunately, this obvious natural path is not easy for people to remember or follow, in an economy dominated and brainwashed by corporate greed rather than organized around improving nutrition and health for all.

In general, cheap industrial food has the least chance of being safe or humane. Killing animals for food never could be humane, but modern practices of mass-producing animals for slaughter remains vastly different from the respect and prayerfulness of a Native American Plains Indians before killing a buffalo. (It is interesting to note here that two historically-based studies showed that sixty percent of all Native American tribes in the U.S. were vegan.[12])

Food irradiation does not solve the problem of food contamination; it only gives the illusion of helping. It actually makes the situation worse, because it makes possible the conditions for lowering hygiene standards even further, based on the idea that we can simply irradiate carelessly handled food.

Whom are we kidding? Food irradiation is not 100% effective. It is already known that food irradiation does not eliminate all the *E. coli* and salmonella bacteria. Food irradiation has become a source of mutant bacteria, and perhaps viruses, that are radiation-resistant. It is the old antibiotic-resistant story, with a new twist. In addition, food irradiation plants themselves are unsafe. Radioactive accidents have already happened at the few food irradiation plants in this country and worldwide. Since 1974, the Nuclear Regulatory Commission has recorded fifty-four accidents at 132 irradiation facilities around the world. In New Jersey, which has the highest concentration of irradiation plants, almost every plant has a record of environmental contamination, worker overexposure, or regulatory failures.

There is no solid evidence to show that eating irradiated food is safe, but there is some evidence to show that it has dangers. The food is irradiated with gamma rays, which break up the molecular structure of the food and create free radicals. The free radicals then react with the food to form new chemical substances called radiolytic products, which include formaldehyde, benzene, formic acid, and quinones—all of which are known to be harmful to human health. In one experiment, levels of benzene, a known carcinogen, were seven times higher in irradiated beef than in non-irradiated beef. Some of these radiolytic products are unique to the irradiation process, and have not been adequately identified or tested for toxicity.

Irradiating food destroys 20–80% of the vitamins, including vitamin A, B1, B3, B6, B12, C, E, K, and folic acid. Amino acids and essential fatty acids are also destroyed. Enzymes, of course, are destroyed, as are the biophotons.

A significant number of studies show some dangers of eating irradiated food, for both animals and humans. Raltech Scientific Services, Inc., after a series of twelve studies on feeding irradiated chicken to various animal species, found the possibility of chromosome damage, immunotoxicity, greater incidence of kidney disease, cardiac thrombus, and fibroplasia. According to *Food and Water Journal,* from which much of this information was received, USDA researcher Donald Thayer concluded, "A collective assessment of study results argues against a definitive conclusion that the gamma-irradiated test material (irradiated chicken) was free of toxic properties." Rats who received irradiated food showed a statistically significant increase in testicular tumors, and possible kidney and testicular damage.

The Organic Live-Food Solution

For those interested in health, what we are looking at is an unsavory situation. We are faced with commercially grown foods, irradiated foods, genetically engineered foods, and government authorities who are choosing, in essence, by not requiring thorough labeling, to make it very difficult to discern whether or not something has been irradiated or genetically modified. This presents a complex problem.

There is, however, a very simple, delicious, healthy, yet powerful solution: Go organic, vegan, authentic—and/or grow your own.

If we follow the guideline to eat only whole, vegan, organic, high-energy, authentic foods, the irresponsible tampering with our nation's main food supply will have little effect on us personally. If these issues pain your heart and conscience such that you want to help others—as they do us—there are many positive steps to take. Find active organizations addressing world issues of food, choose one or more that appeal to you, and support them.

Clearly, growing your own food or buying from a local organic source or CSA (community-supported agriculture) farm is the best way to go. After three days, food begins to loose its life-force and nutritional value. If it looks wilted—even if it is organic—don't buy it. If you don't want any GMOs in your diet, the *Non-GMO Shopping Guide* is available free at www.nongmoshoppingguide.com.

Select only organic produce; the best label is the "USDA Certified Organic" seal. In order to be called organic, a product must be grown and produced according to standardized organic farming methods. The most trustworthy organic food is grown by your local farmer, who should be willing to allow you to personally inspect their farm.

Organic food should be grown in alignment with natural laws, and contain no artificial ingredients or preservatives. This means avoiding anything with MSG, including cooked soy (as all cooked soy contains MSG); corn syrup; artificial sweeteners (Equal, Nutrisweet, Conderel, and Amino Sweet, for instance); sucralose (Splenda, Sweet One); and saccharine (Sweet'N Low, Sugar Twin). The only relatively safe sweeteners are stevia, erythritol, and xylitol.

Organic foods do not contain growth hormones, antibiotics, or other drugs. That is why we choose vegan organic. If one is consuming flesh food, it is best if it does not come from any confined animal feeding operations (CAFOs). Further ecological considerations demand that food be grown sustainably using wise water practices, and measures to avoid soil depletion. All foods should be cleansed in fresh, non-fluoridated water.

The physical development of our children plays a significant role in the realization of their full potential for aliveness and liberation. To walk the Earth as a full human being, we need to have proper body-mind functioning, which is greatly supported by eating authentic food.

Because 50% of our food's protein, 60–70% of its vitamins and minerals, and 95–100% of its natural phytonutrients are lost through cooking, fresh, organic, living foods that remain uncooked (although they may be warmed) offer the highest nutritional support for the developing body. The highly beneficial sunlight energy of chlorophyll, found in living greens and resulting from photosynthesis and life-force energy, is lost in the cooking process as well. Life-force energy, photographed through the use of Kirlian photography, is visibly decreased after high temperatures have been applied to food for more than three minutes.

Another benefit of receiving raw nutriment is that the more alive our food is, the more alive we feel. Leah tells a story that her children love, of a particular day when Leah was enjoying a freshly picked salad infused with appreciation of the children's daddy's gardening services. Levi, who was four years old at the time, happened by and asked her if he could have a salad of his own, "just like hers." Leah practically ran to the garden, as this was Levi's first request for salad at breakfast time. The two then sat and shared savored moments; and just as Levi's plate became leafless he spontaneously threw his hands into the air and exclaimed, "I'm alive!"

Not only are organic plant-sourced foods highly vitalizing and nutritious, but eating this way minimizes the child's exposure to carcinogenic pesticides, insecticides, and herbicides, as well as the harmful growth hormones and antibiotics that are found in most animal products. In a 2004 study by the Environmental Working Group, 287 industrial chemicals were identified in babies' umbilical-cord blood. These include 180 known carcinogens, and 217 chemicals that are toxic to the brain and nervous system.[13] The ingestion of these phosphate chemicals, which were developed from World War II-era nerve gas, has now been linked to developmental problems in childhood, such as behavior problems, delayed motor skills, ADHD, and short-term memory disruption.[14]

Studies also reveal a link between childhood leukemia and increased pesticide use around the home. From the National Academy of Science we read warnings and position papers stating that exposure to pesticides early in life can increase cancer rates down the road, in addition to increased mental and immune system disorders.[15] [16] As featured in the CNN documentary film *Toxic Childhood,* most chemicals in common use today have never been tested for public safety. This is especially true when it comes to the effects of cumulative and prolonged exposures.

Not only do children in this country statistically consume more GM foods than do adults, particularly corn products, soy-based infant formula, and dairy containing the GM bovine growth hormone rbGH, but unnatural changes to foods have more impact on the structure and functioning of a child's rapidly growing body. When a child eats, more of the food is converted to build organs and tissues, whereas adults convert more energy to be stored as fat.

Children under age two are at particular risk, because their digestive system is more permeable. Genetically modified products may be leading to earlier introduction of certain proteins, resulting in food allergies when they leak directly into the bloodstream from the gut. GEs can also be ingested directly, in commercial baby foods or from the breastmilk of a mother who is consuming GE foods. The child is 3–4 times more prone to allergies than the adult, and is at highest risk of death from allergic reactions to food. The introduction of GMOs might eventually be shown to be a factor in the rising rates of childhood food allergies.

Conscious Eating, by Gabriel Cousens, MD, highlights the profound connection between diet and physical degeneration. We have seen that when refined carbohydrates and sugars become heavily used within a culture, the resultant rise in heart disease and diabetes rates appear in the next generation. The famous Pottenger Cat Study of the 1930s and '40s demonstrated this process of intergenerational degeneration from an unhealthy diet. In this scientific study of approximately nine hundred cats, one group of cats—the controls or "normals"—were fed raw meats, milk, and cod liver oil, while the second group—the "deficient" cats—ate cooked meats and cooked milk, and also received cod liver oil.

The results were alarming. From generation to generation the "normals" were uniform in size and development, without any skeletal, tissue tone, or fur changes. The calcium and phosphorus content of their bones remained consistent, and their internal organs showed full development. They were resistant to infections, fleas, and parasites, and showed no signs of allergies. Their mental states were friendly, with purring and predictable behavior patterns. They maintained a high level of nervous-system coordination. They reproduced one homogeneous generation after another, all in good health, and the mothers had no trouble with the birth process or nursing. The average litter was five kittens, with an average weight of 119 grams.

In contrast, cats fed the cooked-meat diet gave birth to heterogeneous offspring with many variations in skeletal structure. By the third generation, their bones became as soft as rubber. Generations of "deficient" cats suffered heart problems, nearsightedness, underactivity or inflammation of the thyroid and bladder, arthritis and inflammation of the joints, inflammation of the nervous system with paralysis and meningitis, and infections of the kidney, bones, liver, testes, and ovaries. There was also a general decrease in the health of visceral organs. On autopsy, the females were found to have ovarian atrophy and uterine congestion, while the males showed a failure in active spermatogenesis. In the first generation of cats who ate the cooked food, spontaneous abortions ran about 25%, and that number went up to 70% in the second generation. Deliveries were difficult, and many females died giving birth. Mortality rates of the kittens were high. The average cooked-food kitten's weight was nineteen grams less than the raw meat-nurtured cats. Vermin and intestinal parasites were numerous. Skin lesions and allergies were frequent, and got worse with each generation. In the third generation, the cooked-meat cats were so deficient that none survived beyond the sixth month.[17] The cats eating the cooked foods were unable to reproduce after the third generation.

Although our children are not cats, a trend of intergenerational degeneration is at least subtly happening.

Living foods also support our children's lives through greater longevity for themselves and their loved ones. The book *Disease-Proof Your Child,* by family doctor Joel Fuhrman, MD, highlights plant-sourced, live foods as being key to not only reducing childhood ailments such as asthma, ear infections, and allergies, but also for providing protection against a future of disease such as diabetes, cardiovascular disease, and cancer.[18] As explained in *There is a Cure for Diabetes,* living foods actually activate our human antiaging, antiinflamatory, anticancer, and antioxidant genes. Seventy-year-old Annette Larkins was dubbed the "ageless woman" when she was featured in a televised news story about her raw-food lifestyle as her "fountain of youth." In the film *Raw for Life,* we also see eighty-three-year-old championship diver Tom Hairabedian attribute his robust state of health to his long-term commitment to living nutrition.

Yet another example is centenarian Bernando LaPallo, who recalls, "My father, a medical doctor, told me 100 years ago, when I was five years old, 'Son, if you want to live a long, healthy life, then avoid man's food and eat God's food, the way He made it—RAW.' I am now 105 years young, and walk for an hour every morning, from 5:00 AM to 6:00 AM. I have lived long enough to have had three careers."[19]

In the book *Raw Knowledge* by Paul Nison, we also read an interview with long-term raw-fooder William Esser, who was not only remarkably youthful in appearance but was still able to go running and play tennis at the age of ninety.[20] Rabbi Dr. Gabriel, now a seventy-two-year-old grandfather, is able to do 601 push-ups and thirty-two pull-ups, and has greater endurance and flexibility than when he was in his twenties, captain of an undefeated Amherst College football team and an awardee of the National Football Foundation's College Hall of Fame. During his football years he could only do seventy consecutive push-ups.

Leah's family recently attended the ninetieth birthday of her daughter's piano teacher, whose small town community marvels at her special ability to love others as well as to still live independently, driving and taking in new students. It was fun to find out that this very special woman, who trades piano lessons for homegrown sprouts, had been given fresh green juice throughout her life, as her herbalist mother was influenced by the late Ann Wigmore. Leah is also very inspired by her own father who, through living nutrition, has been able to drop over eighty pounds of excess weight, avoid all medications in his seventies, and be a shining example for his grandchildren of a vibrant, fasting, juicing, organic-gardening grandpa.

Our children greatly benefit from having healthy, active, and youthful adults in their lives. Sadly, however, many of today's children are in clinical need of age-reversing themselves. As childhood nutrition educator Michael Donaldson, PhD puts it, "It's bad enough that children have sicknesses particular to them, like asthma and ADD/ADHD, but now they are increasingly getting adult-type symptoms—high blood pressure, high cholesterol, obesity, all risk factors for heart disease, type 2 diabetes (which used to be called adult-onset diabetes), juvenile arthritis, colitis, chronic fatigue, and depression. Johnny's life is tough enough in modern times, but does he have to get grandpa's disease too?"[21]

According to Donaldson, fibromyalgia isn't just for middle-aged men and women either. We are now seeing juvenile fibromyalgia, and know that living with chronic pain increases one's risk of dying from cardiovascular disease or cancer by twenty to thirty percent.[22] According to some predictions, we are actually looking at a potential decline in life expectancy in the United States in the twenty-first century. More than a few experts are predicting that parents will actually begin to outlive their children!

In the context of supporting the child's expansion of consciousness, which allows time and space for their development, we can see the eternal value of physical health, regeneration, and longevity. As charted by Maslow's famous hierarchy of needs, it is when the basic physical human needs are met that we have enough stability to give our attention to spiritual development—the very purpose of our being. In other words, if all of our energy must be spent on survival, there is less energy left for the work of self-realization, the work of waking up to our aliveness.

Minerals and Children—Precious Gems

Minerals are frequencies of Light, frequencies of information, frequencies of consciousness, and frequencies of potential.

—Gabriel Cousens, MD, in *Spiritual Nutrition*

Minerals are essential to every aspect of the developing child.

Physically, we see that their bones and teeth are made of calcium and phosphorus, their skin and hair are made of silicon, and iron is an essential element of their blood. Minerals are needed for all enzyme reactions and for all aspects of growth in general. Just as a mother's nutrition is imperative to her nursing baby's immunity, when Mother Earth is depleted of minerals her children—plants, animals, and humans—are also less resistant to disease.

Fortunately, the reverse is also true. When the Earth's soil is replenished with minerals, specifically via seawater solutions, as is done at the Tree of Life Foundation Gardens, we see a resulting increase in growth, vitality, and resistance to disease for both the plants grown from this mineral-rich soil and the animals that have eaten these mineral-dense, disease-resistant plants. Particularly key minerals for children are 1) zinc, needed in over 300 enzymatic processes to build the brain, immune system, and secondary sexual characteristics; and 2) magnesium, needed in over 300 neurotransmitter-enzyme systems. The minerals zinc, calcium, iodine, magnesium, manganese, phosphorus, potassium, selenium, silicon, sodium, and sulfur are key building blocks for the child's developing brain and nervous system. Foods high in minerals such as sea vegetables, sprouts, leafy greens, phytoplankton concentrate, and *shilajit* (a resinous vegan substance from the Himalayas), which is high in fulvic acid, are optimal for enhancing mineral absorption.

How do minerals support the child's **spirit?** As explained in *Spiritual Nutrition:* "Minerals are one of the deep secrets of Spiritual Nutrition.... Each mineral has a vibratory rate that supports different aspects of consciousness and spiritual awareness, as well as chakras and organ systems."[23]

Phosphorus and sulfur stimulate the link between the physical body and the soul as well as supporting meditation, vision, and expansion of consciousness. For the child's **social** and **emotional** development, the mineral manganese is associated with love and compassion. These are only but a few of the approximately ninety minerals available to us from nature. Just as gems, which have long been associated with healing and spiritual qualities, are made up of minerals, so is the child's body made up of these minerals and, when fully mineralized, will become a human gem.

The increased mineralization that we get with authentic live food, supporting the activation of the full enzymatic expression in the body, is fundamental to the optimal health and growth of our children. This is a distinct advantage of authentic food over commercial and, to a lesser extent, organic food. Healthy mineral balance through good nutrition based on authentic live foods is vital for optimum health and healing in humans, and is especially important in serving the nutritional needs of the growing bodies of children.

Minerals such as zinc, magnesium, sulfur, and phosphorous, and particularly microminerals such as gold, cobalt, platinum, and manganese, help the body naturally form unique enzymes and vitamins, mostly through the action of microflora in the gut. An optimal supply of minerals held in their chelated, bioavailable form in raw food helps to form unique enzyme bridges that lead to superior bodily performance and optimum health. Enzymes are catalysts that enhance intracellular biochemical processes. The function of a catalyst is to promote and accelerate biochemical transformations from one chemical form to another without being used up in the process. This is the basis for cellular longevity and rejuvenation.

When combined with a good probiotic supplement to create optimum performance of the gut microflora, optimally mineralized foods may help young bodies avoid, protect, and even *possibly repair* cellular damage that leads to neurological system dysfunction manifesting in such disorders as ADD and autism.

How do we provide our children with a diet rich in minerals? The oceans hold an abundance of essential minerals, partly because minerals from topsoil are constantly being washed by the rains into the sea. One way to get them back from the oceans is to grow our organic land vegetables with soil amendments of sea vegetation and seawater solutions. The Tree of Life Foundation has been exploring how to best do this with organic, veganic gardening and sprouting, and is now teaching workshops on this.

Another way is to add sea vegetation directly into the family diet. Sea vegetables contain more than sixty trace minerals and trace elements. Since the Fukushima disaster, however, we do not advise eating sea vegetables from the Pacific Ocean between Japan and the U.S. West Coast.

Sea veggies include kelp, dulse, hiziki, wakame, laver, alaria, nori, sea lettuce, and Irish moss. These can be purchased dried, in whole or powdered form. Raw kelp noodles can also be found online or in health food stores for soups, spring rolls, and Asian pasta salads. Irish moss is used as a thickener in salad dressings, and lends a light, gelatinous consistency to desserts. Children appreciate nori, dried into thin, paper-like sheets. These can be eaten as is, cut into shapes, crumpled over salads, rolled up with a filling such as avocado slices, or seasoned and dried into chips. (See recipes for Cucumber Boats with Nori Sails, Moon and Stars, Ninja Chips, and Noritos.)

Sea algae: Chlorella and spirulina are available in powdered form. "E-3 Live" from Klamath Lake is a highly nourishing liquid or powder form that is specifically good for brain development. Small amounts of these can be added to smoothies and nut or seed mylks. These can also be mashed into avocados or other soft fruits for baby. (See Leah's book *Baby Greens* for more on introducing living foods to baby.)

Raw Himalayan crystal salt, pink salt, scalar salts, and other high-mineral raw salts are another way to receive the precious gift of minerals. Scalar salts are raw, mined salts (not being from the ocean, they are not radioactive) gathered from the Himalayas, Hawaii, Utah, and the Andes Mountains. Raw salt holds the frequency of the Earth, which enhances both Earth energy and Earth frequency in a growing child. Most regular culinary salts have been heated, and have thus become covalent in structure; this makes them less assimilable, and strips them of essential minerals. One of the best sources of minerals is a resinous vegan substance called *shilajit,* which comes from the Himalayan Mountains. It is high in fulvic acid, a key element that helps plants and humans absorb minerals.

The problem with most mineral supplements is that our bodies are designed to receive minerals in ionic form, in pieces the size of an angstrom. (Named after Johan Angström, an angstrom is one ten-thousandth of a micron, which is one millionth of a meter.) Almost all mineral supplements you can buy are larger than one micron. Angstrom-size minerals are absorbed through the mouth, and are small enough to be absorbed directly into the cells and their nuclei, for optimal absorption.

The roots of plants break down minerals from the soil into angstrom-size minerals for us. By consuming the plants, we are able to receive our vital minerals in optimally absorbable form. Angstrom-size minerals, incidentally, help to rid the body of unhealthy mineral deposits by competitive inhibition (taking up the available spaces). High-quality salts and Angstrom-size mineral supplements are available at the Tree of Life online shop and onsite natural pharmacy.

Living foods and minerals: Remember that when we cook our food, we are removing or deactivating sixty to seventy percent of the mineral content from the meal. Also noteworthy is that dairy products cause depletion of calcium, an important mineral in the body. Mineral-dense plant sources of calcium include dulse, Irish moss, kelp, leafy greens, sesame seeds, and other nuts, seeds, and grains.

Children Need Dietary Fats

Cutting out animal fats, where toxins are most concentrated, and trans fats such as hydrogenated oils or fried foods, is highly beneficial to our children's health; but providing raw, plant-sourced fats is absolutely essential. DHA is the most important long-chain omega-3 fatty acid for brain, neurological, eye, cognitive function, heart health, cancer prevention, skin health, and memory. Omega-3s are required for the healthy development of the growing child. In Dr. Gabriel's medical practice he has found that plant-sourced raw fats are key to a successful living-food lifestyle, as they are key components to brain and eye development as well as a good fuel for the heart, memory, and learning development. It is no accident that mother's milk is fifty-four percent fat.

For this reason, we recommend a moderate 25–45% raw plant-fat intake, supplemented by up to 1,200 milligrams of long-chain omega-3s for the pregnant or breastfeeding mother, and approximately 100 milligrams of DHA from yellow algae oil to be put in the baby's prepared milk or food. We recommend the DHA and EPA directly from the yellow algae (where the fish get it from) in order to minimize ingesting radioactive contamination in fish. We recommend moderate high fat, adequate protein, and moderate-to-low carbohydrates, so that 25–45% or more of one's live-food vegan diet is comprised of fats.

Healthy fats contain ketones that energize the brain better than carbohydrates. In addition to supporting the nervous system and brain, healthy fats support hormonal balance, bone health, and heart health, and fight inflammation. Fats do not turn into sugars in the body, as do excess proteins and carbohydrates. A diet moderately high in raw plant-sourced fats therefore has a naturally lower glycemic index. This is why living plant-based fats help avoid and decrease obesity, while carbohydrates and sugars are the real culprits behind the obesity epidemic.

Overweight adults who eat an avocado a day, for example, have actually been found to lose up to seventeen percent of their weight in one year. It is also interesting to note that while some indigenous diets of the Maoris of New Zealand are comprised of 500% more fat than is generally recommended in the West, among these people we see minimal cancer, diabetes, or heart disease. This is at least partly because the fats consumed are derived raw and eaten from high intake of coconut and coconut oils.

Other healthy, plant-sourced fats include nuts (for ages nine to twelve months and older), seeds, avocados, and olives, coconut products and oil, as well as small amounts of cold-pressed oils such as extra-virgin olive oil, chia oil, hempseed oil, and unheated sesame oil. A particularly beneficial combination is freshly ground flaxseeds or chia seeds mixed with cold-pressed coconut oil, because together these provide adequate long-chain omega-3 fatty acids. One way to combine these is to make dehydrated breads with flaxseed meal, such as the Apple-Cinnamon Bread in the breakfast recipes, combined with Dairy-Free Salted Butter (page 481) made from coconut oil.

Freshly ground flaxseed meal or chia seed meal and coconut oil can easily be added to smoothies if not using frozen ingredients (which will harden the oil). Coconut oil should be blended minimally, to avoid a soapy flavor. We will give more detail on dietary fats and childhood health in the chapter "Supporting the Child's Developing Mind."

Protein for Growing Bodies

Contrary to the message of fad-diet protein scares, plant-sourced proteins are available in abundance, and the scientific evidence shows that they are of the highest quality and not associated with creating insulin resistance, as animal-based protein does. For example, the protein found in spirulina (currently being used to prevent malnutrition among West African children), chlorella, and blue-green algae is 95% assimilable in the human body, whereas the protein found in beef is 16% assimilable, in chicken 18%, and in fish 17%.

Other rich sources of raw protein include nuts and seeds; nut-butters such as almond, pecan, walnut, Brazil nut, and macadamia; seed-butters such as sunflower, pumpkinseed, hempseed, and tahini; and sprouted Nut/Seed Mylks (page 136). These are all concentrated protein sources.

Other sources of raw protein include goji berries, wheatgrass juice, barley greens (the green grass-shoots of wheat and barley are gluten-free), broccoli, and sprouts. Raw plant-based protein powders that are rice-, nut-, or seed-based, or E-3 Live, algae, spirulina, or chlorella products, can also be added into smoothies if desired. As mentioned before, E-3 Live is excellent for brain development and for enhancing overall intelligence. Sprouted or steamed peas, beans, lentils and whole grains such as quinoa, wild rice—which has double the protein of brown rice—teff, buckwheat, oats, amaranth, millet, milo, and organic non-GMO corn (which is difficult to find), also offer quality protein.

While the use of legumes and grains is sometimes desired, these are not required for a healthy vegan diet. But including legumes and grains as protein sources can be particularly helpful for vegans with nut allergies, and supply variation in the cuisine for our children. We do not recommend gluten and glutinous grains such as wheat, spelt, kamut, barley, rye, semolina, and triticale, as these glutinous grains have a strong tendency to inflame the brain and nervous system and to cause or aggravate digestive disorders including celiac disease.

Another protein source to avoid is soy. While soybean products are common replacements for meat, soy is not only unnecessary for a successful plant-based lifestyle, as previously pointed out, but there are some dangers associated with eating it. One current major problem with soy is that ninety-two to ninety-four percent of soy grown in the United States is genetically modified.[24] The issue with soy being genetically modified goes further: GM soy is loaded with toxic pesticides, now containing 2,4-D—an active component of Agent Orange and far more toxic even than the glyphosate in Roundup®.

Keep in mind that, although six to eight percent of soy is organic, we question, in the complex ecological picture of cross-pollination, how "organic" is even this six to eight percent? Genetically modified plants contain genes from bacteria that produce a protein that has never been part of the human food supply before. We cannot even begin to know the implications of this for our health and ecology. The only human-feeding study on GM foods ever published did verify that the gene inserted into GM soy transfers into the DNA of our gut bacteria.[25] This means that we may actually be producing this allergenic protein in our gut with those GMO bacteria.

The GM soy has also been linked to an increase in allergies, which has important ramifications, such as soy having now become one of the top seven allergens. Also important is that the GM soy has a lot more of these toxic pesticides than humans can safely tolerate. In *Rainbow Green Live-Food Cuisine,* it is noted that glyphosate was listed as the most common cause of all forms of pesticide-related illness in California in the 1990s, and with an increased risk of non-Hodgkin's lymphoma, which is considered the third-fastest growing cancer in the U.S.[26]

Is a Plant-Sourced Diet Safe for Children?

Children who grow up getting nutrition from plant foods rather than meats have a tremendous health advantage. They are less likely to develop weight problems, diabetes, high blood pressure, and some forms of cancer.

—Pediatrician Dr. Benjamin Spock, considered America's leading Authority on Childcare

Many ancient societies lived on plant-sourced and living foods, such as the Essenes, the Pelasgians, the rishis, the Daoists, Pythagoras and his followers, and more. A reading of Genesis 1:29 also reminds us that the plant-sourced diet prescribed nearly 5,773 years ago is far from a new food fad, as some who are ignorant of history would have us believe. And yet we are living in a time when there is much fear surrounding humanity's evolutionary return to plant-sourced sustenance.

Given this current cultural condition, parents who choose to feed their children exclusively plant-sourced foods are often unsupported, challenged, and sometimes even threatened. Thankfully, the science of contemporary nutrition is moving beyond cultural fear, addiction, monetary interests, and bias, and is now documenting the health advantages and safety of plant-sourced nutrition for all ages. In 2009, for example, the American Dietetic Association (ADA) issued the following statement:

It is the position of the American Dietetic Association that appropriately planned vegetarian diets, including total vegetarian diets or vegan diets, are healthful, nutritionally adequate, and may provide health benefits in the prevention and treatment of certain diseases. Well-planned vegetarian diets are appropriate for individuals during all stages of the lifecycle, including pregnancy, lactation, infancy, childhood and adolescence, and for athletes.[27]

Another factor to consider when referring to childhood growth charts is that breastfed infants tend to be leaner than formula-fed infants, which means they are generally gaining weight at about the same rate for the first two to three months, and then show slower weight gain from three to twelve months. The sizes and growth rates of breastfed babies tend to vary widely from those of formula-fed babies, as healthy nursing babies are often smaller and have growth spurts at different stages of development.

A healthy plant-sourced diet is not only safe, it has several advantages over non-vegan vegetarian and omnivorous diets. This is substantiated by numerous separate scientific studies and by qualified nutritional experts and physicians. In over forty years of clinical work, Gabriel Cousens, MD, MD(H), has observed that a balanced, carefully thought-out plant-sourced diet, which most conscientious parents can develop, is a most powerful and successful method for achieving and maintaining excellent health for families, especially for children.

Just as both omnivorous and vegetarian parents seeking to raise healthy children must be educated and aware of how to create a well-planned, nutrient-rich, balanced diet for the whole family, so do parents following a plant-sourced approach. Just because a diet is plant-source only does not automatically make it a good one. Research indicates that vegan parents tend to be highly self-educated and knowledgeable about nutrition and health. Additionally, over eighty-five percent of college-educated parents choose to breastfeed rather than feed with formula, and many of those educated parents also choose a plant-sourced diet.

Please note that children as well as adults need dietary supplements on a plant-sourced diet. At the same time, it is important to understand that *the meat-eating diet also requires as much supplementation as a vegan diet.* During this time of extreme environmental soil depletion and toxicity, neither diet is totally complete on its own. Even if meat and dairy are obtained directly from the farm or natural-food stores, animal-sourced foods contain thirty times the carcinogens, radioactivity, and other contaminants than organically grown plant-sourced foods. *When we eat meat, we increase our intake of toxins by ninety-six percent, as compared to a vegan diet; the impact on the ecology is greater by far; there is unnecessary wasting of natural resources; we contribute to animal suffering—and we still need supplements.*

We recommend vitamin B12 and vitamin D supplements for all children. While vitamin-D levels have been found to be higher among raw-food eaters than others, 100% of all children under one year old are deficient in vitamin D. Up to ninety percent of pregnant mothers in the U.S. are deficient in DHA, so many newborns also start out deficient in long-chain omega-3s.

Recent genetic research suggests that up to seventy-five percent of the population needs a higher-protein diet, which is easy to attain with a vegan cuisine. Nuts, for example, are an excellent protein source. When considering protein sources for vegan children, however, nuts should not be given to them until their teeth begin to grow in. After the age of nine months, nuts and seeds are quite protective to children's health, and some nuts are particularly good choices.

Researchers have found that people who never ate nuts, compared to those who occasionally ate nuts, had a seven-percent smaller incidence of dying from any cause during a thirty-year study. The study followed 119,000 Americans over a thirty-year period, and was published in the November 2013 issue of the *New England Journal of Medicine*.[28] People in the study who consumed nuts once weekly had an eleven-percent smaller death rate, and people who had two to four servings of nuts weekly had a thirteen percent lower incidence of death. Those who consumed one ounce of nuts daily had a twenty-percent lower overall death rate. Eating more nuts was linked to lower rates of death from heart disease, cancer, and respiratory disease. This is a strong statement about nuts as a health food in general.

Almonds have been shown to lower LDL cholesterol, and walnuts have shown to be important in protecting against heart disease and in building the intima, the inner lining of the blood vessels. Research found that taking 100 grams (3.5 ounces) of almonds per day lowered total cholesterol levels 21–23%.[29] Walnuts were shown to have the remarkable ability to repair endothelial dysfunction. Eating eight to sixteen walnuts per day decreased total LDL cholesterol by five to ten percent, and reduced incidence of stroke and clogging of arteries up to seventy percent.[30] Five ounces of nuts per week has been shown to cause a 27% decrease in type 2 diabetes. We have here ample evidence of the importance of nuts; after the age of nine months, it is quite beneficial to introduce nut butters and nut milks to a child's diet.

As a culture we are rediscovering living, vegan, organic foods for healing, vitality, and spiritual awakening. This is very positive and exciting. And yet we must still use care and common sense as we make dietary changes for our families. If a child is not thriving on either a plant-sourced or omnivorous diet, it may be that something needs to be adjusted, such as relying less heavily on fruits, adding high-mineral foods, decreasing any processed vegan foods, or increasing living foods, healthy fats and protein.

Going at a balanced pace with dietary transition is also important, as well as insuring that the child has access to as much living food as is desired, with the exception of excessive amounts of dried fruits and high-glycemic fruits.

But Children Don't Like Healthy Food!

In 2006, 44 major companies spent a total of $1.6 billion marketing their food and beverages to children and adolescents; carbonated drinks, restaurant food, and breakfast cereals accounted for 63% of the total amount of marketing spent on youth. The marketers' favorite advertising medium? Television.[31]

Here in Candy Land, children certainly have a reputation for certain food preferences. A friend of ours who was watching cartoons with her son pointed out that every time a child was portrayed as rejecting a particular food, "It was always something green." This is just one example of how children are literally programmed to think that they don't like veggies.

At a closer look, however, we can see that this commonly held, media-programmed belief is not actually based on careful observation of the child. A recent study of middle-school students by researchers at the Harvard School of Public Health, for example, reveals contrary findings. In this study, researchers went into Boston middle schools; some served heavily processed lunches high in white flour, white sugar, animal fats, and foods requiring minimal preparation, while others had switched over to lunches made from scratch from fresh fruits and vegetables, whole grains, and reduced animal fats. The researchers wanted to find out how much food was actually being eaten by the schoolchildren in both groups.

The results? The children that were offered healthier school lunches ate more of their meals than those who were given more processed white flour, sugar, and trans-fat foods. By tracking how much food was being thrown away, it was discovered that the schools that were serving less nutritious fare had more food waste than the schools that had adopted the "Chefs in Schools" program sponsored by "Project Bread," devoted to helping inner-city children at high risk of malnutrition. What's more, the children that were offered fresher lunches ate thirty percent more of their vegetables.[32]

It is true that certain unhealthy foods are addictive; therefore, a child who is hooked may choose the junk over healthier options; but it is important not to confuse this junk-food-addicted state with the normal, healthy desires of childhood. In the book *What's Eating Your Child?: The Hidden Connections Between Food and Childhood Ailments,* Kelly Dorfman, MS, LND, tells us that although picky eating may be a widespread problem, it is not a childhood attribute. Picky eating may be pointing to an underlying health issue such as reflux, colon impaction, zinc deficiency (which deadens taste and smell), or excessive mucus production due to dairy intolerance. All of these may cause a disinterest in food, behavior problems, food allergies such as gluten intolerance, and other symptoms.

According to Dorfman, because finicky eating habits affect the child's development, the child needs parents to proactively help with this, rather than assuming it will be outgrown without support. Dorfman shares stories of children whose diets once consisted of just a few bland, white and/or starchy and refined foods, who were helped to expand their dietary horizons through her EAT program: "E" to first Eliminate any irritants that may be causing a bad reaction; "A" to Add one food at a time; "T" to Try one bite of this food every night for two weeks.[33]

This approach is effective when the child is open to it, and when parents remain calm, patient, and supportive as the child faces his fears. Dorfman also shares that vitamin, mineral, and essential fatty-acid supplementation can be a first step in helping kids to try new foods, if anxiety about new foods is aggravated by an inadequately nourished digestive system.[34]

In our own work with children, we are often reinspired by their own intuitive delight and enthusiasm for vegan living foods rather than junk food, processed food, and foods that carry the energy of a dead, fearful, and suffering animal. In a culture that considers children and vegetables to be at odds, it is very moving to see the children themselves wanting nutritious food.

Leah once had a father enter her preschool classroom after hours, demanding, "What's all this about seaweed?!" Remembering that she had set out nori for the children as one of their snack choices, Leah started to defend the health benefits of nori. He abruptly replied, "Yeah, yeah—what I want to know is *where do I get some?!* My daughter says she has to have it!" Apparently this student's fondness for nori was shared, because after the children had sampled it in the classroom it became difficult for Leah to eat her own nori wrap with the children at lunchtime. As soon as they saw what their teacher had in her lunch, they all started clamoring for some too!

Leah was also very touched by a particular child who often had candy and leftover fast food packed in his lunchbox. On a regular basis, this child would put extra healthy snacks from the classroom snack table into his own lunchbox to later supplement his own meal. This suggests that children are more aware of what is healthy for them than adults may think.

Another student's parent thanked Leah over and over because her son was now asking for raw broccoli at home. In all honesty, it wasn't so much the teacher that had done this magical act but the natural environment calling to the child's own inner teacher. This young boy's new fondness for broccoli was simply a result of experiencing the growth of vegetables in a small raised bed just outside the classroom. Leah also received reports from parents that their children had taken an interest in native, wild edible plants. This new love had unfolded naturally, due to their daily guided nature walks.

When Leah was leading a weekly living-food-prep class for kids, she was very pleased to see the highly positive responses among the children (ages three to fourteen). She heard sincere comments from the children such as, "Food-prep class is so fun!" "That yogurt we made last time was so good!" "I want *all* of the recipe cards for my box." "I think this is the best salad I ever tasted!" and "I love you. Thank you for having this class!"

While some of the flavors and textures were new to many of the children, the overall success rate, based on smiles, requests for more, plate-licking, and parents reporting that food-prep-class was "the highlight of their child's week," seemed to be somewhere around ninety-five percent. What was also very fun was that the children were asking their parents to make living foods at home. One week, for example, a mother called to say that her child was ill and asking for wheatgrass juice with orange juice, "just like we made in class," in order to help her feel better. The mom wanted to know where to get some. The wheatgrass juice that Leah had then taken over to this student's house was shared with her parents. Later, this student told Leah, "My parents liked it too, so we ended up buying a whole tray of wheatgrass."

Leah has also swapped stories with a local mother who received grant money to take fresh, organic garden produce to children attending public school. The children there have responded in a similar way to her program, consistently requesting that she please bring them more salad. It is the children themselves who have taught Leah that sneaking green vegetables into their diet isn't generally necessary. We can indeed trust their wise inner teachers. Children want to know their food intimately, and to be equipped to make healthy choices. The message is clear—a naturally health-educated child will naturally tend to choose healthy food, and also to be an inspiration to parents to move to a more natural and healthy diet.

Soy What? And Other Vegan Foods to be Wary of

Soy in the diet is no longer needed to be a healthy vegan, so promoting veganism does not require defending soy consumption. We are one-thousand-percent committed to helping people achieve success on a vegan diet, and believe this can be easily and more healthfully achieved without soy in the diet.

When a person needs to increase their protein intake, they often think they are craving meat. When they increase their plant protein intake, however, their craving for meat seems to disappear. Dr. Cousens's clinical experience over forty years of working with people to transition to a well-designed vegan, live-food diet has close to a 99% efficacy rate. In other words, this science-based approach to individualizing the diet, in our experience, consistently works.

This approach is significantly different than the traditional vegan diet's low-protein, low-fat, high-carbohydrate approach—which may work for perhaps 30% of people. The emerging field of nutri-genomics and clinical experience suggest that about 70% of us need a higher-protein diet, so we must consider the best sources for this.

According to the science of diet, there is no need for vegans ever to eat fish, as some leaders in the vegan movement have publicly admitted doing. There are also dangers in eating soy. We do not recommend soy except as a transition food for people newly moving into a vegetarian/vegan lifestyle—and even then only organic, fermented soy products, in small quantities.

From a holistic point of view, one major problem with soy currently is that approximately ninety to ninety-four percent of soy is genetically modified. The issue goes further; GM soy is loaded with toxic pesticides and ever-increasing amounts of Roundup® and similar toxic preparations needed to keep up with mutating insects and weeds.

Keep in mind that although approximately six to eight percent of soy is organic, we question, in the complex ecological picture of cross-pollination, how "organic" is this small percentage? Genetically modified plants contain genes from bacteria that produce a protein that has never been part of the human food supply. We cannot even begin to know the implications of this. The only published human-feeding study on GM foods ever conducted did verify that the gene inserted into GM soy transfers into the DNA of our gut bacteria. This means that we actually may be producing allergenic proteins in our gut from those bacteria.

GM soy has been linked to an increase in allergies, which has important ramifications—soy has now become one of the top seven food allergens. And GM soy contains much more of the toxic pesticide Roundup® than humans can safely tolerate. *Rainbow Green Live-Food Cuisine* cites that by the 1990s, glyphosate was listed as the most common cause of all of forms of pesticide–related illness in California, and has been implicated in an increased risk of non-Hodgkin's lymphoma, the third-fastest-growing cancer in the U.S. Now the World Health Organization is saying that glyphosates may cause cancer.

Some soy issues may not be very consequential in the long run, such as the fact that soy contains antinutrients including saponins, soyatoxin, phytates, protease inhibitors, and oxalates that interfere with absorption of minerals, leading to the claim that vegans are mineral-deficient (which is not necessarily the case). It is interesting to note that in 1936 the U.S. Congress declared that ninety-nine percent of Americans were mineral-deficient. Almost everyone that Dr. Gabriel sees—meat eaters and vegans alike—are mineral-deficient, which correlates with this 1936 finding. This cannot reasonably be blamed on soy.

There are some potential health problems associated with soy, however; there are, for instance, toxic levels of aluminum and manganese connected to soy-production procedures. Soy formula has up to eighty times more manganese than we find in breast milk, but there is no research to prove this is detrimental. These are all areas of controversy that may turn out to be more theoretical than clinical.

Whether soy prevents or causes cancer is also debatable. The Japanese, who ingest up to thirty times more iodine than North Americans, have a lower incidence of breast, uterine, and prostate cancer, as iodine helps to protect the reproductive organs, especially the breasts, from cancer. But the Japanese and other Asian soy-eaters have higher rates of other types of cancers including esophagus, stomach, pancreas, and liver—but lower rates of thyroid cancer. The cancer topic has been debated back and forth, and will be resolved in time as the research unfolds; but it must be considered in the overall discussion. We would only add that soy tends to create a dominance of estrogen over progesterone. Progesterone has a general anticancer effect because it stimulates apoptosis, or death of cancer cells. So a high estrogen-to-progesterone ratio has been, at least theoretically, linked with the growth of cancer.

One area of concern that seems to be reasonably well documented is expressed by Mike Fitzpatrick, a New Zealand toxicologist: "The amount of phytoestrogens that are in a day's worth of soy infant formula equals five birth control pills."[35] Another study reported in *The Lancet* found that the "daily exposure of infants to isoflavones in soy infant-formulas is six to eleven times higher, on a bodyweight basis, than the dose that has hormonal effects in adults consuming soy foods." The estrogen dose equivalent to what is in two glasses of soymilk per day was enough to change menstrual patterns in women. In the blood of infants tested in this study, who were on soymilk as a substitute for mother's milk, concentrations of isoflavones were 13,000 to 22,000 times higher than natural estrogen concentrations in early life. This has other unhealthy implications. At some point it will become clear that high estrogen is not good for male nor female fetuses or children, particularly in its potential effects on sexual development, gender identity, and reproductive health.

In 2003, a study was done of the IGF-1 (insulin-like growth factor 1) increase in the body stimulated by forty grams of soy. This is the amount in one soy candy bar and a soy shake, or four soy patties, and its effects were compared to forty grams of milk protein. Soy was found to be almost twice as powerful as milk protein in increasing IGF-1 levels (36% for milk, 69% for soy). This new IGF-1 data potentially places soy in the category of a powerful promoter of cancer of the breast, prostate, lung, and colon.

Although this connection is still controversial, many in the medical world agree that excessive IGF-1 could at least stimulate the aforementioned cancers if they are already present. In essence, this is still at the level of theoretical speculation but it merits a preventive attention. Canada, Australia, Japan, and all twenty-seven countries of the European Union will not accept milk from the United States if it comes from rBGH cows, because of the connection between rBGH and increased IGF-1 levels, which are associated with a potential increase in breast cancer.[36]

Once we move past the controversial aspects of the soy discussion, it is useful to look at the less debatable aspects of our concern. One of these is soy's allergenic quality. In 1986, Stuart Berger, MD, placed soy among the seven top allergens, calling it one of the "sinister seven." Scientists are not completely certain which components of soy cause allergic reactions. They have found at least sixteen allergenic protein components in soy, and some researchers identify as many as thirty.

Allergic reactions occur not only when soy is eaten but even when soybean flour or dust is inhaled. Among epidemiologists, soybean dust is known as an "epidemic asthma agent." From 1981 to 1987, soy dust from grain-silo unloading in the harbor caused twenty-six epidemics of asthma in Barcelona, seriously affecting 687 people and leading to 1,155 hospitalizations. No further epidemics occurred after filters were installed, but a minor outbreak in 1994 established the need for monitoring of preventive measures.

Reports of the epidemic in Barcelona led epidemiologists in New Orleans to investigate asthma epidemics that had occurred from 1957 to 1968, when more than 200 people sought treatment at a charity Hospital. Comparisons of weather patterns and cargo data from the New Orleans harbor with dates of epidemic asthma identified soy dust from ships carrying soybeans as the probable cause. No association was found between asthma-epidemic days and the presence of wheat or corn in ships in the harbor. The researchers concluded: "The results of this analysis provide further evidence that ambient soy dust is very asthmogenic, and that asthma morbidity in a community can be influenced by exposures in the ambient atmosphere."

Another undebatable fact is that cooking soy naturally produces MSG. It matters not whether the soy is organic or GMO—if it is cooked, it contains MSG. All soy products, except raw edamame soybeans, are cooked in processing. Some, such as textured soy protein (TSP), may even contain added MSG. This is a real concern, and not a theoretical speculation. MSG is a brain-damaging excitotoxin that has been conclusively linked with brain damage, endocrine disorders—in particular, disruption of the hypothalamic function—reproductive disorders, behavior disorders, general adverse reactions, and neurodegenerative diseases. This is not something that we recommend exposing yourself or your children to. In essence, all ingestion of soy, whether GMO or not, except for raw edamame, exposes your children to MSG.

Following and perhaps associated with this MSG fact, the most important question about soy is its effect on the brain. There is some suggestion that a twice-a-week soy intake may be connected with a 2.4-times higher rate of Alzheimer's disease, and accelerated brain degeneration.[37] [38] Soy is considered *kaphagenic* in the 3,000-year-old Ayurvedic system of medicine, which means in part that it is associated with increasing the incidence of diabetes. The incidence of diabetes in heavy soy users indeed appears to be 200% that of the general population.

In a major study involving 3,734 elderly Japanese American men, those who ate the most tofu (soybean curd) during midlife had up to 2.4 times the risk of later developing Alzheimer's disease.[39] As part of a three-decade-long Honolulu-Asia Aging Study, twenty-seven foods and drinks were correlated with participants' health. Men who consumed tofu at least twice weekly had more cognitive impairment than those who rarely or never ate it. Going further, higher midlife tofu consumption was also associated with low brain weight, suggesting that soy consumption is associated with brain-cell destruction and loss. Brain atrophy was assessed in 574 men using MRI results, and in 290 men using autopsy information. Brain shrinkage occurs naturally with age, but for the men who had consumed more tofu, according to lead researcher Dr. Lon R. White from the Hawaii Center for Health Research, "Their brains seemed to be showing an exaggeration of the usual patterns we see in aging." This level of epidemiology combined with hard science is a significant consideration in the soy discussion.

This all fits together with a pattern of soy affecting the brain—the MSG exposure, and the allergies causing brain inflammation, as inflammation is a driving force behind Alzheimer's and accelerated brain aging. The association with overall brain shrinkage and brain-cell destruction and loss makes us more than uncomfortable about recommending soy to children or adults.

There are two other points that need to be addressed: One major study from 1997 to 2005, conducted in the U.S. with 4,000 people, showed that of 96% of the American populace is deficient in iodine (compared to 72–74% globally). Besides the fact that only about twenty percent of salt today is iodized, even the iodine in iodized salt is only about ten percent bioavailable; and most commercial iodized salt contains chlorine, toxic stabilizers, and excipients.

Iodized salt is no longer mandated for restaurant or processed foods, and sea salt contains only 1/71 the amount of iodine in iodized salt. Soy, and particularly soy oil, is a major depleter of iodine in the system. Low iodine contributes to hypothyroidism, cretinism, and the diminishing of many body functions including that of the heart and ovaries. Soy has also been noted to have other goitrogenic (thyroid-enlarging) factors that contribute to hypothyroidism.

Though the hypothyroid issue appears to be debatable, Dr. Gabriel sees low thyroid function in nearly all his patients, whether or not they are eating soy, meat, or live vegan foods. Nearly everyone he sees clinically is suffering from subclinical symptoms of iodine deficiency, which certainly correlates with the seven-year study showing 96% deficiency in Americans. Avoiding soy helps to minimize this problem.

The people in Japan, before the Fukushima disaster, had little thyroid trouble, probably related to an iodine intake thirty times that of Americans. However, since Fukushima and its continued radiation spills, thyroid disease is increasing in Japan and worldwide. More disturbing is a recent study that found that children born in Alaska, California, Hawaii, Oregon, and Washington one to sixteen weeks after the Fukushima melt-down were 28% more likely to suffer from congenital hypothyroidism than children born in those same states during the same period one year earlier.[40]

In the Fukushima area, the rate of congenital hypothyroidism was 44%, which seems clearly associated with a buildup of radioactive iodine-131 in the thyroid. If a baby has adequate iodine in the thyroid, it is "full up" and the I-131 cannot get in, so adequate iodine is a key protector against I-131 toxicity. Given that the toxic radiation from Fuku-shima includes so much I-131, it makes reasonable sense to minimize anything that lowers iodine saturation in the body, and to increase iodine saturation as a protection against absorbing I-131.

When we refer to the longevity of pre-Fukushima Okinawans, and attribute it to their soy intake—while others have attributed their longev-ity to intake of coral calcium—we are not considering the cultural and genetic influences on their longevity. It is superficial to correlate their longevity with soy alone; most Americans, of course, are not Okinawans, and this theory is speculative and potentially misleading. We have to be careful in making cross-cultural comparisons.

Another concern about soy is that its isoflavones have been shown to reduce testicular function by lowering the luteinizing hormone (LH) that stimulates the testicles to function. A high soy intake—and poten-tially lower LH—increases the probability of estrogen dominance in men, contributing to hair loss, swollen and cancerous prostates, and insulin resistance. Doris Rapp, MD, a leading pediatric allergist, asserts that environmental and food estrogens are responsible for the worldwide reduction in male fertility. Recent human research has shown that soy intake is associated with a 50% decrease in sperm fertility.[41] This kind of research on humans is very hard to ignore when we consider the survival of the species.

In conclusion, soy was considered an important health-food protein decades ago, as it is 38% protein and 25% carbohydrate; but several changes have occurred since then. The most serious detrimental change has been the introduction of genetically modified soy. Another consideration is that many other high-quality proteins are now available that offer better assimilation and higher protein, with fewer potential health problems. For example, spirulina, chlorella, and Klamath Lake blue-green algae are 60–70% protein—at least 33% higher than soy—a protein that is 95% assimilable in humans. There simply is no higher-quality protein availability, vegan or flesh-derived, than from those algae. Other high-quality, natural, unprocessed raw protein sources are also available, such as pumpkinseed-protein concentrates.

The star role that soy once played has, in essence, become obsolete. What we once considered a great food and protein source is not the same soy that is generally available today. There is a Biblical warning about food selection: If there is a chance of harm with a food, don't use it. This is especially true if better options are available.

In the last forty years, soy has occupied an important place in the transition from an unhealthy meat-based diet to vegetarian and vegan cuisine. Now, however, it may be time for us to upgrade our food choices to those with more benefits and less negative potential. Eliminating soy from your diet can be tough if you are just eating processed vegetarian or vegan food. Many packaged and prepared foods contain processed soy as an ingredient, but it may be listed as "textured vegetable protein" (or "TVP"), "textured plant protein," or "hydrolyzed vegetable protein" (or "HVP"). These all contain naturally occurring MSG (monosodium glutamate), and more MSG is often added as well.

When we look at the whole picture, we see a very strong argument for why an 80% live-food, organic, vegan cuisine is superior in terms of physical health and growth, as well as long-term protection from cancer, diabetes, heart disease, and nearly all forms of chronic physical diseases and brain deterioration.

Can an Omnivorous Diet be Safe?

After learning all the dangers of an omnivorous diet, the real question is: Can an omnivorous diet be safe for children—or for adults?

A typical omnivorous diet today, wherein most calories come from junk food and processed foods containing radiation, pesticides, and herbicides, with a low intake of fruits and vegetables, is unquestionably detrimental. Unfortunately, this commonly consumed omnivorous diet is followed by a majority of omnivores, while the vast majority of vegans do not follow extreme, unbalanced diets such as vegan macrobiotic or fruitarian diets.

The omnivorous, standard American diet (SAD) is the mainstay of the majority of those eating omnivorously follow this unhealthy diet, which is directly connected to the skyrocketing early onset of type 2 diabetes, cancer, hypertension, and obesity in the general population of children and teens. This is quite different from a carefully planned omnivorous diet that contains organic, whole foods and derives only a small fraction (perhaps five to ten percent) of its calories from animal products.

One of the serious downsides of animal-protein products is that they contain minimal to no fiber content, minimal antioxidants, minimal to no vitamins C, B3, B6, E, and K, folate, phytochemicals, bioflavonoids, carotenoids, or lignans. All of these vitamins, minerals, and phytonutrients are necessary for optimal health, but occur minimally in a typical omnivorous "SAD" diet. The phytonutrients, especially bioflavonoids, that they contain make fruits and vegetables the primary anticancer foods over the long term.

In considering the advantages of various diets, we want to choose a diet that will give us the highest amounts of phytonutrients, polyphenols, bioflavonoids, and anthocyanins. A science-based, organic, vegan diet provides all of these, and organic produce has been shown to be higher in polyphenols, antioxidants, and bioflavonoids than conventional produce. In other words, an organic, plant-source diet has a higher concentration of life-force-enhancing micronutrients.

To be scientifically fair, research shows that when comparing vegan diets and a quasi-vegan diet that is limited to five to ten percent omnivorous content, scientifically guided, and made healthy with thoughtful supplementation and nutritional sophistication—particularly if it is high in nuts, seeds, vegetables, beans and other nutrient-dense foods—those who are mostly vegan but "cheat" a little by eating an occasional animal product still have very good long-term health results.[42]

If life is simply about physical health, the discussion of five to ten percent versus zero percent animal products ends with this limited, materialistic worldview: There is little health detriment from consuming a very small amount of high-quality, organic, animal-based food. In this next chapter, however, we address a different way to perceive our diets and our lives: What we are recommending is a way of eating and living that uplifts all parts of the web of life, that sanctifies all of life rather than destroying it.

CHAPTER 5

Holistic Veganism

If we confine our focus to the physical health of the body, we are ignoring the moral, ethical, and spiritual issues of what life is about; we are limiting ourselves to a materialistic viewpoint. This book, and the entire scope of holistic veganism, goes far beyond this limited, physical-health perspective on veganism.

The holistic vegan diet looks beyond the narrow perspective of what is best for the physical body and health, to ask: How can we bring the most light into the world through our dietary choices? This key question gives us the opportunity to teach morals, ethics, and spirituality to our child in the context of diet. Holistic veganism's benefits are not limited to physical health. Holistic veganism is part of an entire worldview for the health of the planet, and the evolution and uplifting of humanity. Holistic veganism is the evolutionary diet of the future. Truly, in each generation, we are given the medicine for the healing of that generation; holistic veganism is the medicine for the healing of our current generation, on multiple levels.

Holistic veganism is a way of life that is a way of love, peace, harmony, and evolution for the planet. The Hindu tradition refers to this emphasis on peace as *ahimsa*—minimizing the amount of harm we cause to other living creatures on the planet. Our mere presence on Earth inevitably creates a certain amount of harm, and the purpose of *ahimsa* is to minimize this negative impact. A holistic vegan diet creates minimal harm in many ways compared with an omnivorous diet.

At its highest octave, the ethic and wisdom of holistic veganism goes beyond the teaching of ethical veganism to ask the questions: How can we eat in a way that enhances holiness and vitality in all of life? How can we eat in a way that sanctifies all of life? How can we eat in a way that heals and uplifts the individual and planetary body, mind, and soul, and the entire planetary web of life? How can we eat in a way that amplifies our ability to be in touch with the central meaning of life? How can we, in essence, eat in a way that enhances the evolution of the planetary web of life?

When we are killing animals, or supporting cruelty and misery by paying those who do, we are not accomplishing this. We are degrading and degenerating life. This is the deeper reason why holistic veganism is so important.

The history of veganism goes back at least 6,000 years. It includes the Pelasgians, were 100% live-food vegans who lived in southern Greece around 3,000 BCE, as reported by the great Greek historian Herodotus. Their average age at death was reported to be 200 years. Some people uninformed about its history say that veganism is untested—but for us, 6,000-plus years seems a pretty good test. Veganism was the original diet prescribed for humanity in Genesis 1:29—it was the Garden of Eden cuisine.

In other words, veganism is not a new idea that began when Donald Watson coined the term in 1944. It is said that Pythagoras studied with the Essenes on Mount Carmel around 500 BCE, and took the teaching of a plant-based raw diet back to Greece. Before the term "veganism" was coined, those who ate a plant-source-only diet were called "Pythagoreans." Prior to this, some of the Pharaohs, including Akhenaten and Nefertiti in 1,300 BCE, also prescribed live-food veganism for the priest caste.

Some anthropological findings from two to three million years ago suggest, according to Robert Leakey, the presence of tree-dwelling humans who may have been ninety-seven-percent vegan. Veganism is not new or experimental; the actually new and experimental diet is the standard American diet (SAD) being eaten by Americans at this point in history. SAD is an approximately eighty-year-old experiment that is already demonstrating a horrendously negative outcome not only for humans but also for the health and survival of the planet. The holistic vegan diet is a cuisine that supports not only personal health but the survival and enhancement of the planet's evolution.

The 2,000-year-old Greek Orthodox Church still has a minimum of 300 days a year when church members are supposed to maintain a vegan diet. The scriptures of almost all the great wisdom traditions offer us much wisdom for choosing the compassion and *ahimsa* of a plant-based diet:

- Psalm 145:9 says, "God's mercies are for all of creation." It appears that the vegan teaching in most traditions was based on avoiding the spilling of blood. A key teaching of *ahimsa* is to do the least amount of harm, and veganism does the least amount of harm while allowing us humans to live fruitfully on the planet.
- Deuteronomy 4:15 says, "Be protective of your lives."
- Sir Arthur Conan Doyle said, "At the moment, our human world is based on the suffering and destruction of millions of nonhumans. To perceive this and to do something to change it in personal and public ways is to undergo a change in perception akin to a religious conversion. Nothing can ever be seen in quite the same way again, because once you have admitted the terror and pain of other species you will, unless you resist conversion, be always aware of the endless permutations of suffering that supports our society."
- The Laws of Manu (Manusmriti) 5.49 says, "Having well considered the origin of flesh foods, the cruelty of fettering and flaying of sentient beings, a person should abstain from eating flesh." The same text (Manusmriti 6.60) further states, "By not killing any living being, one becomes fit for liberation."
- Proverbs 12:10 says, "The righteous person regards the life of his or her animal."
- The Laws of Manu 5.45 says, "He who injures harmless beings from a wish to give himself pleasure never knows happiness in life or death." Verse 5.51 says, "He who permits the slaughter

of an animal and kills it, he who cuts it up, he who cooks it, he
who serves it, and he who eats it, are all slayers."
- Psalm 24:1 says, "The Earth is the Lord's, and everything in it."
- Psalm 34:14 says, "Seek peace and pursue it."
- The famous fifteenth-century Jewish rabbi Joseph Albo, and the
  great twentieth-century visionary mystic Rudolph Steiner, both
  said that people would become vegetarian in the Messianic era.
  We are now entering that era.
- Rabbi Joseph Albo, of the fifteenth century, also said, "Aside
  from cruelty, rage, and fury in killing animals, and the fact that
  it teaches human beings the bad trait of shedding blood for
  naught (lust); eating the flesh even of select animals will give rise
  to a mean and insensitive soul."
- Buddha is quoted as saying, "Him I call Brahmin (priestly) who
  slays no creatures, who does not kill, or cause to be killed, any
  living thing."
- These quotes and spiritual dietary practices attune us to the
  spiritual essence and motivation of holistic veganism. It is no
  accident that ancient Taoist masters and Indian rishis practiced
  live-food veganism to enhance and support spiritual life.

Applying this understanding helps us act as models for our kids. In
the previous chapter, we brought out the fact that, even in pregnancy, the
diet of the mother affects the diet of the child.[1] Research also shows that
the diet of the parents makes a strong impression to guide the children.[2]
By like measure, how we live our lives is a model for how to relate to the
planet, and holistic veganism is a model of how to heal and uplift the
planet as well as ourselves.

When we introduce our children to this way of life, it is something
they can relate to. Children are not naturally cruel. They are not naturally
bloodthirsty or mean. These are negative traits they may derive from their
parents, their society, and/or their social environment. Our role as conscious parents is to create a better world, instead of narcissistically thinking of only our personal health. As conscious parents and grandparents,

it is a blessing to the world to empower our children to create a healthier physical, mental, emotional, spiritual, ecological, and cultural world. They needn't wait to get older to do this, or wait for Congress to pass a set of conscious laws. We can act now.

As holistic vegans, our children can learn to live in a way that uplifts their souls and the world around them, including their peers. Our children can become heroic leaders, because inherently kids want to create peace, and they want to grow up in a healthier, cruelty-free, ecologically viable world. Empowering our children with the understanding of holistic veganism gives them a powerful message about how to do this. Holistic veganism is a way to sanctify ourselves, creating holiness through our daily acts of eating and living.

We have condensed the principles of Holistic Veganism to the following seven teachings, so that one can be focused on as a teaching tool for each day of the week.

The Seven Principles of Holistic Veganism

1) PROTECTION OF THE GERM CELL
AND SURVIVAL OF THE SPECIES

We mentioned the problem of radiation, pesticides, and herbicides, which are fifteen to thirty times more concentrated in foods such as meat, fish, chicken, and dairy that are higher on the food chain. By eating lower on the food chain, we diminish our potential exposure to higher concentrations of radiation, pesticides, herbicides, GMO "frankenfoods," and toxic minerals such as fluoride and mercury. A diet consisting of plant foods, therefore, is best suited for the protection and survival of our germ cells, the sperm and ova.

A high exposure to environmental toxins decreases fertility. This is very important because not only are worldwide rates of infertility escalating, but we also see documented increases in a variety of congenital defects from radiation exposure and GMO foods. From this viewpoint too, holistic veganism is best suited for the healthy survival of the human species.

For example, in considering the issue of the safety of fish for human consumption, this flesh food has been found to be very detrimental to the preservation of the germ cell because of the PCBs and mercury that contaminate the water. PCBs, along with dioxin and DDT, are among the most toxic chemicals on the planet. The tenth annual report of the Council of Environmental Quality, sponsored by the U.S. government, found PCBs in 100% of sperm samples tested, as noted in *Conscious Eating.*

As far back as 1979, PCBs were found to be one of the main reasons that the sperm count of the average American male was approximately seventy percent of what it was thirty years ago. Twenty-five percent of all college males are sterile today, compared to one-half to one percent fifty years ago. The main source of this contamination comes from eating fish from waters high in PCBs. Fish can accumulate up to nine million times higher PCB levels than the water they swim in. Shellfish also naturally concentrate toxins. These include oysters, clams, and mussels, which may accumulate 70,000 times the toxin level of as the water they live in.

Consumer Reports in 2014 pointed out that the mercury levels in the upper layers of the ocean have more than tripled since the Industrial Revolution. Mercury is fat-soluble, and therefore hard to eliminate. Because of this, the FDA has issued new recommendations for pregnant women and breastfeeding mothers and children, to limit their mercury consumption by eating lower on the food chain and particularly by avoiding all varieties of tuna, shark, tilefish (from the Gulf of Mexico), swordfish, and king mackerel, which are larger fish and therefore higher on the food chain. Obviously, there are other sources of mercury, such as amalgam dental fillings, and even vaccines that still contain mercury, including flu vaccines recommended to be taken even during pregnancy by government agencies and many allopathic doctors.

2) ABUNDANT VITALITY

Another way that holistic veganism helps us is through increased vitality and personal energy, which we've discussed in detail as it relates to children and as a template for the prevention of chronic diseases. In general, as noted in *Conscious Eating* and documented in approximately ten research studies dating back to 1917, those on a plant-source-only diet have approximately two to three times the endurance and energy of omnivores.

3) COMBATING GLOBAL HUNGER

Another level in this discussion is the power of a vegan diet to feed the world's hungry. The data on this subject is overwhelming. Twenty to forty million people starve to death each year. According to the United Nations, this includes approximately 29,000–40,000 children who starve to death each day. This is something our children can relate to, because these are their peers.

The grain that is used to feed 100 cows can feed 2,000 humans. An estimated seventy to eighty percent of all grains produced go to support a meat-centered diet through the feeding of cows. Research suggests that if just ten percent of meat-eaters in the U.S. became vegan—or if everyone just reduced their meat consumption by ten percent—there would be enough plant-based food to feed all forty million of these starving people. For perspective on this enormous humanitarian crisis, it helps to know that more people have died of starvation in the last five years than from all wars combined in the last 150 years. U.S. livestock eats enough grain and soy to feed the U.S. human population five times over. The total global livestock population eats twice the amount of calories as the world's human population. If the whole world became vegan, there would be enough food and water to feed the global human population seven times over.

When we run plant protein through a cow or sheep, we glean only one-tenth of the plant's protein yield for human nutrition. In other words, we lose about ninety percent of the plant's protein when it is cycled through cow flesh. In addition, we lose approximately 100% of the plant's complex carbohydrates, and ninety-five percent of the plant's phytonutrients. It is estimated that approximately sixteen vegans can live off the same land and water supply it takes to sustain one meat-eater.

A meat-centered diet, seen this way, is obviously not ecologically sustainable. About twenty times more fossil fuels are needed to produce one calorie of beef as one calorie of vegetable protein. The overwhelming implication here is that a flesh-centered diet represents an unfair distribution and misappropriation of resources, because it requires so much more water, soil, air, and energy to sustain it.

The United Nations estimates that half the world's population suffers from malnutrition, with an estimated 100–200 million people seriously malnourished and twenty-five percent of the world's children suffering from lack of food. As stated earlier, by being vegan we could potentially save the lives of 29,000–40,000 kids daily. Our children can begin to feel heroic about the world service of their veganism. By eating lower on the food chain, we could potentially feed the global human population and all the world's children. If our children, and we as parents, start to understand and feel the compassionate power of a vegan way of life, we can even begin to feel that we are feeding the Divine in feeding those starving children.

This is an incredibly powerful thought for our children to connect with. We can explain that by eating a vegan diet we could attain production of enough food for all the people of the world, which could keep alive the poor and starving. The less the children of the world are malnourished, the greater will be their overall ability to reach their full physical, mental, and creative potential to achieve their life purpose. A plant-sourced vegan diet is a major step toward healthily reorganizing the way that the world's resources are distributed. There is simply no need for anyone to die of starvation in the world today.

We can help our children to understand what an important role we play through the act of eating. We don't need an act of Congress, just an act of conscious eating. If every person became vegan, it would be possible to give four tons of grain to every starving person on Earth. Participating in this idea is an exciting gift we can give our children when they sit down with us to eat.

4) PROTECTING AGAINST CRUELTY TO ANIMALS

Holistic veganism protects against animal cruelty. People engaging in cruel actions also damage their own minds. In eating animals and fish, the eater may indirectly take on the psychology of victimhood. In eating dead animals, one takes the energy of death deep into one's subtle body and mind. From a subtle psychological point of view, then, it is hard to separate the consumption of flesh food from a passive death wish.

It is hard to comprehend how much pain and death we are causing with a diet of meat. The average American meat-eater in one lifetime consumes eleven whole steers, one calf, three lambs, twenty-three hogs, forty-five turkeys, and 826 fish. That's a lot of cruelty and death to digest and assimilate. In the U.S. and Canada, the average adult consumes over 200 pounds of animal flesh each year. That adds up to an estimated total of forty-eight billion cattle, calves, sheep, hogs, chickens, ducks, and turkeys.

As the thirteenth-century rabbi and physician Moshe ben Nachman (Nachmanides) said, "Cruelty expands in a man's soul, as is well-known amongst cattle-slaughterers." As Pythagoras said, "As long as men kill animals, they will kill each other. He who sows the seed of murder and pain cannot reap love and joy."

Part of holistic veganism is being honest about our actions. Every day in the U.S., 60,000 broiler chickens are thrown into scalding tanks, alive and breathing. About 14,000 chickens are killed in the U.S. every minute. The great medieval physician and rabbi Moshe ben Maimon (Maimonides) said, "It should not be believed that all living things exist for the sake of humanity. On the contrary, all living things have been created for their own sake, and not for the sake of another."

This teaching can help children to understand that, like us, all animals have a sacred design and a sacred place in the universe although, according to the Bible, humans have been given dominion over the animal and plant kingdoms. "Dominion," however, does not mean domination; we have not been instructed, nor do we have permission, to dominate, exploit, rape, and destroy for our own egocentric lusts. A conscious vegan focuses on the positive implications of the vegan way of life.

The Link Between Animal Cruelty and Human Violence

Researchers, as well as the FBI and other law-enforcement agencies nationwide, have linked animal cruelty to domestic violence, child abuse, serial killings, and to the recent rash of killings by school-age children.

—Dr. Randall Lockwood, vice-president of Training Initiatives for The Humane Society of the United States (HSUS)

If we are to teach children how to respect their human and natural environment and all its elements, they must be taught they are a part of nature.... One of the objectives of education from nursery school onwards must be to give children a balanced sensitivity to life—a humane education.

—Canadian Senate Committee on Health, Welfare and Science (meeting on the rise of violent juvenile delinquencies in the 1970s)

Teaching our children compassion toward animals aids them in developing empathy, morality, and character development—skills that transfer to healthy social interactions with people. Conversely, violence toward animals is strongly linked to violence toward people. In every highly publicized school shooting where children were killed by a classmate, it is amazing to see that every young shooter had a documented history of abusing or killing animals before turning on their peers.

A sixteen-year-old boy wrote in his journal that he and another child had beaten, burned, and brutally killed his dog, Sparkle, describing the act as "true beauty." He later stabbed his mother to death, shot and killed two classmates, and injured seven others. Another boy, at age fifteen, frequently told others how he tortured animals. This boy ended up killing both his parents, then opened fired in his high-school cafeteria, killing two students and injuring twenty-two others. Another high school student was known to smash the heads of mice with a crowbar and set them on fire, long before he and a classmate killed twelve students and a teacher at his school—Columbine High School in Littleton, Colorado.

Adult violent offenders also tend to have a history of serious and repeated animal cruelty in their childhood and adolescence. Jeffrey

Dahmer, Ted Bundy, Andrew Cunanan, David "Son of Sam" Berkowitz, and Albert "Boston Strangler" DeSalvo were *all* cruel to animals before they started harming people.

These tragic examples show us that cruelty toward animals is not normal or healthy human behavior. The culture of death, which deems the inhumane treatment of animals for food production acceptable and necessary, thus perpetuates a consciousness of brutality, which we have known for millennia to be linked to violence toward humans.

5) PREVENTION AND REMEDIATION OF ECOLOGICAL DESTRUCTION CAUSED BY A MEAT-CENTERED DIET

The ecological destruction of the planet is being greatly accelerated by a meat-centered diet. An estimated fifty to seventy percent of the water in the U.S. is used for livestock feed and production. This is particularly significant in light of the current droughts on the West Coast, in the Southwest, and in other areas of the United States. Many other places around the world are also facing serious drought.

The math speaks clearly for itself: It takes 2,500 gallons of water to produce one pound of meat, compared with twenty-five gallons of water to produce one pound of wheat. A meat-centered diet effectively requires 4,500 gallons of water each day to sustain, whereas a vegetarian diet requires about 300. So vegan families save approximately 1.5 million gallons of water per person a year, compared to an omnivore.

Animal agriculture also uses approximately thirty-three percent of the world's raw materials for the production of livestock, compared to the two percent of the world's raw materials used for vegetarian agriculture.

Every individual calorie of meat consumed requires thirty-two calories of energy to produce. While estimates vary, it takes about forty times more calories of fossil fuel to get one calorie of beef protein, compared to that same calorie of protein from soybeans. Eighty-five percent of topsoil loss is due to animal agriculture. Every five seconds, an acre of trees disappears, mostly to clear land for beef cattle. Rainforests are being cut down at a rate of thirty-one million acres a year, an area roughly the size of New York City.

The livestock are also creating a tremendous amount of excrement. The farm-animal population produces over 230,000 pounds of excrement each second. By comparison, the human population produces an estimated 12,000 pounds of excrement each second. This equates to a huge amount of waste and environmental pollution caused by the livestock, as pesticides, hormones, antibiotics, and pathogens are released into our rivers, lakes, and land—which becomes an even more glaring imbalance in these times when we are facing such a critical shortage of water. Twenty-five percent of all *E. coli* infections can be traced back to fruits and vegetables grown with infected manure. Meat-eating and its byproducts are a public-health issue as well as a global-resource survival issue.

The United Nations and the European Union have reflected that meat-eating could be the primary reason for world deforestation. A 2006 U.N. report titled *Livestock's Long Shadow* suggests that animal agriculture is one of the chief contributors to environmental problems on every scale, from local to global. The reports estimate that animal agriculture contributes to up to eighteen percent of global-warming gases, compared to CO_2 production from industry and transportation contributing just nine percent. This is indeed an inconvenient truth for supporters of animal agriculture. In June 2010 the United Nations and the European Commission called for a shift toward a vegan diet to save the Earth.

The United Nations is not exactly a vegan organization, but they've launched a major report calling for radical change in the way that world economies use resources—because those resources are dwindling. They identified overuse of fossil fuels and animal agriculture as the two leading causes of environmental degradation. The report highlighted the fact that there is an unsustainably large proportion of the world's crops currently fed to livestock. This results in ecological damage from excessively high water consumption and the toxic effects of pesticides and synthetic fertilizers. The report states that a global drop in meat consumption is vital to avoid devastating global-warming consequences. The authors of this report recommend that a substantial decrease in impact will only be possible with a substantial worldwide dietary shift away from a meat-centered diet.

The "cow in the living room" is also a primary source of methane, which has a twenty-seven times greater global-warming effect than CO_2, and of nitrogen from manure, whose effect is 296 times greater. Nitrogen contributes as much as sixty percent of global-warming gases. *Livestock's Long Shadow* also points out that for every kilogram of animal protein produced, livestock are fed about six kilograms of plant protein, a highly energy-inefficient ratio. The report further states that it takes eight times as much fossil fuel to produce animal food than plant food. Some researchers feel that this figure is too conservative, and estimate it takes twenty-two times more fossil fuel to create animal food than plant-source alternatives.

This imbalance creates a serious desecration of our ecology. Animal agriculture represents the worst synthesis of industrialization, capitalism, and technology to threaten the survival of the planet. It creates monumental costs in environmental decay and, ultimately, an overburdened healthcare system as well. Presently, cattle take up a quarter of the Earth's arable land, and about ninety percent of U.S. agricultural land is used for animals. The resultant overgrazing affects everything in the environment including climate, water, and soil erosion.

Animal agriculture and an omnivorous diet are a dramatic, traumatic environmental insult. Each pound of animal feed produced causes the erosion of thirty-five pounds of topsoil. The impact of making one quarter-pound hamburger destroys fifty-five feet of rainforest; and 100 species of animals are estimated to become extinct with every two billion fast-food hamburgers sold.

These are things we can share with our children, so that they can become environmental protectors and heroes for saving the planet and their own lives. One acre of grain yields five times more protein than an acre of beef. One acre of leafy green vegetables yields twenty-five times more protein than an acre of beef. We can illustrate these facts very clearly to children.

Anyone who wants to blame global weather changes on that human-caused nine percent carbon dioxide, while ignoring the far more serious effects of animal agriculture—which has twice the global warming effect as the carbon dioxide from industry and transportation—is in a state of serious ignorance or gross denial. The overall ecological evidence is that animal agriculture is a primary causal factor in climate change, and leads us to the obvious conclusion about how to protect the planet: Go vegan!

The European Journal of Clinical Nutrition notes that "vegetarian diets could play an important role in preserving environmental resources and reducing hunger and malnutrition in poorer nations." *The Lancet* recommended in September 2007 that if people in the industrial world ate ten percent less meat, it would reduce greenhouse-gas emissions and improve human health. The article stated,

> The unprecedented serious challenge imposed by climate change necessitates radical responses.... For the world's higher-income populations, greenhouse gas emissions from meat-eating warrant the same scrutiny as do emissions from driving and flying.

In considering global weather instability, the contribution of the herd of cows in the room is far more significant than the nine percent of global-warming gases claimed to be caused by carbon-dioxide emissions from industry. Those emissions cannot be ignored as a significant cause of global warming. But a vegan driving a Hummer is creating far less ecological destruction and possible global warming than an omnivore driving a Prius. Of course, we must consider all causes of global climate change, rather than seeing it as an either/or proposition.

Our children can reverse the destruction. They can stand up to and transform a meat-eating, cruel, degenerate, culture-of-death world. Part of this requires understanding that heroes are not often the most popular people. But vegan live-food children will have clearer minds, morals, ethics, and a spiritual understanding that supports them in not going along with group-think. We are here to save the planet, humanity, and our spirits. Our children, when imbued with a heroic consciousness that goes beyond fear for our health, become empowered to be ethical, moral, ecological, and spiritual heroes that can inspire their classmates to take on this heroic role as well.

6) PROTECTING OUR MENTAL AND PHYSICAL WELLNESS

Eating lower on the food chain puts fewer toxins into the mind and body. The mind is more capable of focus when it is not agitated by the pain, suffering, and cruelty we take on through eating meat. We create a mind more able to think clearly, pray, or meditate. A holistic vegan diet creates a more compassionate and peaceful mind.

Spiritually speaking, almost all the great wisdom traditions, including Hinduism, Judaism, original Christianity, Taoism, and Buddhism, make the absence of bloodshed a crucial component of a diet that best supports spiritual life. They agree that not eating death is best for a spiritual life.

The general teaching is that those who kill and eat animals are also the ones that tend to kill humans. Our internal subtle bodies—including the yogic *nadis,* and the *sefirotic* vessels of the Tree of Life in Kabbalistic wisdom, which carry the spiritual energy within us—are disrupted when the energy of death enters them and acts as sludge, slowing our inner evolution. A vegan diet is associated with spiritual growth and enlightenment in almost all the traditions.

7) MORALITY, ETHICS, AND SPIRITUALITY

A vegan diet best creates the conditions of *ahimsa* and fulfills the yogic *yamas* (recommended abstinences) and *niyamas* (positive practices) and the Ten Speakings (Ten Commandments). Holistic veganism is not about morality but about being responsible for the total impact of our actions. Eating a vegan diet creates the Sevenfold Peace—peace with the body, peace with the mind, peace with the family, peace with the community, peace with all cultures, peace with the ecology, and peace with the Divine.

The highest directive of the *yamas,* the *niyamas* and the Ten Speakings alike is the directive against violence: "Thou shalt not murder." As of 2009, an estimated fifty-nine billion animals are being killed worldwide each year to satisfy humanity's meat lust. Veganism results in no animal death to feed our egocentric lusts. The compassionate practice of *ahimsa* is the most primary and practical way to live peacefully in the world.

The yogic idea of *yama satya* (truthfulness) correlates with the Hebraic "Thou shalt not bear false witness." Many omnivores do not see the ramifications of their diet as connected to the survival of the whole of life on Earth, so there is worldwide denial and self-delusion at play here. Somehow people think steak comes from the grocery counter rather than from a dead cow, and that Elsie the smiling cow is happy with her babies taken away to be tortured and slaughtered as "veal," and to have her life shortened from approximately thirty natural years to only three to five years, by being milked to death. This lying and deceiving of self and others is a second violation of moral law.

The Eighth Speaking is "Thou shalt not commit adultery," which correlates with the yogic *brahmacharya,* seeking the Divine through self-restraint. The word "adultery" in the Ten Speakings, according to Torah scholarship, is more accurately understood as "sexual perversion," and closer to the literal Hebrew meaning, as described in the book *Torah as a Guide to Enlightenment* by Rabbi Gabriel Cousens, MD.[3] Animal agriculture includes the artificial fertilization of chickens and cattle, and seminal extraction from bulls—all accomplished through human/animal sexual violation, and all constituting sexual perversions. These fertilization techniques require invasion of the animal's sexual cycle by humans—certainly a perversion of the natural order, if not possibly also a diluted, indirect, conscious, or unconscious form of bestiality.[4]

The Ninth Speaking, "Thou shalt not steal," is known as *asteya* in the yogic tradition. This is similarly dismissed in the marketing, sales, and consumption of animal products. The omnivorous diet is based on stealing milk, bodies, skin, fur, and the animals' natural lifecycle itself. In eating this food we become complicit thieves, which undermines us physically, mentally, and spiritually as well.

Aparigraha means nongreediness in yogic terminology. "Thou shalt not covet" is the Biblical correlate. Coopting resources from the rest of the world to fuel our unsustainable lust for meat consumption violates this spiritual law. This covetousness is creating pollution of the public commons—a further violation. Twenty million acres of new desert is created each year, with approximately fifty to seventy million acres of trees cut and plowed under yearly for animal-farming purposes. We are skinning the Earth alive.

Carbon emissions and global warming are also a concern here. Normal CO_2 levels were 280 parts per million, and the levels are currently around 385 ppm, with levels rising by as much as three ppm each year. Carbon dioxide is depleting the oxygen, most notably in the cities. The percentage of oxygen in the atmosphere was thirty-eight percent 200 years ago, and is presently nineteen percent, and in some cities as low as twelve percent. A twelve-percent oxygen ratio begins to create serious health problems. Lack of oxygen contributes to cancer, as cells grow in a reduced oxygen environment, as well as contributing to fungal infections such as candida.

The vegan diet supports a quiet mind, and ultimately spiritual life and liberation, if that is our aim. Patanjali's *Yoga Sutras* states, *"yoga chitta vritti nirodha,"* meaning, "Yoga is the cessation of the fluctuations of the mind." A vegan diet helps accomplish this quieting of the mind. As Rabbi Dr. Gabriel has said, "Each particle of food has its own vibration. Animal foods set up a chaotic vibration, whipping the mind into a state of imbalance as the culmination of the pain, suffering, and distress of the animals being exploited and slaughtered. This makes transcendence of the mind very difficult."

This is part of how an omnivorous diet disrupts spiritual life, and how a plant-based, vegan diet supports a quiet mind. Diet affects consciousness. It affects our thoughts, and ultimately our actions. A quiet, peaceful mind tends to create peaceful actions. As Rabbi Dr. Gabriel has noted, "Food is a love-note from the Divine, and we are an act of divine love powered by that love-note." A plant-based, holistic, vegan, live-food diet is a way of bringing love into all our actions, and bringing love into the healing of the planet.

Abhay Charanaravinda Bhaktivedanta Swami Prabhupada, founder of the International Society for Krishna Consciousness, is quoted as saying, "If one can maintain it, raw fruits and vegetables are the best diet for human spiritual life." Holistic veganism is a diet for the sanctification and healing of ourselves and the planet, and for purifying our spirits. It is distinct from a diet for strictly physical health. It is distinct from both omnivorous and vegetarian diets that are not necessarily based on morals or ethics. Holistic veganism works on every level for uplifting ourselves and the planet.

A holistic, vegan, optimally healthy diet is organic, plant-source-only, moderately low-insulin index, low-glycemic, high-mineral, nutrient-concentrated, well-hydrated, and deriving at least 80% of its calories from live foods, with moderate amounts of plant-source-only, raw fat, including short- and long-chain omega-3s for optimal brain and cognitive development and prevention of cancer and heart disease. It is individualized to one's unique constitution, without overeating, and made with love.

The general macronutrient base of this diet is approximately 10–20% protein, depending upon age and constitution, 25–45% raw plant fat, and 25–45% carbohydrates, depending upon constitution. Our future, and the survival of the planet, depends upon a conscious application of the wisdom and practice of holistic veganism. Holistic veganism strengthens clarity and expanded consciousness. The consciousness that emerges from holistic veganism is the spiritual force pushing us toward a millennium of peace. Holistic veganism is the turning of the tide. By living this way, we are creating the preconditions for our children and grandchildren to be creative, heroic, alive, alert, conscious visionaries leading this transformation.

As Rabbi Dr. Gabriel points out in his lectures, *"In each generation, we are given the medicine needed for the world's repair. Holistic veganism is the medicine for healing today's world. It is the wave of the present and the future on every level."*

CHAPTER 6

Supporting the Child's Emotional Development

It's all right to feel things, though the feelings may be strange.

—Carol Hall

Living Foods and Freeing Up Emotions

As shown in extensive detail in *Depression-Free for Life,* and as animated by the story of Levi's breakfast salad, living foods help us to feel good as they raise neurotransmitter production. Tryptophan-rich foods like hemp seeds, cashews, sunflower seeds, pumpkin seeds, bananas, and avocados, for example, well-chewed, as described in *Depression-Free for Life,* can increase serotonin levels in the brain 500%, helping the brain to produce this neurotransmitter that increases our sense of well-being.[1]

Likewise, antioxidant-rich foods such as berries, pomegranates, dark leafy greens, red beets, nuts and seeds, chili peppers, cloves, ginger, and green tea extract, also help reduce stress. According to two studies on food and mood, there appears to be a direct link between a meat-free lifestyle and decreased stress, anxiety, depression, and negative emotion.[2] Among other factors, this has been attributed to the arachidonic acid found in meat and animal foods that is known to cause inflammation in the brain. By receiving the essential vitamins, minerals, and fatty acids that we need—far higher in living foods—we are not only nourishing the family's physical health and mental wellness, we are also supporting the EQ (Emotional IQ) of the home. By receiving the living elements of earth, air, water, and fire (sunlight), we can actually feel the greater connection; we can feel the emotions of coming alive. In a study of 525 people on a diet of 80% vegan live food for two years, conducted by a masters student in the Cousens' School of Holistic Wellness, 87.5% felt more creative and more mentally and spiritually alive on this diet.

This sounds pretty good—but what about when other, less pleasurable, emotions start coming up? As addressed in the book *Raw Emotion* by Angela Stokes, and in *Spiritual Nutrition* by Rabbi Gabriel Cousens, MD, when we eat living foods we are no longer suppressing our emotions with food, as happens when we eat cooked junk foods. This is why when we transition from eating foods that numb us to those that sensitize, energize, and empower us, we start to feel the emotions that we have been "swallowing."

Junk foods create a junk consciousness, which creates literal physical as well as mental toxins that block our access to unconscious suppressed emotions. These toxins block clarity and refined brain functions. When Appleton High School eliminated processed and GMO foods from its cafeteria, the students' minds got so clear that there was a major shift toward inner peace, which was so strong that they stopped needing police to patrol the hallways. The surfacing of the suppressed emotions helps us face them in a healthy way. As the somewhat crude saying goes, "You can either face your stuff, or stuff your face."

Do you mean the kids are going to feel even more emotions than they do now?! Wait—before you drop this book, run for cover, and never turn the next page—remember that we can help prevent exaggerated mood swings through proper hydration and a natural, moderately low-sugar diet. This is because omega-3 and omega-6 fatty acids in proper balance, with adequate mineralization, support the child's developing brain and create a neurotransmitter and hormonal balance that tends to decrease anger and hostility caused by an inflamed and irradiated brain, and to bring about the more healthy and mature emotional expression called EQ (emotional intelligence).

It is also important to realize that supporting our children with spiritual nutrition is not necessarily going to intensify their emotions. Instead, we are supporting their awareness of the noncausal joy already present inside them! We are also helping to bring greater awareness to unpleasant emotional responses that hinder the child's innate joyous expression, such as anger, grief, hurt, and guilt. We are giving them the emotional power and training to express these feelings in more constructive and healthy ways.

Part of our job as parental mentors is helping our children and grandchildren learn to safely process their emotions. With greater awareness, all of us are better equipped to appropriately release pent-up emotions that tend to promote disease, and to learn how to change our emotional responses to life's stimuli. This is a wonderful family process.

Fortunately, there is support for healthy emotional development for families. For grown-ups, there are "Zero Point" workshops. This self-inquiry process was developed and facilitated by Rabbi Dr. Gabriel at the Tree of Life Center U.S. In this life-changing process, adults learn to access the seeds of their own negative thought forms, and to dissolve them. They learn that the personality is a case of mistaken identity.

For the child, whose still-developing ego needs to be honored, there are other resources, as the Zero Point Course is only offered to those in their mid-teens or older. Once we parents have improved our EQ, we are empowered to actively support our children in becoming emotionally literate, and to teach EQ to our children according to their EQ at the moment.

The *Emotional Literacy* series of booklets for parents by Enchanté Innertainment can also be useful for helping the child to find healthy ways to release strong emotions. Emotional Literacy materials are designed to aid both parent and child in accepting, understanding, and being the boss of one's own feelings, so that emotions aren't running the home. These EQ materials are beginning to be taught in some public schools in the U.S. as well.

Another resource is *The Journey for Kids: Liberating Your Child's Shining Potential* (book and workshop). The Journey, which is a therapeutic metaphor process, was developed by Brandon Bays after her natural and complete healing of a basketball-sized uterine tumor. While Brandon was on a 100% living-foods diet, she experienced the emotional healing of a cellular memory of trauma that had been stored in her uterus. Brandon has shared her Journeywork for adults worldwide, and has modified it for use with children. In her book *The Journey for Kids*, there are testimonials from parents and other stories of deep healing that have taken place with the help of this forgiveness-based process. Some of these include healings of the physical symptoms of ADHD and even life-threatening allergies (see "Resources," page 485).

Stop Reacting and Start Responding: 108 Ways to Discipline Consciously and Become the Parent You Want to Be, by Sharon Silver of Proactive Parenting, is a highly insightful resource for understanding childhood behaviors based on stages of development. Silver also provides practical pointers for day-to-day positive parenting via on-line webinars.

Listening to How your Child Feels about Eating Animals

As you've perhaps observed, many children find it very disturbing that they are eating an animal when they first find out that a hamburger is cow's flesh, or that a drumstick is a chicken's leg. Many children experience profound feelings of compassion and connection with farm animals, as well as a strong sense of ethical treatment of animals, even when they are very young.

An example of this is an endearing home video of a small Brazilian boy as he makes this discovery at the table. This lovely conversation between Luiz Antonio and his mother has been translated into English and has received millions of views on YouTube.

In a popular homeschool science curriculum, the textbook author sympathizes with its young readers as they learn about predator-prey interactions, acknowledging the child's feelings as spiritual promptings, and providing scripture verses about all species' plant-sourced origin and prophesied return.[3] Our culture of death, by contrast, rather than validating these intuitive feelings in appreciation of the child's sensitivity, teaches tuned-in kids to ignore their own hearts and thus fragment themselves from their natural compassion, love, and morals, each time they eat.

As part of Leah's rural upbringing, she went to animal auctions with her dad—who incidentally is also now a vegan. At an early age, Leah could see clearly that these animals were not being respected, and that they were very frightened. She also recalls in detail a grade-school fieldtrip to a local meatpacking plant. While Leah did not witness animal slaughter there, she has a vivid memory of the sights, smells, and general feeling of death, as well as her own feeling of uneasiness in that setting. Had the class gone to a vegetable farm and harvested tomatoes and cucumbers, the experience of course would have been completely different.

When a child's eyes are opened to animal suffering, misery, fear, and death, they may very well opt on their own to become vegetarians. Fortunately, parents now have access to information about supporting this choice with whole-food nutrition. Listening to the child's objection to participating in the animal industry is one way to support the child's emotional development. In so doing, we are sending the message that the child can come to the table as a whole person, able to listen to his own inner teacher.

Thoughts, Emotions, and the Preparation of Food

How about we bless this food?

—Levi Chrisemer, an almost two-year-old nursling
with a hand on each of his mother's breasts

Not only are the emotions of animals stored in the flesh and the milk that we consume, but all the food we eat also transmits the energies of those who have prepared it. This is why the wise practice of blessing the food before we eat is found in all of the great cultural and spiritual traditions.

When we bless the food that we prepare for the family, we are very truly blessing the whole family. Conversely, when we experience negative emotions while preparing the meal, our loved ones are also affected, as those emotions become imbedded in the water of our food. To introduce this teaching to children, the following story as shared in Dr. Gabriel's book *Conscious Eating* can be enjoyed together. It can be read aloud, memorized and retold, or performed as a puppet play:

> Once upon a time there was a monk who lived in the forest of India. He lived in a simple setting, meditating regularly and eating pure food that he gathered from the land. It was the custom in this region for the kings and wealthy people to invite the monks to live with them during the monsoon season. It was considered a blessing for the king to invite this particular monk to stay with him.
>
> The king, being of a greedy nature, also had a greedy cook. During the time of the monsoon, the monk ate the food prepared by the greedy cook of the greedy king. Over time, the pure mind of the monk began to have greedy thoughts as a result of eating the food that had taken on the greedy thoughts of the cook.
>
> One day, near the end of the monsoon, the monk impulsively stole a necklace belonging the queen. The palace was in an uproar about this and, of course, no one suspected the monk. After a short time, the monk announced that he was leaving, and returned to the forest with the necklace. After a few weeks of eating his own food, his mind began to clear.
>
> One day, he looked at this necklace and could not figure out what he was doing with this useless piece of jewelry. When it became clear to him what had happened, he returned to the palace with the necklace. The king, of course, wanted to know why he had taken it. The monk explained that the food he had been eating while he was in the king's palace had been permeated by the greedy consciousness of the cook, and had temporarily infected his mind with that greed. When he began to eat his own pure food, prepared with love, his mind cleared and the greed left him.[4]

When we grow and prepare our child's food with consciousness, we are supporting their emotional, social, and spiritual development, as well as modeling for them how to do it for themselves.

RAISIN EXERCISE

The following exercise is loved by many children. This can be done with one or two children at home, or in a classroom setting during circle time:

Tell the children that you will be giving them each a raisin, and not to put it in their mouths until you give them the signal. After everyone has received a raisin, ask the children to close their eyes. Then calmly lead them through the following series, briefly pausing between thoughts to give the children a chance to fully take in the experience:

"Place your raisin on your tongue. Move it around your mouth to feel it, but be careful not to bite into it. Now hold the raisin still on your tongue, and with your eyes still closed, see the grapevine full of grapes being ripened by the sun and kissed by a gentle breeze. These are the sun and the wind's gifts to you.

"See the stem of the grape, and follow it all the way down the vine, and to the roots. See the roots taking in water and nutrients from the soil. These are the Earth's gifts to you.

"You may want to say a silent thank-you to the sun, the air, the water and the soil for this gift, as you now bite into your raisin and slowly eat it. If you eat slowly enough, you might just feel the gifts of sun, the air, the water and the Earth inside your raisin. Keeping your eyes closed as you feel the raisin going into your body, feel now what it is like to be one raisin heavier. Now open your eyes."

The singing of blessings before mealtimes also appeals to the child's spirit, uniting the hearts of family members and supporting the child's growing sense of rhythm. Whether we sing songs of blessing, take a moment of silence, or utter a prayer, what makes the blessing real is when we ourselves become the blessing.

A simple mealtime blessing might go like this:

Blessings on the blossoms,

Blessings on the fruit.

Blessings on the stems and leaves,

Blessings on the root.

Blessings on our family, friends, and food. (The last line is spoken.)

—Learned from teachers at Pleasant Ridge
Waldorf School in Viroqua, Wisconsin

Each time a family sings this song together, they can close their eyes, see, and feel vibrant and abundant blossoms, fruits, stems, leaves, and roots covering the living planet, and making their way into the happy hands and mouths of children everywhere. At the end of the blessing, there should be a feeling of gratefulness and self-esteem.

Self-Esteem

The hunger for love is much more difficult to remove than the hunger for bread.

—Mother Theresa

We're a culture of low self-esteem. That is really the disease that we're talking about.

—Sharon Gannon, cofounder of Jivamukti Yoga
Center, in the film Raw for Life

Keeping self-esteem alive is as necessary for each human being as water is for plants. Self-esteem is the daily food of emotional health.

—Patricia H. Berne and Louis M. Savary,
in Building Self-Esteem in Children

By their nature, plants know what nutrients they need to grow and develop. So it is with children, and what they need to be fed is love. Love is the "life-force" food they need.

—Peggy Jenkins, PhD, in *The Joyful Child: A Sourcebook of Activities and Ideas for Releasing Children's Natural Joy*

The greatest gift we can give our children and grand-children is a healthy self-esteem. Our enduring love for them is the basis of a healthy self-esteem.

—Rabbi Gabriel Cousens, MD

Mom, you and Dad need to savor me as a child.

—Leah's daughter Quinn, at age four

The self-esteem of the child plays a vital role in the five domains of childhood development—social, emotional, physical, mental, and spiritual. To love and to value oneself is pivotal for engaging in healthy relationships and other lifestyle choices, for being able to take safe risks, and for bouncing back from life's difficulties. A healthy self-esteem is pivotal to children's journey of discovering their full potential for aliveness throughout their life.

The foundation of self-esteem is to feel loved by one's parents. This is the greatest gift a child can receive. It lasts for a lifetime.

The first step in supporting the child's self-esteem is to look at how we value ourselves. This is the true basis of how we love the child, for children's self-esteem is inherited. As they grow, they unconsciously absorb the parents' expressions of self-esteem—through both self-love and love shown toward others. What the child receives from the adults around them helps to form their interpretation of every life experience they have.

As a result of parents' own childhood experiences, we may feel at times as if we're on training wheels when it comes to self-love. By incorporating the Six Foundations and Sevenfold Peace practices discussed above, we can gain momentum. These foundations help us give ourselves permission to receive and to share Divine love. This profound heart-opening in turn becomes a blessing to our children. As we live by these foundations of spiritual life, the illusion of separation from the Divine naturally begins to fade. So may we as parents be blessed with an alive environment and diet that supports the organic unfolding of our wholeness and true self-worth.

How we offer feedback to our children also transmits messages about how we view them. Educational methods that pay careful attention to such subtleties help us show our children that we trust in their innate ability to self-correct. In the Waldorf Schools tradition, for example, we see daily storytelling used to help children become more aware of their own actions and the effects of those actions. Rather than delivering a lecture, Waldorf teachers thoughtfully select a story based on careful observations they have made about students and their social process together.

In the Montessori system, we see that each lesson given to the child has a built-in error control. When the child finds that they have spilled water droplets on a tray, for example, or that there aren't enough spindles left to use as counting sticks for the next numeral, the work itself gives the child the needed feedback.

These types of supports tell children that we acknowledge their inner teacher, rather than training them to be dependent on us to make all of the adjustments. This is a subtle way of honoring the child's sovereignty. By finding gentle and indirect ways to offer direction, we also show care for our children's feelings, so as not to embarrass them, sending the false impression that they are somehow less than we are. Seeking to correct the child, when needed, with respect, humility, and kindness has far-reaching effects.

Another way to support our child's positive sense of self is by considering what they are ready for when we offer guidance. For example, when first taking her daughter to preschool, Leah was touched by the thoughtfulness in the drawings that marked each child's cubby. It wasn't just that they were soft and lovely images carefully handcrafted by the teacher, but the children were able to identify which place was theirs, since they didn't yet know how to read.

Likewise, when we slow down to show a young child how to use a tool such as scissors, step-by-step, and allowing time for their mastery of this skill before we present a multi-stepped project involving tracing, cutting, and gluing, for example, we also nurture self-confidence. When we offer a project that is too advanced for a child's ability, and then offer to do it for them when they find they are unable to do it, we undermine the child's self-confidence.

This is true of our older children as well. We often see this with teens who, because they look like adults, are commonly expected to behave like adults. However, when we fail to meet our children, big or small, where they are, we experience greater disconnection and their disappointed alienation. Conversely, as we begin to observe our children without judgment, appreciate where they are in their individual journeys, and offer discreet direction, we find greater fulfillment in our relationships.

As self-help author Byron Katie once commented about spending time with her grandchildren: "It was heaven. They didn't have to be more grown up than they were." Rabbi Dr. Gabriel supports the self-esteem of his three granddaughters by listening very attentively to them no matter how long it takes for them to express themselves. He also invites their participation in various spiritual ceremonies with adults, in active, age-appropriate roles. And—most important of all—we must continually remind them that they are loved, in ways they can understand, so that they always feel loved and listened to. Small, silent heart-to-heart touches through the day make powerful connections that transcend maturity levels.

Another way that we model self-esteem for our children is by setting appropriate boundaries in our lives. There is a place for compassion within those boundaries, and yet clearly there are times to take a firm stand. An example of this is when it comes to protecting our lives and control over our bodies, with accessibility of supplements, organic nutrition, and such things as the right to refuse vaccination. When we esteem our own lives and the lives of others, we are teaching our children to esteem themselves and others as well.

When we set appropriate boundaries with our children, they may initially protest; but so long as we demonstrate that we are still there for them, they receive, on some level, the respect underlying our stop signs. Modeling self-esteem in this way also teaches our children how to set healthy boundaries with their peers. Sometimes it can be difficult to allow our children to experience the consequences of their actions, and yet these lessons are essential to their developing ability to read life's feedback and make their own adjustments.

The key to setting healthy boundaries is to remember that our children are learning and developing, and doing their best in this process, as their idea of boundaries continues to evolve. We want to always send them the message that they aren't bad just because their actions have brought about undesirable results. Being lavish with our affirmation helps the child to get a sense of being ok, even though there is always much to be learned in life.

Lily's Story: There once was a preschooler we'll call Lily. There was a time when Lily used to laugh and run away from her teacher, who we'll call Leah, every time she would call. This is only one example of Lily's consistency in doing the exact opposite of what she knew the teacher wanted, right in front of the teacher, while wearing a big grin on her face! This was happening multiple times a day, disrupting other children in the classroom.

The scenario was a source of frustration for her puzzled teacher, until one day Leah got it: Although her efforts were misguided, they were trying to thrive! How could that be? A study conducted on plants, mentioned in *The Hidden Messages in Water* by Dr. Masaru Emoto, helps to piece it together: In this study, one group of plants was told positive, loving statements with their daily watering, while another group was told negative, hateful statements, and a third group of plants was watered but otherwise left isolated, without any additional attention. The plants in all three groups were of the same species and received the same amount of water.

The results? The plants that showed most signs of thriving were the ones who received love with their water. However, the plants that got no attention other than water did even more poorly than the plants that received the negative attention.

Ok, so Lily is not a plant—but her innate intelligence was going for the best that she'd known so far, which was negative attention. Hey, it's better than nothing! What Leah found to work was to refuse to play the negative attention game. That meant no running after Lily, no lectures, no pleading, no getting upset, and no sidestepping the consequences of her actions. But the exciting part was teaching another possibility—positive attention! When Lily was not misbehaving, Leah would ask her if she would like to ask the teacher for a hug. "Yes!" Lily would exclaim, so Leah told her, "Ok, Please say, 'Can I have a hug?'" Lily took a turn, received a hug, and beamed like the sun.

When Lily would lapse into old patterns, Leah would ask her, "Lily, would you rather ask for a hug?" and as the other game was getting her no attention, Lily would stop the misbehavior and ask her teacher for a hug. Lily started making the connection that positive attention is even better than negative attention—and how to ask for it. For us adults, it is important to try to decode the child's communication in order to give them positive support for who they are, and help them feel valued as a unique expression of the Divine.

CHAPTER 7

Supporting the Child's Social Development

A healthy social life is found only when in the mirror of each soul the whole community finds its reflection, and when in the whole community the virtue of each one is living.

—Rudolf Steiner

Living Foods and the Child's Social Development

Mom, don't pack kale chips in my lunch anymore! My friends always want them.

—Quinn Chrisemer, at age eight

Mom, will you pack more kale chips in my lunch? My friend really likes them.

—Levi Chrisemer, at age eight

Most people don't look inside a slaughterhouse because they know if they did, they might be compelled to make different choices. It is our fear of change—our attachment to old habits—that drives us to keep eat-ing animals and their products. It is our fear of doing something different that keeps us stuck in old behavior. This is what I mean when I say that this habit harms our relationships. Our ability to compartmentalize our emotions and justify the pain of other living creatures in favor of momentary pleasure cannot but affect us at the most fundamental level.

—Colleen Patrick-Goudreau, in *The Vegan Table*

We've looked at how living foods support the child's unfolding aliveness by nourishing the body-mind and emotional IQ; now we'll discuss liv-ing foods and the child's social development. First of all, let's clarify what is meant here by social development. What we are referring to, in the context of the culture of life and liberation, is supporting the child in the unfolding of their Divine expression as a confident, strong, positive, thoughtful, cooperative, respectful, honorable, responsible, compassion-ate, spiritual, loving, whole, and helpful member of our interdependent global family, positively supporting the overall evolution of humanity.

We are talking about raising the next generation of healers, builders, leaders, problem-solvers, and holy ones who, because they are in touch with who they are as children of the Divine, may potentially usher in the next Golden Age or Messianic Times. These are children who naturally shine their light. This ideal is worlds away from teaching the child to seek to be like everyone else in order to fit in.

To support the enlightened socialization of all children, it is our job to model social responsibility for the child, including in their relationship to food. This need is evidenced by the 2.2 trillion dollars the U.S. spends per year on healthcare—five times what we spend on the defense budget, and more than any other industrialized nation spends on healthcare. We realize that, according to the AMA in 1968, ninety-seven percent of all chronic disease such as type 2 diabetes, heart disease, and cancer are related to diet, and that our individual dietary choices are indeed a social issue.

Even though the U.S. spends the most on health care of any nation in the world, it ranks about forty-fifth in the world in healthcare quality. In *Diet for a New America* by John Robbins, we can see clearly the social implications of our individual food choices. A plant-sourced diet, for example, inherently shares planetary resources of clean air, water, and food with the whole global family, in contrast to an animal-sourced diet which, by its necessary consumptions, selfishly appropriates and pollutes these priceless resources.

If all people became vegans, we would save enough resources to feed the planet at least seven times over. If we were all live-food vegans, in fact, there could be enough food resources to feed the planetary population at least ten times over, because cooking food coagulates fifty percent of the protein, and destroys sixty to seventy percent of the vitamins and minerals and ninety-five percent of the phytonutrients. With a live-food vegan approach we would need to eat about fifty percent less to get proper nourishment from the food. As Thich Nhat Hanh, author of *Being Peace,* has said:

> If you do not eat mindfully, you are eating the flesh of your son and daughter; you are eating the flesh of your parent. Every day, 29,400– 40,000 children in the world, according to the United Nations, die for lack of food. We who overeat in the West, who feed grain to animals to make meat, are eating the flesh of these children (Speech at Riverside Church, New York, September 25, 2001).

By sharing the world's resources, the veganic living-foods lifestyle pro- motes social peace. As the ancient Greek philosopher and mathemati- cian Pythagoras predicted in a debate against introducing meat into the human diet, when we graze cattle for food the result could be a scarcity of land and water, which could result in wars over resources that are being diminished by the cattle.

We have also seen that when the pain, suffering, and violence of animal slaughter, which enters the meat, is consumed by humankind, we perpetuate this vibration of pain, suffering, and violence with one another. In this context, we repeat Pythagoras' great teaching,

> As long as man continues to be the ruthless destroyer of lower living beings, he will never know health or peace. For as long as men massacre animals, they will kill each other. Indeed, he who sows the seed of murder and pain cannot reap joy and love.

People eating living foods often report experiencing greater mental clarity and emotional health as a result. There is also a visible tendency for people to direct their attention more toward a spiritual life, whatever their tradition, once established on living plant-sourced foods. A strong case could be made, especially now with our mounting weapons of mass destruction, that heightened mental clarity, emotional stability, and proactive spirituality are very important attributes for our world's leaders to possess. Along these same lines, the book of Isaiah offers us an inspiring prophecy, "They shall beat their swords into plowshares, and their spears into pruning hooks; nation shall not lift up sword against nation; neither shall they learn war anymore" (Isaiah 2:4).

Living veganic foods inherently promote social peace because living foods are not filled with the bloodlust of death, and thus connect us with life and the living soul of the planet. Like a good Internet connection, living foods carry the energy signals, sometimes called *chi, prana,* or *nefesh,* that we all want to pick up. They increase the vital life-force, which empowers our cells to throw off our toxic loads. On a diet of living foods, our reception gets really clear, so that we are better able to tune into our interconnectedness with the wondrous web of life.

As our arteries and digestive tracts get a literal cleaning-out, we also experience an unclogging of more subtle connections to our source, which equips us to have more flow from it. The illusion of separation begins to dissipate, and the experience of our oneness gets stronger and stronger. This is highly valuable in the context of peace with our community as well as our shared social responsibility for the ecology.

Once we have a cleared-up connection, it becomes unacceptable to live on the Earth as if we were at a liquidation sale, with every person for themselves. Everything we buy, eat, and drink has an effect on the rest of the whole, living planet. The question about eating becomes: How can I eat in a way that uplifts the web of life on the planet? Awareness about the social, economic, ecological, humanitarian, and spiritual implications of our diet is a primordial exercise in social responsibility, as we become human copartners for the survival of our species and the planet as we know it today.

A conversation overheard at the preschool lunch table illustrates this idea well: One little girl turned to her friend and said, "I don't drink milk because my mom says that it hurts the cows." The other girl, appearing surprised at such a silly notion, said, "No, you just get milk at the store!" This may be rather cute coming from a four-year-old but, sadly, until adults outgrow this immature perspective we will continue to inflict suffering upon the entire ecology and animal kingdom, and thus upon ourselves.

Fortunately, connections are now being made. We are starting to understand that pharmaceutical substances, such as the synthetic hormone in our birth-control pills, aren't just personal decisions. These get excreted into the communal septic systems, re-entering public drinking water and even rivers, affecting other humans as well as fish. Ordering chicken nuggets in the drive-through isn't just a once-in-a-while unhealthy choice for your child, but has dire consequences for other sentient beings and all chickens who suffer inhumane conditions for their entire lives and deaths.

As the oft-quoted Paul McCartney saying goes, "If slaughterhouses had glass walls, we would all become vegetarians." The culture of life and liberation is a lifting of the veil that keeps us from seeing social evils, allowing us all to see our way clearly to ways of living that uplift our children, our global family, and ourselves.

By raising our children with plant-sourced nutrition, we are guiding them to live compassionately. This tone of heartfelt compassion, as well as the physical benefits received from the food, tend to also enhance our relationships within the home. In an interview for the Raw Mom Summit, Valya Boutenko of the Raw Family recounted that, when everyone in her family switched to raw foods, there were fewer arguments between her and her brother, both of whom were children at the time. Live-Food Parent Educator Kelly Bailey shares a similar story in one of her teleseminars. Bailey notes that although prepackaged foods had been really convenient, replacing them with fresher choices was followed by a noticeable decrease in sibling fighting and other behavior problems, which for most parents are less than convenient.

Positive Socialization Within the Home

Peace with the family is key to the child's social development. Intimate relationships enhance our character development, provide a reflection of ourselves within another, provide an opportunity to nurture and be nurtured, and deepen our experience of oneness. In his book *Creating Peace by Being Peace,* Rabbi Dr. Gabriel says:

> Family exists not only for propagation, but also to provide a training ground for learning how to develop intimacy and a mature emotional body. This function is true for all long-term relationships. Life in the family is designed by its very nature to help our feeling body mature.
>
> Intimacy is one of the last frontiers of human consciousness. In true intimate relationships, one experiences durable love, steady trust, and a willingness to be vulnerable. Durable intimacy requires a continual willingness to keep one's heart open under any circumstances. Intimacy is not about having a fixed and secure relationship. It is being willing to leap into the unknown with your intimate other; it is about being willing to face all the issues of the human condition with one's partner, from birth to death; it includes healing patterns from one's family of origin.
>
> Relationship in this context is not about shaping the partner into your idea of who he or she should be, but supporting the partner in reaching full potential as a mature and aware human being. It is about helping your partner to be the full wild woman or man each of us is meant to be. At the highest level, each inspires the other

to move deeper into unity with the Divine. In this way, a durable commitment to intimacy in relationship is a powerful spiritual path.

Because the level of intimacy experienced between a child's parents has a profound effect on the child's ability to overcome fears of intimacy, and to maintain and build healthy relationships later in life, the parent-to-parent connection is a primary way of supporting the child's social development. The idea of developing a sacred relationship, as taught at the Tree of Life Center U.S., in which intimacy is seen as an enduring, radiant love underlying a safe and spiritually evolving relationship, is a powerful way to understand the value of one's relationship as a spiritual commitment and spiritual path.

Peaceful Conflict Resolution

The child is always looking to us to learn conflict-resolution skills. While today's big-action media inundates the child with violent solutions, most situations in life require other skills and strategies to solve problems. These include listening, impulse control, patience, understanding one's own emotions, negotiation, and compassion for others. Facilitating "peace talks" can oftentimes be helpful in developing these skills. As depicted in the book *The Peace Rose* by Alicia Jewell, it may be helpful to have a tangible item such as a rose or a "talking stick," as in Native American tradition, for the child to hold when it is their turn to speak and be listened to, and to pass to another child when it is their turn.

In *Honoring the Light of the Child,* Sonnie McFarland suggests that each child be asked how the other person feels after that child has stated their feelings, as a way to draw forth empathy and raise awareness of how our words and actions affect the feelings of others. This model works well in the classroom; often, after a few facilitated peace talks, children follow the "peace-talk" format on their own, and come to peaceful resolution without any teacher guiding them. The model works for families, teen groups, and in a variety of community settings.

Sura Hart and Victoria Kindle Hodson have also created a cooperative board game called "The No-Fault Zone" as another model for developing conflict-resolution skills in the home and classroom, by helping children take responsibility for their own feelings rather than focusing on blame and judgment.

A family "make-up box," as shared by Sharon Silver in *Stop Reacting and Start Responding,* can also work well. This offers a format for times when a parent or child needs to make amends to another family member. The box contains index cards for each family member, each one listing a meaningful way to make up for hurtful words or actions. Each family member writes or draws pictures of what they want on their own card. The person who needs to make amends then has the choice of which card to use.

Choosing affirmation, connection, and other positive experiences together as a family helps everyone better handle the stresses and frictions that arise in day-to-day life. The point is that there is a variety of conflict-resolution options that children, adults, and families can choose to fit their own style.

Other Opportunities for Positive Socialization

The healthy social-interactive patterns we create within the home are a template for our interaction with the community at large. By providing a loving home, we create a foundation for the child's healthy socialization outside the home. Interacting with peers from differing lifestyles can sometimes be a bit of a dance; however, when we stay positive—seeing this as a spiritual challenge—it helps us to remain in the light. Positive social interactions help the child learn about the feelings and needs of others, gain a sense of community and social responsibility, and discover their own individual role within it. Here are some possibilities to explore in support of this process:

Provide spiritual community: Spiritual community gives children an environment for drawing forth positive character-development traits, as well as teaching them social ethics and morality. The primary spiritual community starts in the home. The Pioneer Study of 1930–1940 showed that the physical, emotional, mental, and spiritual health of the child directly reflected the health of their family.

Community gardens, music, theatre, art, team sports, and intentional playgroups can help the child to learn how to be part of a team.

Volunteering on an inspiring service project with a nonprofit organization is a wonderful way to further learn cooperation skills, and sets the stage for heart-opening throughout life.

If there is not a living-foods potluck in your area, start one! Or, if you're so inspired, create a food-prep class for kids in your area. Many of the recipes in this book have been used successfully in the "I'm Alive! Food Prep Class for Kids," taught by Leah and her daughter Quinn, as well as at the Tree of Life Center, U.S.

Minimize undermining influences: Not everything is under our control, but there is a lot we can do to proactively remove stumbling blocks in our children's social impressions. The most important socialization training is the atmosphere of our own home. Caring for companion animals in the home can be a beautiful opportunity for the child to learn tolerance and compassion for others, including another species, and to explore what needs another may be attempting to meet through sometimes perplexing behavior.

Be open to social changes: As you make life-affirming changes for your family, you may very well find yourself attracted to new social settings. Go with the flow! For some families, this may even be a important factor in a decision to relocate for greater social support. Just as seedlings and saplings need protective care while young and vulnerable, there are times when we all need a positive environment surrounding us, as we grow stronger. This may be especially true when we are first coming into a new and healthier lifestyle. As we become more established in our lifestyle change, we can generally handle more interface with opposition, and a little opposition at the right time can actually serve to strengthen us even more.

Advocate for healthy changes at school: For example, you can be part of the exciting trend of bringing healthier foods into school systems. Many Montessori schools in this country have sugar-free campuses, and some, such as Khalsa Montessori School of Tucson and Phoenix, Arizona, also have a meat-free wellness policy. Desert Garden Montessori in Phoenix offers an organic, vegan hot-lunch option to students, and Martin Luther King, Jr. Middle School of Berkeley, California, has integrated an organic lunch program called "The Edible Schoolyard" into the school's curriculum, in which middle-school students participate in growing and preparing their own lunch. Pleasant Ridge Waldorf School of Viroqua, Wisconsin, is another example of a school that has opted to serve a vegetarian lunch daily, emphasizing organic and local produce.

Especially with the timely legislative policies for increased wellness programs in our nation's public schools, more educators are now finding creative alternatives to candy sales as fundraisers, for example—some schools sell garden-vegetable starts that the children grow (see "Resources," page 485, for fundraising with the *Mitch Spinach* book series), as well as offering alternatives to sugary foods as classroom rewards.

We are also now seeing nonprofit organizations dedicated to helping schools transition into healthier lunch programs. If your community school could use some help in coming more alive, consider getting a copy of the documentary film *Impact of Fresh, Healthy Foods on Learning and Behavior* for your administrators, and request that your school board put childhood nutrition on their agenda. Chances are that there are other parents who will join you in your efforts. Add their signatures to your letter to the school board, etc. Even small steps, such as the removal of soda/espresso machines and the addition of a salad bar, can make a difference in children's social and learning environments.

Holidays and birthday parties: These offer spaces and places for veganic creativity, flexibility, trust, compassion, and a positive outlook; courteous rebellion will generally get you through any opposition. Here are a few more helpful tips:

- Plan ahead whenever possible. Some families explain dietary differences to the host when they RSVP, mentioning that they generally bring their own treats to parties. With this information, a host will likely not be offended and may even offer to accommodate you with plant-sourced options.
- Talk about party food with the children ahead of time, educating them on food choices. For the very young child, who can

feel overwhelmed with too many choices, the decision is generally best left up to the parent, whereas it is generally appropriate to allow for increasingly independent decision-making by older children. When Leah's daughter Quinn was the only vegan in her classroom, for example, she was provided with her favorite vegan treats during parties. Quinn also knew that she was allowed to sample other offerings if she so chose.

Leah finds it interesting that both of her children feel very strongly about eschewing meat because of their love for animals. Quinn told her mom that she had once spooned onto her plate something that she thought was vegan at a potluck, but that when she took a bite, "It tasted good, but something didn't feel right, so I spit it out." Come to find out, the dish had meat in it. This was a prime opportunity to talk about the vibrations of food, helping Quinn to understand her experience in discriminating food energies.

• Throw live-food parties as a way to develop social context. They may catch on! These don't have to be big productions. Keeping things simple, and placing value on the quality of sustenance and togetherness, has a lot of appeal. When we gather to celebrate, things can get so complex that the actual purpose is lost in the shuffle. If it is our child's birthday, for example, we may have remembered the cake, candles, invitations, and confetti—yet are we relaying a clear message that the overall purpose is to honor the life of the child?

One idea to help to set the tone is to invite guests to bring a written blessing for the child's upcoming year. Some parents and teachers tell stories of the child's birth and growth throughout the years, highlighting how the child's life has been a blessing. Perhaps, when all has quieted down, you can follow the annual tradition of a bringing out a memory box wrapped like a present. As you look through old photos, or read strips of paper recording events from the past year, you and your child might enjoy reflecting on how each and every memory has been a gift. It can be a profound teaching to also include life events that were challenging, in order to find more hidden gifts.

At Levi's fifth birthday celebration, Leah quietly went around asking guests what they were most thankful for about her son, jotting down their responses to read to him before bed that night. Not only is this a happy transition into bedtime after a stimulating day, but other parents can be inspired by such positive self-esteem and self-love approaches.

- Here is a birthday blessing song you might want to include:

Happy Birthday, Happy Birthday! We love you.

Happy Birthday, and may all your dreams come true!

When you blow out the candles, one light stays aglow;

It's the love-light in your eyes where'er you go.

—Lyrics by Tom Chapin; melody is the theme from
"The Merry Widow Waltz" by Franz Lehár

Have You Ever Heard of the Candy Fairy?

Sometimes well-meaning grown-ups give our kids candy without first asking our permission. What do we do? If the little guy/girl has already eaten it, don't freak out. Why add toxic negativity along with the Tootsie Roll? Who knows, it might be an opportunity to tune in, observe, and talk about the experience together. But if the candy is still in sight, see if your little one wants to play Candy Fairy. It's like the tooth fairy, but in this game she helps you to keep your teeth by taking off with the sugary treat!

Here's how you play: Decide on a place to leave your candies overnight as a gift to the Candy Fairy, and in the morning check the same spot for a present from her—something small that your child wants even more than candy. This game turns an awkward moment into sheer delight. When the child is ready, it is good to explain that it is a pretending game, so that they don't later feel deceived. The Candy Fairy is a gentle conflict-resolution approach to this common issue that pops up in a variety of ways, such as on Halloween.

All these thoughtful approaches that you as a parent create for your children are powerful socialization processes for developing both intimacy skills—which seem to be diminishing in our world society—and healthy social interactions among different groups and societies. All that we have shared involves respect for the other. These are dramatically different approaches than beheading men, women, and children of different religious cultures, as we have seen in recent years.

Part of the learning exercise is to critique the approaches of different societies and their leaders, as it is important to counter the lying, cheating, negotiating through raw power, and other negative models displayed by our leaders. Because these dysfunctional social responsibility and activities are so predominant in our world today, it is important to teach our children not to accept them as normal social interaction.

CHAPTER 8

Supporting the Child's Developing Mind

The Heart and the Mind

What will our children do in the morning? Will they wake with their hearts wanting to play, the way wings should? ... I know the ways of the heart—how it wants to be alive.

—The great mystic Rumi, from the poem
"The Way Wings Should"

Don't let your brain interfere with your heart.

—Albert Einstein

Trust in the Lord with all your heart. Lean not on your own understanding.

—Proverbs 3:5

With every beat of the heart, a burst of neural activity is relayed in the brain.

—Pam Montgomery, in Plant Spirit Healing

> *Agni,* whose name means fire, is said to be all-seeing,
> the fire symbolizing Brahman, the Revealer; the two fire
> sticks which, being rubbed together, produce the fire,
> represent the heart and the mind of man.
>
> —The Upanishads

While the culture of death operates from a standpoint of separating the heart and the mind, emphasizing the intellect and mental prowess while suppressing the role of the heart, in alive parenting we are coming from a perspective of unification. We see the heart and the mind as one, together expressing heart-wisdom. In Judaic tradition, this unfolding awareness is referred to as the merging of the Heavens and the Earth, and symbolized by the Star of David. Holistic support for the child's development thus differs from a purely academic approach focusing primarily on cognitive function while neglecting the heart and emotional IQ and well-being of the child.

Supporting the child's mind, body, and spirit is not such a new idea. We read in Deuteronomy 6:5–7, for example, that when Moshe (Moses) received the sacred teaching of, "Love the Lord your God with all your heart and with all your soul and with all your strength", he was also advised to impress this and the other Ten Speakings upon the children.

In more recent history, we see that the work of eighteenth- and nineteenth-century educational theorists Jean-Jacques Rousseau, Johann Pestalozzi, and Friedrich Froebel was the foundation for the holistic-education movement in the United States. From this movement sprang the magazine *Holistic Education Review* (now *Encounter: Education for Meaning and Social Justice*) in the 1980s, drawing from the works of Steiner and Montessori. These leaders in holistic education hold a view of education that is consistent with its Latin root—"leading-out or drawing forth" of life-energies and personal potentials from within an individual.

Steiner education is careful to support the child holistically rather than rushing them into formal study before they show readiness. As writers of Oak Meadow Waldorf School's inspired homeschooling curriculum put it,

> Parents who are eager for their children to display their mental talents should remember that a child is more than just an intellect. A brilliant intellect is useless without a focused will, and dangerous without a loving heart.

Waldorf parents are also encouraged to share their full presence with their child, rather than operating strictly from the head because, especially in the early years, the child responds best to physical and emotional energies. Physical demonstration of what we wish to teach while coming from a place of the heart, for example, works much better than simply giving verbal instruction.

Dr. Parker Palmer, a senior leader in higher education and author of the book *The Courage to Teach: Exploring the Inner Landscape of a Teacher's Life,* describes his experience with clinical depression:

> … partly due to the way (he) was formed—or deformed—in the educational systems of this country to live out of the top inch and a half of the human self; to live exclusively through cognitive rationality and the powers of the intellect; to live out of touch with anything that lay below that top inch and a half—body, intuition, feeling, emotion, relationship.

Palmer then goes on to share that part of his healing process was to reconnect with his emotional body, and to become more grounded in the physical as well.

Dr. Montessori's holistic view of the role of the intellect is revealed in her personal interpretation of the classic painting "The Madonna of the Chair" by Raphael. This painting, which Montessori requested hang in all classrooms that follow her methods,

> … is an homage to the mother, and an homage to the child who brings the light. See that person in the background? That is John the Baptist. He represents the intellect. He says, 'I am not the light,

I prepare the way for the light.' The intellect divides to make things clear. But do not stay at the level of the intellect. Go above it to spirit, which unites everything (Direct quote from a personal conversation between Maria Montessori and Elisabeth Caspari, which is now shared with students of Caspari Montessori Institute).

From the perspective of supporting the child's aliveness, supporting healthy mental function is important—not for a competitive filling of the mind with facts and figures, but for the purpose of supporting integrated awareness and the unfolding of a quiet mind. In the strictly academic approach, which is all about the mind, knowledge is not merely a tool to use on the path to enlightenment, but is sought after as the end in itself. From this limited viewpoint, knowledge is mistaken as a god to be worshiped and served.

In a holistic approach to education, by contrast, we are supporting the relationship between the heart and the mind—thus supporting an unfoldment that takes one beyond the mind. In the words of Parker Palmer,

Education at its best—this profound human transaction called teaching and learning—is not just about getting information, or getting a job. Education is about healing and wholeness. It is about empowerment, liberation, transcendence—about renewing the vitality of life.[1]

Education should not be limited to job-training preparation. It is about helping our children become awake and healthy people on every level, including their emotional and relationship IQ.

Movement and the Mind

From his very earliest days, the young child tries to make sense of the real world. Whether this process is explorative and imitative, or based on fantasy and the imagination, it is all "learning." Whatever kind of play the child is engaged in, they learn best and most easily through active participation: They must do it themselves; it is their "work."

—From Natural Childhood by John Thomson

Life is like riding a bicycle. To keep balance, you must keep moving.

—Albert Einstein

Here in the West, where we now have the option of a sedentary lifestyle, we are experiencing the natural consequences of this behavior. Lack of activity, together with unhealthy eating habits, has led us to an alarming nationwide epidemic of childhood obesity. With at least twenty percent of our children now obese, this is considered America's number-one pediatric and general public-health concern.

We have long known of the importance of exercise for our physical health—but what are the effects of inactivity on the child's mind? Following are quotes from Maria Montessori, whose classroom methods incorporated the child's need for movement:

If muscles that should normally be functioning are dormant, there is not only a physical but a psychic depression as well. This is why action can have an influence also upon one's spiritual energies.[2]

Movement is of great importance for a child. It is the functional incarnation of the creative energy.

Through movement, he acts upon his external environment and thus carries out his own personal mission in the world. Movement is not only an impression of the ego but it is an indispensable factor in the development of consciousness, since it is the only real means that places the ego in a clearly defined relationship with external reality. Movement, or physical activity, is thus an essential factor in intellectual growth, which depends upon impressions received from outside. Through movement we come in contact with external reality, and it is through these contacts that we eventually acquire even abstract ideas. Physical activity connects the spirit with the world, but the spirit has need of action in a twofold sense—to acquire concepts and to express itself exteriorly.[3]

While children may have learning-mode preferences such as auditory, visual, or kinesthetic, all children need to be in physical interaction with their environment for integrated understanding. As Aristotle put it, "There is nothing in the intellect that was not first in the senses." And as the late Dr. Elisabeth Caspari (cofounder of the Caspari Montessori Institute, and personal friend to Maria Montessori) would often say of the young child, "Movement is the law of their being."

Childhood Depression

In our culture of sedation and junk food, depression among children is on the rise. The fastest-growing market for antidepressant drugs is among preschoolers. At least four percent of the nation's preschool-age children—over one million of them—are clinically depressed.[4] This is a sobering statistic, considering the damaging effect that antidepressant drugs have on psycho-social-spiritual development.

The good news is that both movement and living nutrition are highly effective for the prevention and the treatment of depression. It is common for children and adults to feel more uplifted and energized on live foods. On this healthy diet it is not natural to be depressed.

We have twenty times more mentally disabled adults in the U.S. now than we had in 1850. There are a variety of reasons for this, including ever-increasing social and mental stress; the use of antidepressants, antipsychotics, and antianxiety drugs; a diet of white sugar, white flour, and junk food; vaccinations; environmental toxicity; nutritional deficiencies; pesticide and herbicide exposure; EMF brainwave disruption; illegal drug use; allergies to dairy, gluten, soy, and other common foods; and a variety of other factors. The use of psychotropic drugs, including those for hyperactivity, have been linked to interference with normal brain function and psychosocial and sexual development.[5]

According to depression specialists, additional causes of childhood depression include trauma such as family conflict, violence—whether in the home and neighborhood or viewed on TV—yelling, criticism, inappropriate or unclear expectations, neglect (which can occur even when neither parent is working), maternal separation, divorce, and abuse.

Happily, when children are in a consistent, highly supportive environment free from trauma, their bodies and brains can heal and develop. There are simple, healthy ways to actually repair the brain—an organic, vegan, and raw diet; exercise; and basic adequate nutritional supplements are some of these ways. *Depression-Free for Life* offers a ninety-percent successful approach to healing depression naturally.[6] Time in nature and with pets, yoga, and other forms of spiritual practice, as well as spending time with supportive adults, are also recommended for the safe treatment of childhood depression. Activities that support the child's self-esteem are also highly beneficial.

The great gift from parents to their children is to create a family environment in which they feel loved, appreciated, validated, and safe. The more children feel loved, the stronger and healthier their adult self-esteem will be.

Nature and Learning

That direct experience in nature, we now understand,
is nothing short of vital to our children's intellectual,
emotional, physical, and spiritual development.

—from "The Green Hour" by Todd Christopher,
Creator of the National Wildlife Federation's GreenHour.org

The bestselling book *Last Child in the Woods,* in which Richard Louv coined the term "nature deficit disorder," has brought to public attention the imbalances created by minimizing childhood experiences in nature. Partly as a result of this insightful writing, nature clubs for families as well as outdoor resources for educators are now cropping up around the nation. This is encouraging, as time in nature is for the healthy development of our children, who will inherit the social responsibility of caring for the ecology.

In addition to the overall physical benefits from fresh air and sunshine, a study published by the *American Journal of Public Health* (2004) reveals that time with nature is also therapeutic for symptoms of ADD/ADHD.[7] In the book *The Green Hour,* Todd Christopher, creator of the National Wildlife Federation's GreenHour.org, tells us:

> Frances E. Kuo and Andrea Faber Taylor found that "green" outdoor settings appear to reduce ADHD symptoms in children; even in individuals not diagnosed with an attention disorder, time in nature had the effect of reducing ADHD-like symptoms such as inattention and impulsivity. In a carefully controlled test in a follow-up study, they found that children professionally diagnosed with ADHD enjoyed greater levels of attention and concentration after twenty-minute nature walks in a green setting.

In other words, the effects of nature were comparable to and considered to be as effective as methylphenidate (Ritalin), a heavily prescribed medication, which pharmacologically acts as a time-release cocaine. The use of Ritalin in children has been linked to increased cocaine use in the teen and later years. Christopher also refers to a study conducted by Cornell researcher Nancy Wells, which showed an increase in attention and in psychological well-being for children who have nature in and around their homes.

Wilderness therapy organizations also find positive results in their work supporting social and emotional healing for troubled teens and their families through experiences in nature.

Waldorf Schools around the world integrate experiences in nature with other aspects of their curriculum, understanding that the ecstatic energies of that which is alive offer a more holistic education than classrooms relying solely on books and other manmade objects for learning. Rather than providing the usual back-to-school supply list of pencils, paper, glue sticks, or tissue boxes, Waldorf preschoolers' parents are often responsible for providing their child with a raincoat, rainpants, puddle boots, and rainhat as well as other outdoor clothing items, for romping in all types of weather. Observing nature can be a part of children's science as well as social studies, geometry, and art lessons. Waldorf as well as many other types of schools are also incorporating gardening as a part of the daily rhythm of educational community life.

Nature uplifts our children's spirits, evoking a sense of awe, wonder, and inspiration. In the great mystical Kabbalistic work *Sefer ha-Behir ("The Book of Brightness"),*[8] it is said that the Divine is in nature as a hand is in a glove. When we spend time in nature, we find greater connection to the Divine expression within all of creation, enhancing our connection to the Divine expression within ourselves. "In order to serve God, one needs access to the enjoyment of the beauties of nature, such as the contemplation of flower-decorated meadows, majestic mountains, flowing rivers, and so on," said the thirteenth-century Rabbi Avraham ben HaRambam, "for all these are essential to the spiritual development of even the holiest of people."[9]

Emotional Safety and Learning

> For the child ... it is not half so important to know as to feel. If facts are the seeds that later produce knowledge and wisdom, then the emotions and the impressions of the senses are the fertile soil in which the seeds must grow.
>
> —Rachel Carson, author and ecologist

Brain research shows us the closely knit relationship between emotional safety and learning. As reported by Sura Hart and Victoria Kindle Hodson in *The Compassionate Classroom,*

> When infants or children of any age experience a physical or emotional threat, they become anxious and afraid. Hormones are secreted that automatically shut down the thinking, learning, and reasoning zones of the brain to prepare the child to defend himself or to run

away from the danger. These are primitive fight, flight, or freeze responses that are triggered daily in the lives of children who don't feel safe. When, from very early ages, major portions of the brain shut down under emotionally stressful conditions, a child's brain development, success in learning, and ability to relate to others can be seriously affected.[10]

This process of stress-hormone secretion also happens with other species when undergoing inhumane living conditions, having their young taken from them and slaughtered, and the experience of being slaughtered themselves. These secretions remain within the animals' flesh and milk, which then tends to aggravate the mind of the humans who consume these foods.

Deficient Diet and Mental Degeneration

As parents, what we eat even prior to conception has an effect on our child's mental development. As explained in *Conscious Eating*, "With poor nutrition, the germ plasm is weakened, and we produce children with physical congenital changes and diminished brain function."[11] In this same text we read of Dr. Weston Price's work in the 1930s, documenting a deterioration in the younger members of American families in the same generation when white flour, white sugar, and junk food were added to their diet.

Price estimated that between twenty-five and seventy-five percent of our nation's children were affected even in the 1930s by this shift to junk, processed, and empty-calorie foods. Not only did these children show structural changes, but their IQs were lower, resulting in inferiority complexes, and they had poorer immune systems, and more congenital defects.

VITAMIN B COMPLEX-DEFICIENCY SYNDROME

One of the major causes of violence, depression, anxiety, feelings of impending doom, hostility, mental confusion, and murder by teenagers is most likely a generalized B-complex deficiency in the standard American teenage diet. This deficiency is particularly damaging to young brains. This deficiency in a variety of B vitamins, including B1, B2, B3, B6, B12, and folic acid, interferes with normal brain development and brain function even in adults.

These same "psychological symptoms" are noted in a variety of ways in B-vitamin-deficient adults. These nutritional deficiencies are caused by the standard American diet of white flour, white sugar, junk foods, and soda pop. This is compounded by a diet low in healthy fats, which further debilitates the brain because of a lack of long-chain omega-3s and cholesterol needed for proper brain development and daily function. This deficiency has been associated with severe anxiety, depression, violence, confusion, feelings of impending doom, suicidal feelings, and homicidal feelings, and some believe it may be associated with the teenage mass-murders in Oregon and Colorado.

The key solution to this deficiency is to eat a diet high in natural B vitamins. Regular consumption of nuts, seeds, leafy greens, whole grains, and beans can go a long way toward preventing B complex-deficiency syndrome, and can support natural and normal brain development, which is dependent on B vitamins.

We also recommend giving children a natural-food B-vitamin concentrate. This is a subtle kind of support that is, in fact, not so subtle. It is important for parents to develop a diet for their children through their teen years that is naturally high in B vitamins. That will help protect our children from this deficiency syndrome that is playing such a significant but widely unrecognized role in mental and brain development and behavior, and allow us to prevent a range of emotional and mental disabilities such as schizophrenia and psychosis.

Living Nutrition for the Living Brain

Do a child's eating habits affect cognitive development? A scientific study of identical twins and their diets has answered this question: While identical twins share the same genetic makeup (and those included in this study were from the same home), when one twin was a "good eater" and another was a "picky eater," there were measurable developmental discrepancies. "The picky eaters consistently did worse across the board as they developed and performed in school."[12]

What nutrients are particularly helpful to the developing brain? This is an especially relevant question in light of our rising concerns over learning disabilities, autism, Asperger's Syndrome, and ADD/ADHD. As we face an alarming rate of neurodevelopment problems, how do we best support the healthy learning of the whole and living child?

"VITAMIN O" (OXYGEN)

Let's look first at oxygen, our primary source of energy. Our brain, which makes up only two percent of our body weight, uses twenty percent of our oxygen intake. This is likely an important contributing factor in the success of nature therapy for children with ADHD. It is also interesting to note that fresh living foods and rain/spring water contain more oxygen than cooked foods and stagnant water. When we eat a plant-based diet, we are receiving more oxygen on the micro level; we are also choosing an alternative to the clearcutting of the world's rainforests for cattle grazing.

WATER

When we don't drink enough water, we get "prune-brain." When our brains lack adequate hydration, they literally begin to shrivel. Not only are living foods helpful for hydration, as they have the highest water content, but meat consumption also requires more bodily fluids to digest than the moisture it contains. Not surprisingly, we see this same theme on a macro level, as the meat industry requires at least ten times more water than the farming of plants.

FOOD FOR THOUGHT

Living foods help with oxygen to the brain and body. Living foods also help with hydration for the brain. As we serve the child's aliveness, it is exciting to see that living foods also offer optimal nutrition for the healthy functioning of the child's developing brain.

There have been some very exciting findings about omega-3 fatty acids and brain health. The National Institute of Mental Health and many scientific journals report that omega-3s can improve brain development and memory functioning, as well as bipolar disorder and depression. This has been clinically demonstrated, as described in the book *Depression-Free for Life* by Gabriel Cousens, MD.

Additional studies are showing that babies who are breastfed have less chance of developing ADHD than formula-fed babies. This is believed to be because, up until recently, infant formula did not include omega-3 long-chain fatty acids DHA and EPA, which are naturally present in breast milk.

In addition to ADHD prevention, a clinical study conducted by Australian researcher Natalie Sinn Parletta, indicates that omega-3 fatty acids have also been used to successfully treat ADHD. In this study, one group of ADHD children was given daily omega-3 supplementation, while another group of ADHD children were given a placebo. After fifteen weeks, almost half of the children who had received omega-3 supplementation showed a significant reduction in core ADHD symptoms of inattention, hyperactivity, and impulsivity. The placebo group, however, did not experience these results until they also were switched over to omega-3 supplementation. The original group taking omega-3s showed continued progress as their supplementation continued for another fifteen weeks, experiencing less cognitive difficulty, inattention, restlessness, impulsivity, and hyperactivity.[13] These are very encouraging results, and point to natural, healthy, and brain-building ways to ameliorate ADHD and ADD.

Long-chain omega-3 fats are also found to be antiinflammatory, which is very important for children recovering from autism-spectrum disorders. These essential fatty acids, so essential for healthy mental function, also support the nervous system and make fat-soluble vitamins A, D, E, K, and beta carotene more absorbable.

THE MYTHICAL DANGERS OF
HIGH CHOLESTEROL AND HIGH FAT

We would like to dissect the "high-cholesterol danger" myth in depth here because it has resulted in dangerous low-fat dietary practices. Adequate long-chain omega-3s and cholesterol are important for optimal brain development and maintenance in children as well as adults. In contrast, the carbohydrate excess in our children's diets is a primary driving force behind the epidemic of childhood obesity.

This is additionally important since research in the last few decades years shows that a serum cholesterol below 159 is unsafe and not optimal for brain and nerve-tissue function. Serum cholesterol as high as 260–270 is not only perfectly safe but actually increases longevity in women by 28%.[14]

Excess carbohydrates are addictive as well, and yes—carbs make you fat. Fat does not make you fat. This has been scientifically understood and proven since the 1700s. An increase in healthy fats supports the macronutrient calorie shift away from carbohydrates, particularly glutinous grains, non-complex carbohydrates, and all forms of sugar. All carbohydrates, in excess, including grains, fruits, and all sugars and sugar substitutes (except stevia and birch tree-based xylitol and erythritol) often result in increased insulin resistance, obesity, increased triglycerides, and increased levels of small, pathogenic LDL cholesterol particles.

One study showed that fifty-six percent of Americans have a fear of fat and cholesterol. What is the worry, and is it justified? Many people have mistakenly taken the earlier research of the 1950s to 1970s to be absolute truth, rather than a phase in the research on heart disease and other chronic diseases. The high cholesterol-heart disease connection is no longer taken as truth in holistic medical circles, or even among many progressive allopathic cardiologists and, more recently, members of the informed public.

Serious, large-scale, post-1970s studies have shown that the high cholesterol-heart disease correlation is not a valid causal or even correlative theory. Some of the more recent research that significantly nullifies the earlier speculative research gives us a new perspective, in which we see why a diet that is 25–45% raw plant-fats, depending on constitution, is optimal. It is also why we feel, based on clinical experience and more recent epidemiological studies, that cholesterol levels of 160–260 and healthy levels of omega-3s are essential for the development and the healthy, optimal, long-term functioning of our children's brains and nervous systems throughout teen years and adulthood.

In a 1992 editorial published in the *Archives of Internal Medicine,* Dr. William P. Castelli, the former director of the Framingham Heart study, made an amazing statement: "In Framingham, Massachusetts, the more saturated fat one ate, the more cholesterol one ate, and the more calories one ate, the lower the person's serum cholesterol was." It is easier to appreciate Dr. Castelli's observation when one understands that the liver makes at least seventy-five percent of its own cholesterol.

The liver produces three to four times more cholesterol than one eats, and is always adjusting for the amount of cholesterol taken in orally. A low-cholesterol diet will increase cholesterol production by the liver, and endogenous (internal) cholesterol production decreases with increased dietary input. There's a homeostasis at work, creating a balance. In addition, when one has a healthy insulin level, one tends to have a healthy cholesterol level, because insulin mediates cholesterol. This remarkable and important statement is validated in the book *The Cholesterol Myths* by Uffe Ravnskov, MD, PhD, which offers many scientific arguments invalidating the idea that saturated fat and cholesterol in the diet cause heart disease. His data, and the data, in general are overwhelming on this point.

The demonization of saturated fat most likely began in 1953 with Dr. Ancel Keys's paper linking saturated-fat intake and heart-disease mortality. The research, when fully examined, is quite weak and biased. Keys based his theory on a study of six countries in which higher saturated fat was associated with his heart-disease theory. However—and this part can emphatically be called *misinformation*—he chose not to report data from sixteen other countries he also studied that did not fit his theory. The data from the other sixteen countries did not show any correlation of a high-cholesterol diet with heart disease. Combining data from all twenty-two countries would have shown that increasing calories from fat actually reduces deaths from coronary heart disease. Many studies since then have validated the point that high cholesterol levels (160–260) are not associated with heart disease. It's shocking, but somehow Ancel Keys's misinformation caught on in spite of its poor science.

There is some truth to the fat concern, but it's not about cholesterol, omega-3s, or omega-6s. Looking at the literature up to 2011, it is about intake of trans fats, which are unquestionably cardiodamaging. Trans fats are found in margarine, vegetable shortening, and hydrogenated vegetable oils, as well as oils that are highly cooked. They are also found in junk foods, and they are damaging to body and brain. Trans fats are not the same thing as raw, plant-source-only, unsaturated, polyunsaturated, omega-3, omega-6, or saturated fats. Trans fats have been identified as definitely dangerous to health in general for a variety of reasons, and should be entirely avoided.

In contrast to the danger of eating trans fats, the actual data about high and low cholesterol reveal no danger associated with a total cholesterol level up to 270 in adults. These data strongly support the currently evolving theory that inflammation, not high cholesterol, is the primary cause of heart disease and cardiac mortality, and the amount of cardiovascular inflammation, not the level of cholesterol, determines the degree of heart disease. As we set future dietary patterns for our children, it is important that these patterns are healthy. We can start with mother's milk, which is high in fat, especially the long-chain omega-3 fatty acid DHA. This is one way mother's milk differs from cow's milk, which is also much higher in protein.

Again, saturated fats come from animal fats, which are cooked, and also from tropical oils such as palm and coconut oils. Raw palm and coconut oils are not a problem if they are not cooked or hydrogenated. Trans fats, by contrast, are cooked at high temperatures, and are often hydrogenated.

Monounsaturated fat from olive oil, and polyunsaturated fat from omega-3 and omega-6 sources like nuts and seeds, are also not a problem. As pointed out previously, nuts after nine months of age are very health-protective. Primary sources of healthy, vegan plant-source fats are olives, raw nuts, seeds, almonds, pecans, walnuts, coconut meat, coconut oil, palm oil, and avocados. Avocados have actually been experimentally shown to be cardioprotective, and to even lower cholesterol in some cases, as previously discussed.[15]

It is important to eat high omega-3 fat foods such as chia seeds, walnuts, flaxseed, and hemp seeds, because they help shift the ratio of omega-6 to omega-3 fats toward 2:1 or 1:1, away from the average and pathological ratios of up to 20:1. To minimize an excess of omega-6, we do not recommend high omega-6 fats such as corn, canola, safflower, or sunflower oil, which further imbalance omega-6 to omega-3 ratios and may be associated with increased cardiovascular disease.

Saturated fats are health-promoting and important because they are needed for the proper functioning of cell membranes, especially those of the neuronal cells, heart, bones, liver, immune system, lungs, hormones, and those that control hunger, calcium balance, and general genetic regulation. We're not recommending polyunsaturated oils, which are high in omega-6 fats, because they have been associated to a certain extent with accelerated aging.

More than one set of major research projects show that people with high cholesterol (from 200–260) developed the same amount of heart disease as people with low cholesterol. One large and significant meta-analysis of twenty-one studies, on a total of 347,747 individuals, showed that people who had heart attacks had not eaten significantly more saturated fat, or more polyunsaturated oil, than other people.[16] Another fact revealed by several large studies is that women with higher cholesterol live longer and have less cardiac mortality than their lower-blood-cholesterol peers.

There are other studies that clarify the confusion and dispel the myth about high cholesterol. For example, Dr. Harlan Krumholz and his coworkers at Yale University's Cardiovascular Medicine department did a study on 997 elderly men and women living in the Bronx during a four-year period. The study showed no difference between lower and higher cholesterol levels in terms of heart disease, except that the women with higher cholesterol lived longer and had less heart disease.[17] The studies overall show that people with total cholesterol levels of 160 or lower develop just as many cholesterol plaques as those with higher cholesterol, up to at least a total cholesterol of 260.

In all the international studies, there was only one citing high cholesterol as having a slight association with increased risk of heart disease in men in the United States, but no such association for men in Canada. Dr. Henry Shanoff at the University of Toronto studied 120 men ten years after they recovered from heart attacks. He found that those with low cholesterol had a second coronary incident just as often as those with high cholesterol. In Russia, low cholesterol is actually associated with an increased risk of coronary heart disease.

In summary, high cholesterol may be slightly pathogenic for American males under age thirty-eight, but not for Canadians, Stockholmers, Russians, or Maoris at any age. The fact that it is maybe slightly dangerous for men in America (but not for men in other nations), or Americans over the age of thirty-eight, raises some questions as to the validity of the American study. High cholesterol has not been shown by any study to be dangerous in U.S. men older than thirty-eight. Paradoxically, the American studies suggest that high cholesterol may be marginally pathogenic for healthy men under thirty-eight—but not for coronary patients—and may even be slightly beneficial for older men.

As stated earlier, the protective benefits of higher cholesterol are clearer for women. In one Norwegian study of 52,287 people between from age twenty to seventy-four, women with total cholesterol levels of 270 or higher had a twenty-eight-percent lower mortality rate than women with cholesterols of less than 193. This is a significant finding that strongly supports the cardioprotective and general longevity qualities of cholesterol for women. In general, girls and women need more fat in their bodies. It should be mentioned that there is a genetic defect called familial hypercholesterolemia, in which people do have significantly raised cholesterol, often above 365, and a higher risk of heart attack.

Additional major research contradicting the myth of high-cholesterol danger is the MONICA (Multinational Monitoring of trends and

Determinants in Cardiovascular Disease) Project, monitoring trends in cardiovascular disease. This large body of research found that mortality rates in coronary disease show a great variation among people with the same blood levels of cholesterol.[18] Other contradictions to the myth include the issue of the French Paradox, which shows how the French were the most "deviant" from a low-cholesterol diet among various nations, but still had lower coronary mortality.

It isn't just the French, however. High cholesterol intake and lower coronary mortality were also observed in Luxembourg and Germany. This supports the critical point that there are too many paradoxes here. Fundamentally, if a theory is to hold, it can't have multiple exceptions, which is what almost all the research is revealing. There are too many discrepancies to give the high-cholesterol/cardiomortality connection any weight.

A key principle of science is that, *if a hypothesis is sound, it must be supported by all observations.* The validation of a scientific hypothesis is not like a sports event, where the team with the highest points or best public relations wins the game (although studies showing a disconnect between cholesterol levels and heart morbidity are now in the majority). One observation that doesn't support a hypothesis is enough to disprove it. In this context, however, there are no real exceptions to support the "danger" of a high cholesterol-cardiac mortality link.

With this perspective it is interesting to note that on the low (ten-percent)-fat Dean Ornish diet, the average total cholesterol level was 173, whereas on Dr. Cousens' "Diabetes Recovery Diet—A Holistic Approach," which recommends twenty-five to forty-five percent fat (with no animal fat, but no restriction on plant-source fats), the typical cholesterol was 159. Cholesterol is internally regulated according to one's needs and level of health. Yet cholesterol can be affected to some extent by stress and other factors.

In the three-week, plant-source-only, one-hundred-percent live-food program (Dr. Cousens' "Diabetes Recovery Program—A Holistic Approach"), there was a sixty-seven-point drop in LDLs, from 149 to 82—a nearly 45 percent decrease—and a total cholesterol drop to 159.

Again, the only restriction on fat intake was avoiding animal fat. The theorized explanation is that when people return to a healthy diet including no white sugar, white flour, or junk, processed, and GMO foods, their bodies return to a normal noninflamed state, and naturally move toward optimal cholesterol production.

The safety of a moderate- to high-fat diet was further confirmed by a study sponsored by The Women's Health Initiative in 1994, of 49,000 middle-aged women, 20,000 of whom who were chosen to eat a low-fat diet.[19] After six years, the women who had cut fat consumption and saturated fat by twenty-five percent did have cholesterols and LDLs somewhat below that of the 29,000 women who did not change their fat consumption, but the change had no effect on their rate of heart disease, stroke, breast cancer, colon cancer, or fat accumulation. It is significant that there was no difference in overall morbidity between the two groups of women. There was no science to support the idea that saturated fats clogged arteries if there is higher cholesterol in the diet.

It is interesting to note that another women's study did find that older women with higher cholesterol lived longer than their lower-cholesterol female counterparts.[20] This, of course, supports the efficacy and safety of a moderate plant-source-only fat intake versus a general low-fat intake diet There have been more than thirty studies, on a total of over 150,000 people, showing that those who did not have heart attacks had not necessarily eaten less saturated or unsaturated fats than those who did.[21]

A study by the Cochrane Collaboration, which is known to be free of all corporate pressures, assessed the benefits of eating less fat and less saturated fat in 2001. They reviewed twenty-seven clinical studies going back to the 1950s. Their conclusion:

> Despite the efforts and many thousands of people and randomized studies, there is still only limited inconclusive evidence of the effects of modification of a total unsaturated and polyunsaturated diet on cardiac morbidity.[22]

This is an important statement that a low-fat diet has not been found to be a significant or even marginal factor in preventing heart disease.

A final concluding point is a survey of all the literature on the cholesterol topic. The April 13, 2009 issue of the *Archives of Internal Medicine* contained a very important study titled "A Systemic Review of the Evidence Supporting the Causal Link Between Dietary Factors and Coronary Heart Disease," considered to be the definitive study on the cholesterol question. This study indicated several important ideas. It showed that the most harmful dietary factors usually related to cardiovascular disease included: 1) the regular intake of trans-fatty acids; and 2) foods that had a high-glycemic index or high-glycemic load—in other words, higher in carbohydrates. So trans fats and carbohydrates were the most dangerous factors associated with increased heart disease.

Their bottom-line conclusion, after looking at all the studies, is that there was no evidence to support the widespread mythical belief that limiting saturated-fat intake benefits heart health. What is interesting is that the methodical research over time has answered the cholesterol question in a way that significantly shifted researchers' position away from the initially very popular low-fat thesis.

Researchers also found that increased consumption of polyunsaturated fats was not associated with relative protection against heart disease. The current research does not recommend increasing polyunsaturated omega-6 fats, as most of these are damaged trans fats, found in highly processed corn, soy, cakes, biscuits, processed vegetable oils, package-ready meals, nondairy creamers, soups, salad dressings, fried foods, sauces, and chocolates. Non-omega-3 vegetable oils were not found to be cardioprotective.

In summary, according to this major review of the literature as of 2009, a high intake of carbohydrates and trans fat was found to be bad for heart health. One need not be afraid of eating the appropriate amount of healthy fat in a diet that is energetically sustaining and optimal for building our children's brains and nervous systems.

The overall research is clear that lowering cholesterol does not correlate with a lengthened life or cardioprotection; for women, low cholesterol seems to shorten the lifespan and increase cardiac mortality rates. A plant-source-only diet yields longevity of 4.42 years longer in women, and 7.28 years longer in men, regardless of cholesterol levels.[23]

As we have examined the literature, we feel very confident in prescribing our 25–45% carbohydrate diet and 25–45% plant-source raw fat diet for our children because, although this diet lowers cholesterol to normal and healthy levels, it doesn't take it into the danger zone (below 159 in almost all cases). It also provides the healing, balancing, and building power of long- and short-chain omega-3s for the brain, nervous system, and for healing diabetes. It appears safe in all areas for protecting mental and physical good health.

THE HEALTH DANGERS OF LOW CHOLESTEROL

The greatest actual concern about cholesterol is the significant and pathological danger of total cholesterol levels under 159. Dr. Gabriel, as a psychiatrist, has been quite aware since the late 1960s of the serious danger of mental illness associated with low cholesterol. Recent research has shown that there is a much higher occurrence of depression, suicidal tendencies, and anxiety when cholesterol levels are less than 159.

Several cohort studies on nondepressed subjects have assessed the relationship between plasma cholesterol and depression. A direct relationship was found between low cholesterol and rates of high depression. It became clear among patients with major depression that there was a strong causative association between depression and low cholesterol. Clinical recovery was also causatively correlated with increases in cholesterol.[24]

Several epidemiological studies have also shown increased suicide risks among subjects with lower cholesterol. Although there are some contradictory findings, it is supported by several cohort studies that there is also a connection between major depression and low polyunsaturated acids and low omega-3s. The overall hypothesis that emerges is that maintaining optimal membrane fluidity and optimal ratios of saturated, monounsaturated, and polyunsaturated fats in the cell membranes in general, and the neuronal cell membranes in particular, positively affects neurotransmitter production and function, which are essential to normal brain development.

Low cholesterol is also associated with a decrease in serotonin receptors in the neurons or brain cells.[25] Another study about cholesterol, called "Low Serum Cholesterol Concentration and Risk of Suicide,"[26] found that those with the lowest serum cholesterol concentrations, adjusting for age and sex, had more than six times the occurrence of suicide attempts. Another study found that if cholesterol levels were equal to or below the twenty-fifth percentile, the risk of a suicide attempt doubled.[27]

When one realizes that the primary causes of death among teenagers are accidents, homicide, suicide, and cancer, this becomes especially important. With all the trans fats in junk food, the false belief in a low-fat diet as healthy, and a lack of healthy plant fats, we have a dangerous setting for our teenagers. Once study found that suicide among soldiers in Iraq and Afghanistan was highest in those with the lowest long-chain omega-3s. Obviously, from a holistic and psychiatric perspective, this is highly significant. And researchers found that the depressive effect of low cholesterol levels persisted for up to five years.

In summary, the data indicate that low-serum cholesterol is associated with increased risk of suicide and depression. A *Psychology Today* article on evolutionary psychiatry by Emily Deans, MD, links low serum cholesterol to increased incidence of suicide, accidents, and violence, as do numerous other papers.[28] It isn't entirely proven, but this may be related to the fact that the brain's dry weight is sixty percent fat, and that cholesterol plays a vital role in neuron signaling and brain structure. One-fourth of our cholesterol is found in the nervous system. It makes sense, if cholesterol drops too low, that our brains and nervous systems can be adversely affected.

Low blood cholesterol (under 159) obviously creates problems on many levels. One needs cholesterol for the brain and cell membranes to work effectively. To again emphasize the point, neuronal and in fact all cell membranes are constructed from fat, and a proper combination of cholesterol and omega-3 and omega-6 fatty acids is key for optimal cell-membrane function.

Trans-fatty acids, on the other hand, significantly disrupt membrane function. Cholesterol depletion is also known to affect serotonin receptors and reduce serotonin release from the synapse.[29] It is also noteworthy that low serotonin in the spinal fluid is associated with aggressive behavior, and is also associated with low cholesterol. Cholesterol is needed to make myelin, the insulating cover for nerves and various other signaling processes associated with anxiety and depression.

A total cholesterol level less than 159 is also associated with a 21% increase in premature births, as compared to only 5% premature deliveries in mothers with cholesterol of 160 to 261.[30] So low cholesterol is not safe for pregnant mothers or their embryos. This is a particularly important reason why we recommend a twenty-five- to forty-five-percent fat intake from plant-source-only live foods, because low-fat, vegan, live-food diets tend to lower cholesterol generally.

It is interesting that in both public and private communications, Dr. Neal Barnard has stated that subjects in his diabetes studies simply avoided all animal fats and cooking oils, which is the same protocol as in my study. This is a practical and easy guideline to follow. A higher fat intake, with plenty of coconut oil, is often effective in raising healthy cholesterol; it is also an added assurance against possible low-cholesterol problems. As concerned parents and grandparents, we don't want to encourage suicide, depression, aggression, and violence by advising a diet with ten-percent or less fat.

THE IMPORTANCE OF OMEGA-3S FOR HEALTH

Adequate omega-3s are also vital to health, in contrast with a low fat (and consequently low-omega-3) diet. General health-protective effects from adequate omega-3s are associated with a reduced risk of death from all causes. In a five-year study, it was discovered that those with an omega-3 index of less than four percent aged much faster than those with indexes above eight percent. And, yes, we do want our children to live healthier and longer!

The same study showed that those with higher omega-3 levels died at a slower rate, or were less likely to die within the study period, than those with low omega-3s. Omega-3 deficiency was considered to be a possibly significant underlying factor in up to 96,000 premature deaths each year, including those from coronary heart disease and stroke. Adequate omega-3s appeared to decrease the risk of premature death by up to 85% when maintained at optimal levels.[31]

Adequate omega-3 contributes to a healthy brain in a variety of important ways. They are important for supporting and improving memory, cognition, sleep, and neuromuscular control, and for reversing the mortality rate of neurodegenerative diseases. Omega-3s also support the new manufacture of acetylcholine, an important neurotransmitter needed for memory. They stimulate release of gamma-aminobutyric acid (GABA), which protects against anxiety, depression, pain, and panic attacks.

Omega-3s are major components of brain tissue. They also help with brain and eye development in babies. An adequate long-chain omega-3 supply also helps prevent and treat postpartum depression.[32] In our society, particularly among teens, it is a good thing to reduce aggression, hostility, and impulsiveness; so adequate omega-3s is even more important. This is hard to achieve with a low (ten-percent or less)-fat diet.

Omega-3s are essential for prevention and treatment of all depression, including bipolar disorder. As pointed out earlier, recent studies investigating the epidemic of military suicides in Iraq and Afghanistan found that those who committed suicide had the lowest omega-3 levels in the military population. Low DHA in particular was associated with a sixty-percent increase in suicides, making the clear point that adequate brain DHA is necessary for healthy brain and mental-health functions.[33] Considering the current increase in depression among children, it would be very interesting to correlate their omega-3 levels with their rates of depression. We recommend being on the safe side, and supplying children of all ages with plenty of omega-3 foods in their diet.

Adequate omega-3s improve mood regulation, and ameliorate impulsivity, hostility, and aggression.[34] They improve dysfunction in monoaminergic (monoamine neurotransmitter) systems including 5-hydroxytryptamine and serotonin.[35] They help prevent cortisol, epinephrine, and norepinephrine elevations that occur with biological or emotional stress. They appear to reduce the risk of Parkinson's disease, and assist in proper nerve-signaling.[36]

Omega-3 fatty acid levels that are too low contribute to many disease dysfunctions including increased heart disease,[37] liver-[38] and kidney-function instability,[39] and general mental disturbances,[40] specifically those that result in suicide.[41]

It becomes obvious that another danger of a low-fat diet is omega-3-deficiency. Adequate omega-3s are important in counteracting or preventing cardiac arrhythmia.[42] They are not only important for our children's brain development and emotional health, but also support good heart health, liver health, immune system, lung, and kidney health.[43] Omega-3s constitute fifty percent of our cell membranes, and give our cells optimal flexibility, integrity, and function.

Omega-3s also have anticancer benefits: They protect skin cells from the cancer-causing effects of the sun, and help decrease prostate-cancer risk as well. In premenopausal women, a high omega-3 to omega-6 ratio was associated with a 50% decreased rate of breast cancer.

From an Ayurvedic perspective, deficient omega-3s, as well as inadequate cholesterol, create an imbalanced *vata* mental state with poorer cognition, memory, and functioning. This results in lower life-force, lower vitality, and generally a lower reserve of vital life-force and sexual energy. Along with this there may be depression, violence, anxiety, and even suicide. The Ayurvedic term for this is vital reserve is *ojas,* which means deep primordial vigor and reserve. Low *ojas* results in a generally weakened physical, emotional, mental, and spiritual condition. In this larger context, the overall effect of a low-fat diet has serious negative ramifications for the quality of life and life-force vibrancy for our children. In today's world, in which our children are getting weaker and less healthy by all parameters, adequate omega-3s are very important. This is why we strongly recommend a moderately high plant-based fat diet, rather than a low-fat diet, as very important for all aspects of our children's physical, emotional, and mental health and development.

In summary, low-cholesterol and low-omega-3 fats have been shown through overwhelming scientific evidence to be dangerous to the general health, vitality, brain development, and emotional and mental function of our babies, children, and teenagers, and to the longevity of the individual.

Saturated fat and omega-3 intake from plant-based fat actually protects the cardiovascular system, brain, mental health, general health, and life-force. Higher healthy-fat intake creates a macronutrient balance with the shift to a 25–45% carbohydrate diet, with its higher fat content derived from vegetables, nuts, and seeds.

This holistic approach to diet is not just for heart disease or diabetes but for overall well-being, and for physical, neurological, brain, and mental development. It is a lifelong enhancement diet for health and longevity in general, which is good for every stage of a child's development.

Cholesterol also seems to be very important for normal brain development and high-level physical, emotional, and mental functioning. The best vegan sources of long-chain omega-3 fatty acids include purslane and AFA *(Aphanizomenon flos-aquae)* algae, found in products such as "E-3 Live" and "E-3 Live Brain-On."

Short-chain omega-3s are found in hemp seeds, chia seeds (Salba® brand is an organic source), flaxseeds, and walnuts—which even look like little brains. Other plant sources of omega-3s include okra and leafy greens. The short-chain conversion to long-chain is approximately doubled by adding a tablespoon of coconut oil to each three tablespoons of the seeds.

What about fish and fish oils, such as the cod-liver oil capsules sold "for kids"? While fish is indeed high in omega-3 fatty acids, these are risky to ingest because our polluted waters contain high levels of mercury and other heavy metals that poison the nervous system and the brain. Especially when it comes to neurodevelopmental disorders, we want to help the body rid itself of toxic metals such as mercury and lead. Concentrated amounts of these metals are found in animal flesh, particularly its fatty tissue—and even in artificial food colorings—but not in vegetarian seafood such as sea veggies and algae.

Unfortunately, today's fish are also carrying dangerous amounts of radiation. As a result of the Fukushima disaster, for example, it has been reported that 300,000 gallons of radioactive water are being dumped into the ocean each day. For this reason, Korea has threatened to sue for injury to its fishing industry.

Where do the fish get all of their beneficial essential fatty acids? They eat yellow algae! While plant-sourced foods have a significantly lower concentration of radiation than flesh foods, we recommend researching where your sea veggies and algae are sourced. The long-chain omega-3 supplements should be obtained from sources away from Fukushima. Such omega-3s from yellow algae—DHA and EPA—are available from Dr. Cousens' Online Store.

To summarizing the overwhelming cholesterol and omega-3 data: Cholesterol levels up to 260 have been shown to have no effect on heart health. On a vegan diet, no matter how much fat one eats, it would be extremely difficult for cholesterol to go above 260. However, deficient cholesterol and omega-3s have a significantly deleterious effect on brain development and on many levels of brain-mind-emotional function. The low-fat craze starting in the 1950s represents an allopathic, single-disease (heart disease) perspective that has been disproven. The key is a holistic approach that supports the health of the total organism, especially the brain, mind, emotional, and intellectual functions, as well as anticancer protection and enhanced longevity.

What else does nutritional science tell us about food and the brain? There are indeed dietary obstacles to our children's healthy synapse development. It has been documented since the 1970s by Dr. Benjamin Feingold that approximately half of children suffering from ADHD experience a decrease in symptoms after changes are made to their diet alone. The Feingold diet involves the elimination of dairy and other common childhood allergens such as soy, peanuts, eggs, wheat, corn, and yeast, as well as artificial colors, processed meats, salicylates found in certain fruits, and other products containing preservatives, MSG, high-fructose corn syrup (HFCS), and artificial sweeteners such as aspartame. These cofactors, plus a high sugar intake, are the leading nutritional causes of hyperactivity. Vaccinations have also been strongly linked to hyperactivity, but not fully proven at the causal level.

Medical practitioners such as Dr. Gabriel and Dr. Joel Fuhrman have successfully treated hundreds of ADHD children through whole-foods nutrition for the whole family, with specific supplementation. The approach includes a nutrient-dense, organic, non-GMO and non-irradiated vegetable, nut/seed, and fruit-based organic diet without any white flour, white sugar, processed food, or junk food. There is an emphasis on walnuts, which contain long-chain omega-3s, DHA supplementation (100–600 milligrams per day), which repairs and improves brain function, and the elimination of trans fats and cooked animal fats.

It is best to avoid dairy and gluten grains—wheat, barley, kamut, spelt, and bulgur. Combining this approach and the Feingold Diet with allergy testing and heavy-metal testing as needed further increases the success rate. Dr. Cousens and Dr. Fuhrman have observed successful outcomes in approximately ninety percent of the children treated in this way for ADHD.[44] Others have had about a fifty-percent success with a more basic approach.

A full holistic approach to rebuilding a child's brain and life includes:

- vegan diet
- 80% live-food cuisine
- organic foods
- avoid all white sugar, white flour, processed and junk food
- gluten-free foods
- low-allergen foods
- appropriate supplementation, including vitamin B12 and long-chain omega-3s
- green algae powders, or products such as E-3 Live from Klamath Lake, which act specifically to improve many levels of brain function (Dr. Cousens once observed a four-year-old child who had not yet spoken begin to speak within four months of taking it regularly.)
- homeopathic remedies
- time in nature
- love
- minimal TV and video games
- adequate sleep
- heavy-metal detoxification

- healthy bowel flora (Leading research in the dietary treatment of autism is helping us to make the connection between a healthy gut and brain function. One of the common threads among children with autism is the presence of an intestinal microbial imbalance, so appropriate probiotics are highly recommended to normalize and upgrade the bowel flora.)
- avoiding vaccinations (which may cause brain swelling and inflammation)
- appropriate family counseling to minimize stress and fear and maximize love and safety in the family dynamic. This can often make a big difference.

This approach is in dramatic contrast to the use of drugs like Ritalin, or antipsychotic, antidepressant, and antianxiety agents that may actually cause an impairment of normal brain neurodevelopment, structure and function that could last a lifetime. Although these psychotropic drugs may create some degree of behavior tranquilization or suppression, they have not been shown to increase learning or heal the condition.

What's the connection between the digestion of food and the digestion of information? First, remember that our intestine has its own nervous system, which is connected to the brain. Secondly, it produces ninety percent of the body's serotonin, and all other classes of neurotransmitters found in our brain are also in our gut.[45] Seeing this synergistic relationship within the whole living body helps us understand how treating candida overgrowth (a fungal imbalance in the gut) also produces positive results in the treatment of autism.

What dietary changes promote a healthy intestine? First of all, we want a strong immune system, as about eighty percent of our immune system resides in our gut. This means replacing immunity-suppressing foods such as heavily processed foods, white flour, and refined sugar with immune-system boosting foods such as organic, high-mineral, low-sugar, living foods, appropriate probiotics, and selected immune-enhancing herbs.

One of the jobs of our immune system is to keep unfriendly fungal and bacterial growth under control. Candida thrives in a toxic acid environment, and feeds on sugar. This is also why a pure, nutrient-dense, moderately low-glycemic diet is so important. In addition to these dietary changes, coconut oil in particular helps to treat candida. Coconut oil is antifungal, as it contains lauric acid, also present in human breast milk to help provide immunity support for baby, as well as caprylic acid, both of which are found in many candida remedies.[46]

Probiotic supplementation can be helpful for maintaining friendly intestinal bacteria, particularly after antibiotic use, but these don't have to be consumed with dairy products. A key principle is that no more than fifteen percent of the bowel flora can be pathogenic. This is especially true regarding the specific dietary needs of children with autism, who commonly experience the inability to digest proteins such as casein (found in dairy) and gluten (found in wheat and many other grains). Sauerkraut and kimchi (Korean pickled cabbage) are excellent maintainers and builders of bowel flora. High quality probiotics for adding into other foods such as nondairy yogurts and smoothies are also available at www.DrCousensOnlineStore.com.

The profound effect of improved nutrition on what is considered a normal child's learning is illustrated well in the exciting story of Appleton, Wisconsin's Central Alternative Charter High School. In 1997, an organization called Natural Ovens began a program to bring healthier foods into area schools, starting with Central Alternative High. At the time, discipline problems and weapons violations on campus were so substantial that a police officer had been brought in on a daily basis to supplement the staff.

When the school removed vending-machine junk-food snacks and sodas, however, in exchange for whole, non-GMO food lunches made from scratch, emphasizing fresh fruits and vegetables, it was not just lunchtime that changed for students and faculty. An unexpected, positive, peaceful social transformation for the entire school environment emerged. Discipline ceased to be a major issue, truancy rates went down, athletic performance went up, and grades improved. The school counselor reported that angry outbursts had stopped. Their school superintendent, Dr. Thomas Scullen, said, "They have learned that healthier foods are going to make them a better person. It keeps them more focused, and makes them happier."[47]

Principal LuAnn Coenen also spoke of her amazement at the change. As part of her responsibilities each year, she reports to the state of Wisconsin how many students at the school have been found using drugs or carrying weapons, or who have dropped out, been expelled, or committed suicide. Since the food program began, the number in each of these categories has been "zero."

Despite their expectations that students would complain about the change, staff members observed an overall acceptance of the wellness policy on campus. When interviewed for an ABC News story, a student at Central Alternative High named Taylor said that he was "able to concentrate better," that he was "not as tired," and that he had "more energy." When asked what it would be like if the school went back to sodas and junk food, Meagan, another student said, "It would probably be crazy. People would be bouncing off the walls." This inspiring story of Central Alternative High School has been documented in the film called *Impact of Fresh, Healthy Foods on Learning and Behavior* (see "Resources," page 485).

Media Effects on the Child's Mind

Television is biased towards death.

—Jerry Mander, former advertiser and author,
in *Four Arguments for the Elimination of Television*

Children see television much the same way they see a refrigerator or a stove—it's something that parents provide. In a young child's mind, parents probably condone what's on the television, just as they choose what's in the refrigerator or on the stove. That's why we who make television for children must be especially careful.

—Reverend Fred Rogers, known as
"Mr. Rogers" (who was also a vegetarian)

Just as what goes into the mouth affects the workings of the developing brain, the decisions we make regarding television, internet use, movies, books, and music also play a significant role in creating impressions that positively or negatively affect the mental health, overall consciousness, and spiritual development of our children. While these communication tools can be used to uplift, educate, and inspire, there are many factors that need to be considered as we make crucial decisions about the mental and spiritual diet that is placed before the child.

Stages of childhood development are an important consideration in such decisions. For the very young child, for example, the medium and electronics of television itself are disruptive to healthy brain development, regardless of content matter. For this reason, the U.S. Surgeon General as well as the American Academy of Pediatrics (AAP) have issued statements that children under the age of two should not be exposed to any television at all. Despite child-media advertising claims, scientific studies are now showing us that "educational" programming for young children can actually hinder language development.

Television consumption under the age of two is also being linked with learning difficulties in the schooling years. The Walt Disney Company, which produces the *Baby Einstein* video series—once promoted as an early-learning tool for infants—has in fact offered full refunds to parents who purchased these scientifically unsubstantiated products. From a holistic learning point of view, this makes sense because, as we've discussed, children are not having an integrated learning experience if their forces of will, in connection with the physical body, are not also engaged in the stimuli.

While television was not a cultural factor in either Steiner or Montessori's lifetime, contemporary leaders in early childhood development from both Montessori and Waldorf traditions are recommending zero television viewing for preschool-age children, based on Montessori and Steiner's insights. The absence of television encourages greater bonding experiences among family members and peers, which are key to socialization. The choice to wait before introducing film also supports the child's development of creativity, concentration, and the ability to self-calm. It also encourages more time in nature, and is supportive of the child's need for physical movement.

Over 1,000 studies, including a Surgeon General's special report in 1972, as well as a study by the National Institute of Mental Health in 1982,[48] have also explored the correlation between television viewing and violent behavior in preschoolers and older children as well. One study of 1,266 four-year-olds, published in *Pediatrics and Adolescent Medicine* (April 2005), has linked television watching at age four with bullying behavior in grade school. Thirty percent of our nation's kids are directly affected by bullying.[49] A University of Michigan study of 354 children ages two to four has also found that preschoolers who spend time in front of the television and playing video games are more prone to eat sweets and salty foods rather than fresh fruits and vegetables.[50]

Additionally, young children who are still learning to distinguish between fiction and nonfiction can be confused by animation and trick photography, making their task of assessing physical reality more difficult. Not only do children reenact the violence that they have been exposed to on the screen, but young children also reenact other dangerous stunts because they are still developing awareness of the natural laws of cause and effect. Understanding that the child is not a miniature adult also helps us to understand that movies that may have inspiring messages for teenage or adult viewers may be very inappropriate for younger children who are at a very different stage of mental development.

Another vital consideration regarding the media and our children is the saturation of advertising in children's television programming, movies, video games, and Internet sites. Ever since the deregulation of children's programing by Congress in 1980, we have seen zero boundaries on the targeting of children for corporate material gain. Child-influenced sales are now estimated at $700 billion in annual revenue. To achieve these results, corporations are hiring child psychologists to conduct studies of children's behavioral responses to marketing stimuli to advise the creation of their advertisements.[51]

How does neuromarketing affect childhood development?

Physically: The child is bombarded with influential messages that blatantly undermine healthy eating practices, a healthy body image, and abstinence from alcohol. The Center on Alcohol Marketing and Youth (CAMY) at Georgetown University found that in 2003, the top fifteen primetime programs most popular with teens were all shown with alcohol ads.[52] Additionally, the U.S. is the only country other than New Zealand that allows advertising for pharmaceutical drugs on television.[53]

Emotionally: The child's need to bond in relationships is being abused for material gain. For example, one basic strategy is to encourage the child to become attached to a cartoon character whose primary role is to befriend the child in order to sell products.

Socially: The child is sometimes pitted against the parent, to make sales through "pester-power." The child's peer environment is made commercially competitive, as the child feels pressured to buy certain toys, clothing, and electronics in order to be accepted by a peer group.

Cognitively: The child is being purposely dumbed-down in order to be more easily manipulated.

Spiritually: The child's self-esteem is affected by advertising. For a marketer to convince consumers that they need something, they must first convince them that they are incomplete or inferior without it. The child is given the underlying message that they, and their healthy development, do not matter to the greater community—only their money and what it can purchase. The child is given the message that life is all about buying things—about having rather than being. Descartes said, "I think, therefore I am." Our modern culture seems to believe, "I have, therefore I am."

Rather than supporting the child's quest to seek wisdom and esteem from within, these culture-of-death media practices keep the child enslaved in materialistic idolatry. Neuromarketing is a blatant violation of children's emotional, intellectual, moral, ethical, and spiritual health and individuation, as well as the natural unfoldment of their aliveness.

Unfortunately, it isn't just ads that undermine the child's holistic development. Subtle and even subliminal messages from the culture of death are also being fed to young viewers. In the case of the *Twilight* movie series, for example, popular cinema is sending the message to our children that to align with the dark side, symbolized by vampires and werewolves, is a cool and sexy way to meet the teenage need to express one's individuality. A comprehensive review of the spiritual implications of this film can be read on Dr. Gabriel's blog (www.drcousens.com).

The dire consequences of death-culture glamorization can be seen in studies linking television viewing among children with a rise in risky behaviors such as smoking cigarettes, drinking alcohol, and promiscuous or unhealthy precocious sexual activity. Although cigarette ads on American television have been banned, researchers have found that, even after adjusting for other risk factors, kids who watch television are more likely to start smoking at an earlier age. The relationship between television viewing and age of starting smoking was even stronger than that of peer smoking and parental smoking.[54]

Studies are also showing that exposure to drinking in movies increases the likelihood that viewers themselves will have positive thoughts about drinking.[55] Alcohol is the most common beverage to be portrayed on television, yet the sobering consequences of consuming it—including physical toxicity, impaired judgment, potential lethality when mixed with driving, weapons, or drugs, and greater vulnerability to demonic influences—are almost never depicted.[56]

As published in the *Journal of Pediatrics* (November 2008), one study has also linked teen pregnancy with television viewing. This study showed that adolescents who have a high level of exposure to television programs containing sexual content are twice as likely to be involved in a pregnancy (as the mother or father) in the next three years as their peers with less exposure to such programming.[57] Just how common is sexual content in popular TV shows? Seventy percent of the television programs most viewed by American teens include sexual content averaging five sexual scenes per hour, and fifteen percent of TV scenes with sexual intercourse depicted characters who have just met having sex.[58]

Understanding this TV exposure, it is no coincidence (although not necessarily causal) that U.S. teens and young adults lead the world in sexually transmitted diseases (STDs), comprising nearly half of all new STDs reported. While the medium of television itself has the potential to help educate teens about conscious sexuality, today's popular media unfortunately does far more to undermine the positive efforts of parents and spiritual community than to support the child in this way.

Another clear example of death-culture glamorization on television and in video games is the prevalence of violence as entertainment. By the age of eighteen, the average American child will have viewed 200,000 acts of violence and 100,000 murders on TV.[59] As previously noted, exposure to violence, even on television, can be a source of trauma for the child, and contribute to childhood depression and anxiety.

Peace is not merely the absence of war, as the ancient warriors taught—one can be in a state of peace even while in physical combat. What we are seeing today, however, is an unconscious bloodbath of violence masquerading as entertainment, which is having highly negative effects on childhood development, amplifying negative thoughtforms in the collective human consciousness, and creating the illusion that random acts of violence are normal.

The amount of time that the American child spends watching television is also alarming. In 2009, children ages two to five watched TV for more than thirty-two hours a week, and children ages six to eight averaged twenty-eight.[60] Also of concern is how much time children are now left at home by themselves, with no parental presence to guide their TV viewing or other activities.

What can be done? It is helpful to use online movie reviews for parents. Such sites give parents useful information for making decisions about which films to put before the child. Internet-filter software for families can also be purchased, which protect the child from graphic imagery that may randomly appear on the computer screen. While these do not replace a proactive parental relationship, filters can help tip things a bit in favor of imagery that is better for the child's mental health.

Additional parent resources include the Center for Media Literacy, MediaSmarts, and the Center for SCREEN-TIME Awareness. We can also educate our children about our mental diet by explaining that, just as we have the choice to fill our bodies with healthful foods or junk foods, we also have a choice to fill our minds with healthy media or junk media.

We can also take an honest look at why we may be permitting media influences that go against our better judgment:

"I feel overwhelmed as a parent (especially a single parent), and need a break!" TV, movies, and video games may mesmerize our children while we get some work done, or some needed rest—but how else might we provide ourselves the necessary breather? What did parents do before the days of the electronic babysitter? Leading early childhood specialists remind us that when we are working, the young child also wants to be working. They want to be included in our lives, contributing to them, and learning about the world in which we live, rather than being dismissed as simply needing to be entertained.

As Peggy Jenkins puts it in her book *The Joyful Child,* "If we teach our children to participate in life, to be active and involved, they will choose doing over watching others do." In addition to involving the child in the work that we do, we can also reach out for community support. In some Waldorf communities, groups of parents have emerged who take turns going over to each other's houses to help with meal-preparation, cleaning, laundry, or any other needed support. Children can help with the work, and/or play together. Anyone is invited to join in, and there is a collective agreement that no one will judge another's home or situation.

Another option is to hire a trusted older child to be a "mother/father/grandparent's helper" as a companion for a younger child with no older siblings. Asking for—and accepting—help from family and friends can be difficult for many parents. Sometimes we get the message from our culture that we need to go it alone. Our interest as parents and grandparents, however, is to build communities that emphasize a culture of unity and support, not isolation and separation. And part of our children's development is to gain that sense of healthy community interaction.

"My child will be the only one who doesn't engage in these activities." You may be pleasantly surprised! There are more and more parents from diverse walks of life that are creating a home environment entirely free of television and video games. This is a time to be strong, and to model for our children that, if we discern something to be an unhealthy influence, we will choose to live authentically rather than follow the herd, so that we can be people rather than "sheeple." It is very powerful to live in alignment with one's own inner compass rather than valuing "everyone" else's opinion above our own. This alone is a great inspirational lesson for our children.

"My child complains of boredom when he's not plugged in." Boredom serves a purpose in the child's life. It can be a motivation for the child to create his own story in imaginative play; to set up a lemonade stand; to reach out to a friend for companionship; to make a drawing or a painting; to take up a new hobby; or to go exploring in nature. Boredom can be understood as their internal prompting to enter into creative, healthy activities, to take on new challenges, and to connect with the world around them.

Media dependency gives the child an electronic drug to numb the boredom. This is similar to an adult taking a pill to cover up bodily symptoms that could prompt and motivate them to make healthy lifestyle changes. Boredom is a state of mind that may occur when we think the world is there to entertain us. When a child realizes they *are* the entertainment, there is no place for boredom to reside, and life becomes what it always was—the joy of the inner expressing itself in the outer world. This is called aliveness. When the Biblical matriarch Sarah left her body, it is said that she was "alive all the days of her life." In aliveness, there is no place for the illusion of boredom.

As with any drug, you can expect a period of withdrawal in a child coming off of media dependency. It may be fairly uncomfortable for the child; there may be a bit of complaining; and yet this is a highly positive change. During this time, the child may need a lot of extra support in finding alternative activities. They may also need support for their developing self-esteem and self-confidence, because media addiction can also cover up feelings of insecurity or inadequacy that keep a child in the comfort zone of inactivity. Liberating our children from media dependency opens up the door to a self-loving self-esteem, and independence that will serve them well throughout their life.

The child may also need extra love during this time, as media addiction can mask hurts within family/friend relationships. Take heart! This is a time of opportunity. Just think—you can use all the money that you save from bypassing the new and improved television set, cable/HBO, DS, iPad, video games, Netflix/Red Box subscription, cinema tickets, or whatever the latest media method that may appear, to support healthy ways of engaging in a life that is a major upgrade from virtual-life. Get something on your wish list—bicycles, music lessons, a new garden, or a family vacation to a scenic wonder of nature. Unplug from any virtual dependency, and do something you've always wanted to!

"It's hard to explain, but something feels uncomfortable when the TV, CD, radio, and computer are turned off." In addition to substituting for full participation in life and relationships, excessive media also keeps us from feeling the pain of our own emptiness. Once again, there is no quick fix for this; however, when we craft our lives around the Six Foundations of Spiritual Life, the emptiness that we once felt begins to be filled with the incomparable experience of the Divine. We will go into greater detail about how to support this process in our "Supporting the Child's Spiritual Development" chapter (page 345).

While it may require more effort to find, we can also include some positive media once the child is of an appropriate age. While today's films may be biased toward the culture of death, some inspirational family films are being produced. Like nourishment for the body, positive and conscious imagery can be highly uplifting for the emotions in support of EQ (emotional IQ), mind, and soul. It is encouraging to see media's potential for promoting positive social change. When there was a significant drop in bacon sales ten years ago, for example, marketing researchers discovered that the movie *Babe* (a popular film about a pig) had just come out, and children throughout the U.S. were refusing to eat bacon.[61]

The Harmful Effects of Pornography

With the Internet now providing unprecedented access to pornography, its harmful effects on the developing mind are an extremely serious concern. In a culture of death, where animals are treated as machines without feelings, needs, or a divine purpose simply to satiate human lusts for flesh and monetary gain, we see this same consciousness in the industry of pornography. Men, women, and children are depicted as "pieces of meat" whose life-force and dignity are prostituted to gratify the insatiable and misguided desires of their dominators.

The consequences of this death-culture media phenomenon are grave. Not only is the viewing of pornography linked to depression and social problems—particularly the ability to be in loving intimate relationships—watching porn is also strongly linked to violence toward women and children. In his final interview before his execution, serial killer Ted Bundy spoke of pornography as the primary influence that led to his numerous acts of murder. He issued the following warning:

> Pornography can reach out and snatch a kid out of any house today. It snatched me out of my home twenty, thirty years ago. I'll tell you, there are lots of other kids playing in streets around the country who are going to be dead tomorrow and the next day and the next day and next month, because other young people are reading the kinds of things and seeing the kinds of things that are available in the media today.

Despite being raised with good morals in the home, Bundy reported that these values were weakened by discovering softcore (less explicit) pornography outside his home as a preteen. His addiction for that then led him to view violent pornographic materials, of which he said the following:

> The wedding of those two forces (pornographic sexual stimuli combined with violence)—as I know only too well—brings about behavior that is too terrible to describe. Those of us who have been so influenced by violence in the media, particularly pornographic violence, are not some kind of inherent monsters. We are your sons and husbands. We grew up in regular families. There are those loose in their towns and communities, like me, whose dangerous impulses are being fueled, day in and day out, by violence in the media in its various forms—particularly sexualized violence. What scares me is when I see what's on cable TV. Some of the violence in the movies

that come into homes today is stuff they wouldn't show in X-rated adult theaters thirty years ago. That is the most graphic violence onscreen, especially when children are unattended, or unaware that they could be a Ted Bundy, that they could have a predisposition to that kind of behavior.

In this interview, Bundy stressed his full accountability for the murders, yet made clear that *his addiction to pornography ignited and fueled the crimes that otherwise would never have happened.* He also insisted that, of others he had met with a similar tendency to violence, "without exception, every one of them was deeply involved in pornography." Pornography has indeed been found in the possession of almost every killer where sex was the motivation.

Pornography tends to twist the minds of all who watch it. Pornography is not normal, nor appropriate for normal development, although in our society today it is active as a common though mentally corrupting and degenerating force. While the link between pornography and violence described by Bundy continues to be debated, there is enough confirming data that the Attorney General's Commission on Pornography has made the following statement:

> …(C)linical and experimental research … (has) focused particularly on sexually violent material, (and) the conclusions have been virtually unanimous. In both clinical and experimental settings, exposure to sexually violent materials has indicated an increase in the likelihood of aggression. More specifically, the research … shows a causal relationship between exposure to material of this type and aggressive behavior towards women.[62]

Numerous studies show a clear link between the viewing of child pornography and sexual crimes against children. A recent example is the clinical work of psychologists Michael Bourke, PhD, and Andres Hernandez, PsyD, whose highly publicized paper suggests that men charged with Internet child-pornography offenses and those who commit hands-on child sex offenses are, in many cases, one and the same.[63]

Tragically, the perpetrators of sexual violence towards children are sometimes other children who have been exposed to Internet porn. An abuse-survivor charity called One in Four reports that many young sex offenders in treatment began offending as adolescents by downloading child pornography.[64]

Because pornography, like animal cruelty, is strongly linked to violence towards people, it should not be misunderstood to be a normal, healthy part of childhood or adolescence. To protect children from these dangers, we recommend vigilant monitoring of media, particularly Internet use, and educating children about virtues such as modesty and respect towards bodies. When you deem it age-appropriate, discuss how sacred and loving sexuality gives rise to joyful and fulfilling relationships. This approach is in stark contrast to the deceptive trap of pornographic exploitation.

The healthy development of our children's brains, emotions, and minds is one of the most important aspects of their holistic development, which we as parents need to consciously protect. Not only do we need to protect our children's fragile, developing consciousness from "liberal" degenerative and destructive societal forces, but it is also important to actively provide them with the wisdom and street skills to self-protect, to avoid and defeat these ever-present dark societal forces that are becoming a "normal" part of life. Pornography and explicit TV violence and sex are only the more blatant aspects of these forces.

CHAPTER 9

The Great Vaccine Question

Vaccination—Pro and Con

ARGUMENTS IN SUPPORT OF VACCINATION

There are many strong opinions on the vaccine question. The general consensus of pro-vaccine doctors is that vaccines are safe and effective, have ended epidemics of infectious disease, and are needed to promote "herd immunity":

> Vaccines save lives and protect against the spread of disease. If you decide not to immunize your child, you put your child at risk. Your child could catch a disease that is dangerous or deadly. Getting vaccinated is much better than getting the disease (American Academy of Pediatrics, August 21, 2014).

> As anti-vaccine activists continue to push more states to allow for easy philosophical exemptions, one thing is clear—more and more children will suffer and occasionally die from vaccine-preventable diseases (Paul Offit, MD, Chief of the Division of Infectious Diseases at the Children's Hospital of Philadelphia, January 20, 2007).

To prevent large segments of the population from disease exposure, vaccination must occur at an early age. It is particularly crucial to immunize young children, since their bodies are still developing, leaving them often incapable of fighting many diseases. Yet over 20 percent of preschool children do not receive all needed vaccines, leaving them vulnerable to many vaccine-preventable diseases ("Closing the Vaccination Gap: A Shot in the Arm for Childhood Immunization Programs," Every Child by Two, August 2004).

Immunization is one of the most important steps you can take to ensure your baby's current and future health (Paul Roumeliotis, MD, Medical Officer of Health at the Eastern Ontario Health Unit, August 21, 2014).

Generally, vaccines are safe and very effective. In my mind, the benefits of immunization far outweigh any risks (ibid.).

Physicians and other healthcare providers should simultaneously administer as many vaccine doses as possible, as indicated on the Recommended Child and Adolescent Immunization Schedule (Centers for Disease Control, December 1, 2006).

Vaccines are safe. All vaccines must be tested by the Food and Drug Administration (FDA). The FDA will not let a vaccine be given unless it has been proven to be safe and to work well in children.... (American Academy of Pediatrics, August 21, 2014).

ARGUMENTS AGAINST VACCINATION

Those opposed to vaccinations have dramatically different opinions:

Live-virus vaccines against influenza or poliomyelitis may in each instance produce the disease that they are intended to prevent (Jonas and Gerald Salk, Science, March 4, 1977).

There is a great deal of evidence to prove that immunization of children does more harm than good (Dr. J. Anthony Morris, former Chief Vaccine Control Officer and Research Virologist, U.S. FDA).

The greatest threat of childhood disease lies in the dangerous and ineffective efforts made to prevent them through mass immunization.... There is no convincing scientific evidence that mass inoculations can be credited with eliminating any childhood disease. (Robert Mendelsohn, M.D., pediatrician, student of Dr. Benjamin Spock, and author of How to Raise a Healthy Child in Spite of Your Doctor).

The "victory over epidemics" was not won by medical science or by doctors—and certainly not by vaccines.... The decline has been the result of technical, social, and hygienic improvements, and especially of improved nutrition.... Consider carefully whether you want to let your children undergo the dangerous, controversial, ineffective, and no longer necessary procedure called vaccination, because the claim that vaccinations are the cause for the decline of infectious diseases is utter nonsense (Dr. Gerhard Buchwald, senior physician at the Klinik Franken of the Bundesversicherungsanstalt für Angestellte and the Klinik am Park in Bad Steben, Germany).

Except for a ten-year period between 1955 and 1965, when the mortality rate was essentially flat, mortality rates have declined at a relatively constant rate of 1–2% yearly since 1900 (David Francis, researcher, National Bureau for Economic Research).

The vaccines are not working, and they are dangerous.... We should be working with nature (Lendon Smith, MD, "The Children's Doctor," American obstetrician, gynecologist, pediatrician, author, and television personality).

I no longer believe that vaccines have any role to play in the protection of the community or the individual. Vaccines may be profitable but, in my review, they are neither safe nor effective. I prefer to put my trust in building up my immune system (Dr. Vernon Coleman).

From my perspective, the idea of compulsory involvement in vaccine trials "for the greater good of society" is not only outlandish, it's a complete abomination. It's tyranny of the worst kind, and the epitome of a heartless system based on broken ethics. Sadly, there are signs that we're already sliding in that direction. For example, consider the fact that the US government has already ok'd the testing of the incredibly controversial and dangerous anthrax vaccine on infants. And the fact that when fourteen babies died in an Argentinian vaccine trial, the drug company, GlaxoSmithKline, was fined a measly $250,000 (Joseph Mercola, MD).

The anti-vaccine position is that:

- Vaccines are neither safe nor effective.
- "Herd immunity" (the idea that all children must be vaccinated in order for vaccinations to be effective) has been proven to be a myth.
- Vaccinated individuals may become carriers and infect both vaccinated and unvaccinated individuals, as indicated by years of research.
- There was a 98–99% drop in acute infectious diseases before vaccines were introduced.
- Informed consent is a right of political, ethical, moral, and spiritual importance in a free country.
- Vaccines cause a significant number of deaths, severe chronic debilitating effects, and acute adverse reactions.

This chapter examines these controversial vaccine positions, and also looks at the potential dangers of vaccines, so that we as parents can have fully informed consent, according to the Nuremberg Code of medical ethics established after World War II. It is secondarily aimed at providing scientific, moral, and ethical perspectives on the great vaccine debate.

After more than 200 years since the first vaccine was introduced, why is the question of vaccination still a debate? This needs to be answered if we as parents are to make an informed decision about something with such potentially powerful consequences in our children's and our own lives. It is not our intent to discuss the issue at the level of vaccine efficacy, vaccine politics, or vaccine economics (although some material inevitably appears as background information, such as the discussion of the Disneyland scare).

A CONFLICT OF PROFESSIONAL OPINIONS

The CDC employees, many allopathic physicians, the FDA, pharmaceutical companies, and the WHO are adamant about the need for vaccinations, but there are hundreds of studies that refute or at least challenge their position.[1] There is also a growing group of allopathic physicians and researchers, holistic physicians, and homeopaths, as well as a significant and expanding number of parents and members of the general public, who are beginning to question the validity of the practice of routine vaccinations as safe and effective.

Just as the question of whether smoking causes cancer took at least thirty years to resolve because of politics and power economics (despite the truth of the research), the vaccine question has not been definitively resolved in over 200 years. In the case of vaccines, there are compelling issues that cloud the decision-making process, such as a complete lack of double-blind studies or other high-quality research in the United States by the CDC, FDA, WHO, or any independent federal government agency. Other factors include fear, ignorance, and economic, political, and scientific influences.

As the data unfolds, however, responsible professionals are moving toward resolving the question.[2] A recent international medical council on vaccination released a document containing over eighty signatures by family physicians, brain surgeons, experts in pathology, chemistry, and immunity, that essentially said: Vaccines pose a significant risk of harm to the health of children, and there is no real scientific backing for the vaccine mythology claiming that vaccines are good for children.[3] This third-party medical position cannot be washed away by denigrating medical professionals around the world as "vaccine deniers."

Is there really a consensus on the safety of vaccines? At some point a parent needs to decide whom to trust. There are a variety of organizations that are against vaccinations, and focus instead on building internal immunity by taking such supplements as vitamin D, vitamin A, vitamin C, zinc, herbs to build the immune system, supplements, healthy diet, and a holistic lifestyle. One of the problems in this decision-making process is the unfortunate effort by key agencies like the CDC that are "doctoring" the information so there is no longer access to the truth about evidence-based findings, which thus contributes to blocking the informed-consent process.

Fortunately, there are people like Dr. William Thompson, a senior researcher at the CDC who in mid-2014 exposed the fact that he was part of a direct coverup of the link between the MMR (measles, mumps and rubella) vaccine and autism in African-American boys. This admission by Dr. Thompson raises the devastating question whether CDC research and opinions are just another sophisticated PR program that governs the CDC's "science." As Peter Doshi, MD suggests (*Harper's*, March 2006), we may be looking at a case of literally "viral" marketing.

Dr. Peter Doshi wrote an article, published in the *British Medical Journal*, in which he charged that vaccines are less effective and have more side effects than the medical profession communicates to the public. He questioned the quality of pro-vaccine studies, particularly of the flu vaccine. Dr. Doshi analyzed the CDC data in 2001,[4] and points out that, according to this data, "influenza and pneumonia took 62,034 lives in 2001; 61,777 were attributed to pneumonia, and only 257 to flu. And of those 257, in only 18 cases was the flu virus positively identified."

There are many causes for pneumonia. Since only eighteen deaths were flu-virus isolated, all we can say with scientific integrity is that these were the only deaths clearly caused by the flu virus. The average CDC estimate of deaths per year from flu is 36,000. There is quite a credibility gap between eighteen documented cases per year and an estimated 36,000 deaths. But those numbers, Dr. Doshi suggests, are communicated as PR for pushing flu vaccines. The CDC's own statistics for flu (separate from pneumonia) from 1979–2001 only found 1,348 flu deaths per year, rather than their publicly stated 36,000 deaths per year. But all they *really* had in 2001 were eighteen positively confirmed viral deaths from flu. In other words, the CDC's estimate of 36,000 "flu" deaths is far in excess of their real data, and even of the 1,348 average annual flu deaths they recorded.[5] This is an embarrassing discrepancy for the CDC.

Ultimately, as parents and grandparents, we have a moral, ethical, and parental responsibility to look at these questions and statements and come up with a personal decision based on the safety of our children, both long- and short-term. What are we protecting against? Measles, mumps, chickenpox—they all have their dangers, but they also seem to play important ecobiological roles, which will be discussed later. And it must be noted that—whether because of children becoming healthier, or receiving better health care if infected, or because the virus is less virulent, or even because of vaccinations, as vaccine proponents argue—no one has died from the wild measles virus since 2005, while at least 108 people have died directly from MMR vaccinations. The data raises the question of risk/benefit trade-offs.

The death rate for measles is 0.2%, which is approximately one's chance of dying in a car accident. It is easy to get caught up in the highly promoted fear about how dangerous these diseases are, and lose our perspective. Unfortunately, fear often controls mass consciousness, rather than a well-thought-out, scientific, evidenced-based perspective.

In the 1940s and 1950s, it was common to get measles, chicken pox, or mumps at an early age. Almost everyone got these diseases, then recovered, and consequently had lifelong immunity. A few did not, however, and now the medical PR is hyperfocused on the "serious" dangers of these illnesses. Yes, there are potential serious complications from all normally benign diseases—but they are rare, and often associated with poor nutrition. It is true that there are dangers, but when we look at the risk-to-benefit ratio of vaccines, we have to ask, "Could I live with myself if my child is the one who is harmed by vaccines—or dies?" A similar question, of course could be asked by parents who do not vaccinate and whose child contracts a serious infection. Raising children is never risk-free—but thoughtful, informed choices are the best we can ever do.

A SUBTLE SHIFT IN ATTITUDES ABOUT VACCINATION

The majority of allopathic physicians and medical organizations, including the CDC, still strongly recommend vaccinations to the extent of calling parents irresponsible if they don't vaccinate their children. A shift has been occurring, however, in the professional community's attitude toward vaccination. Virtually 100% of homeopaths, a very high percentage of holistic physicians, and an increasing number of allopathic physicians are either opposed to vaccination or at least no longer severely criticizing parents for questioning or choosing not to vaccinate; or they are giving parents reasonable alternative options as trustworthy data emerges on this question.

Multiple cracks in the apparent "consensus" are appearing, even at the risk of professional ostracism. The Disneyland measles outbreak (discussed below) and the extreme media response that resulted, have helped force both health practitioners and parents to take more mature positions. Doctors and nurses are beginning to speak out against vaccines, or at least speak privately against it. Survey research shows that the percentage of nurses and a percentage of doctors who do not vaccinate their own children or themselves may be as high as 70%.[6] That is a very revealing but not very publicized piece of information. As one medical doctor put it, "I feel forced by my colleagues to vaccinate my patients; but what I do for my own family is private, and I will not vaccinate my children, in my role as a responsible parent."

Another revelation of the fear-creating falsehoods that conscientious doctors are beginning to admit is a statement by Dr. Diane Harper, the lead researcher/developer in the Gardasil® and Cervarix human papilloma vaccines. Dr. Harper made a public speech at the Fourth International Public Conference on Vaccination in 2009, in which she essentially explained that the Gardasil® and Cervarix vaccines do not work, are dangerous, are not needed, and were not fully tested. Dr. Harper said she was speaking out so that she might finally "be able to sleep at night."

Dr. Harper explained that the risk of cervical cancer is extremely low, and that these vaccinations were unlikely to have any effect on the rate of cervical cancer in the US. She further pointed out that 70% of the cases of HPV (human papilloma virus), an infectious sexually transmitted disease, resolve themselves without treatment in one year, and 90% are naturally healed in two years. And the vaccine works on only four strains out of forty for this specific STD (sexually transmitted disease). Some testing of the vaccine has been done on subjects fifteen years of age and older, but not on nine-year-olds, who are now also receiving the vaccines.

Dr. Harper points out that there is no actual evidence that the vaccine can prevent any cancer. She pointed out that it is misleading for vaccine companies to "report" that these "untreated" cases "can" or "may" lead to cervical cancer.[7] This is a hypothetical statement rather than a scientifically proven correlation between vaccinations and prevention of these rare cancers. She points out that there is only a theoretical conjecture that the HPV vaccines will prevent cervical cancer. What is not theoretical is that one hundred girls in the United States have already died from the vaccination as of 2014, and more than 15,000 adverse effects have been reported including Guillain-Barré syndrome, seizures, blood clots, brain inflammation, and severe autoimmune reactions such as lupus. And these reported adverse effects may represent only a fraction (estimated at 1–10%) of the actual number.

The risks are clearly more serious than any theoretical "benefits." Dr. Harper essentially said that the emperor has no clothes, exposing the false-fear messages used by agencies and pharmaceutical companies to persuade parents to vaccinate their children.

Debunking the Myths about Vaccination

THE MYTH OF "HERD IMMUNITY"

Anti-vaccinators risk not only the lives of their own children, but also those of others who are too medically fragile to get vaccinated and must instead rely on "herd immunity" (David M. Perry, PhD, July 11, 2013).

The best way to reduce vaccine-preventable diseases is to have a highly immune population. Universal vaccination is a critical part of quality health care and should be accomplished through routine and intensive vaccination programs implemented in physicians' offices and in public health clinics (Centers for Disease Control, December 1, 2006).

Vaccines work by protecting individuals, but their strength really lies in the ability to protect one's neighbors. When there are not enough people within a community who are immunized, we are all at risk (Kristen A. Feemster, MPH, MSHPR, MD, March 23, 2014).

The theory of herd immunity, expressed in the quotes above, maintains that if a certain percentage of the population is immunized against a particular disease, epidemics can be prevented. No one is able to specify the exact percentages in this theory. Initially it was thought that a 68% vaccination rate would create this mass immunity. Now they are saying 92–94%, and some suggest 95–100%. In reality, the facts are revealing that herd immunity is an unsubstantiated myth that has been unethically used both to socially stigmatize parents who have refused to vaccinate their children, and as a rationale by the government and pharmaceutical industry to vigorously promote vaccinations.

While it is common for parents of vaccinated children to blame and criticize parents of unvaccinated children, the fact is that if anyone should be upset, it should be the parents of unvaccinated children. It is a scientific fact that recently vaccinated children could be carriers of the viral disease they are vaccinated against for at least two weeks. This may explain why there could be a measles outbreak in schools where 98–100% of students had been vaccinated. The real danger of contagion from these vaccinated children is that, once vaccinated, they may become temporary disease carriers, or vectors, from one to three weeks afterwards, depending on the vaccination type. The scientific data continues to grow on this question, and none of it seems to support the validity of the herd-immunity theory.

An event on February 14, 2014 was reported on October 24, 2014: A U.S. Navy mine ship, whose crew was 99% vaccinated for flu, had a flu outbreak in which 25% of the crew contracted flu of some sort; sixteen of these cases were documented as influenza.[8] The fact that 99% of the crew had been vaccinated and 25% of them got the flu anyway highlights the point that herd immunity is a myth, and that these vaccines are not doing their job.

It may also be that flu vaccinations, in some cases, impair the immune system. A 2011 study in South Korea raises the concern of "breakthrough," or infection with the same disease the vaccinated children were supposedly being protected from. In South Korea, despite near-universal vaccination rates of 97% by 2011, instead of a reduced number of chicken pox (varicella) cases there was a significant increase. The South Korea Centers for Disease Control and Prevention reported a more than threefold increase in chicken pox, from 22.6 cases per 100,000 population in 2006 to 71.6 cases per 100,000 in 2011.[9]

A South Korean research team conducted a case-based study, a case-control study, and an immunogenicity and safety study to identify the reasons for the failure of the vaccine; their findings were published in the journal *Clinical and Vaccine Immunology*.[10] This study suggests that most cases of varicella occurring in South Korea are caused by "breakthrough" infections with the very disease the vaccine was intended to prevent. These infections were either from the vaccine strain or a wild-type strain. Earlier polio-vaccine studies showing that polio vaccine was causing vaccine-induced polio represent the same principle at work.[11] These clinical examples create a serious challenge to one of the biggest and most detrimental myths in the vaccine discussion—the theory of herd immunity.

It is fascinating that vaccine-promoting agencies such as the CDC still have the audacity to talk about herd immunity as a scientific fact. As of 2015, there is no clinical or epidemiological evidence to support the theory; and, as already demonstrated, there is a lot of epidemiological evidence to debunk it. A high percentage of people, for instance, who have been vaccinated for pertussis are getting pertussis—up to 90% in some cases—as also happened with the polio vaccine.[12]

These "unexpected" observations contradicting the herd-immunity theory are also happening in China, which has one of the most vaccination-compliant populations in the world. The vaccination rates for measles, mumps, and rubella are reported to be higher than 99% in Zhejiang province; however, the incidence of those diseases not only remains high but is actually increasing significantly since 2009.[13] It is shocking to find that the rate of measles in vaccinated Chinese children in 2013 was approximately three times greater than the number of measles cases in this same population in 2012.[14] What is even more interesting is that 93.6% of those cases tested seropositive for the measles antibodies that supposedly provide immunity—a percentage that is higher than what is theoretically needed to achieve so-called herd immunity.

These Chinese findings challenge two vaccination claims: 1) the herd-immunity speculation, which has been used as a so-called "fact" in a socially vicious way against parents who have chosen not to vaccinate; and 2) that being seropositive after vaccination ensures that one is immunized, or protected, as opposed to merely "vaccinated." True immunity comes from being exposed to diseases naturally, which creates a natural immunity and actually does protect one from getting the disease again, often for a lifetime.

Another argument for "herd immunity" is that near-universal vaccination will protect those with damaged or compromised immune systems. Besides the fact that herd immunity has not been proven to exist—and therefore cannot protect immune-compromised persons—it borders on the unethical to require unvaccinated people to risk their own health to protect people with compromised immune systems. A more practical approach would be for vaccine companies to develop vaccines specifically for immune-compromised people. The initial chicken pox vaccine was designed to do this, but their market was too small to be cost-effective, so they are now marketed to everyone.

Do vaccinated children put unvaccinated children at risk? This question is seldom asked due to lack of awareness, but it is an important question. When a child has been injected with live viruses of measles, mumps, rubella, varicella (chicken pox), or H1N1 (swine flu), that child has been put at risk of infection by those very same communicable diseases. When Leah was running a home-based childcare program, she saw firsthand that out of the ten families she served, two of the five vaccinated children got the measles, while none of the five vaccine-free kids did. The mother of one of these children told Leah that her daughter's measles had begun almost immediately after receiving her measles shot.

In the case of H1N1, the recipient of the vaccine is a highly active carrier of the H1N1 or other flu viruses for three days, and moderately communicable for three weeks. Research has found these flu viruses active in their bodily fluids and throats for approximately one to three weeks, which means that they can be spread by vaccinated children who serve as active carriers during this period. In other words, it is scientifically documented that vaccinated children can become carriers of a disease for several weeks following a vaccination.

This documentation forces us to reevaluate the idea of herd immunity, and indicates that the recently vaccinated kids may actually be the ones exposing everyone else to the diseases they are being vaccinated against. In reality, it is they who should stay home from school in voluntary isolation for at least two weeks following vaccination. At least one animal pertussis study observed this phenomenon: "When you are newly vaccinated, you are an asymptomatic carrier, which is good for you but not for the population."[15] This was also demonstrated in a Canadian study led by Todd Merkle. When exposed to pertussis via the vaccine, vaccinated children became asymptomatic carriers for one to three weeks.[16]

Parents who are not vaccinating their children should feel empowered by this real science instead of intimidated by paranoia-generating media myths, so that they can stand up against ignorant ostracism and social "mobocracy" attacks by parents who believe the fear-based, ignorant, and/or profit-driven media.

The theory of "herd immunity" is also crumbling in the face of serious outbreaks of pertussis in heavily vaccinated populations where individuals are contracting pertussis at high rates, according to a study published by Oxford University. Another study in *Clinical and Infectious Diseases* reviewed data on every patient who tested positive for pertussis between

March and October of 2010 in California. Out of 132 people who had the disease, 81% were fully up-to-date on their shots.[17] We cannot blame unvaccinated kids for this, just as in China. If the vaccine actually worked at a high vaccination rate, one would not see 81% of the "fully vaccinated" population contracting pertussis. On the contrary, it appears that either vaccinations are causing the disease, or are ineffective, or both.

These scientific reports make it undeniably clear that vaccinated individuals may still contract the disease they have been vaccinated against. The study above also suggests that people who are vaccinated may be more prone to contracting those diseases than the unvaccinated population. In alignment with the pertussis study's findings, according to Dr. James Howenstine, measles outbreaks have occurred in schools with vaccination rates over 98% in all parts of the U.S. as well as China, including areas that had no cases of measles for years.[18] He points out that, as measles immunization rates rise to high levels, measles is becoming a disease seen only in vaccinated people. Dr. Howenstine even cites an outbreak of measles in a school where 100% of children had been vaccinated.

These facts are forcing us to look at some inconvenient truths, more of which come from earlier studies. After the introduction of diphtheria vaccinations in England and Wales in 1894, the number of deaths from diphtheria rose by 20% in the next fifteen years. In Germany in 1939, when diphtheria vaccinations were compulsory, the disease spiraled to 150,000 cases that year. Norway, a geographical neighbor that didn't have compulsory vaccinations, had fifty cases of diphtheria.[19]

The inevitable question arises: Do vaccines such as polio, diphtheria, measles, and pertussis protect people—or do they actually contribute to the spread of these diseases? The statistical data from many countries is now beginning to more clearly answer this question, but it needs a more definitive answer.

An additional voice addressing this question came in the year 2000. Upon reviewing the polio vaccine data, the famous Dr. Jonas Salk said that the vaccine he created was actually the leading cause of the spread of polio. It takes a real scientist and an honest, humble person to make this sort of statement. In the March 4, 1977 edition of *Science*, Jonas and Gerald Salk warned, "Live-virus vaccines against influenza or polio-myelitis may in each instance produce the disease that they are intended to prevent." They went on to say, "The live virus against measles may produce such side effects such as encephalitis [brain inflammation]."[20]

MEASLES MADNESS—ANOTHER FAILURE OF "HERD IMMUNITY"

The "measles outbreak" at Disneyland (December 15–20, 2014) has unfortunately been used as an opportunistic political football to pursue the government and pharmaceutical companies' political and economic goals by creating a climate of fear, intimidation, and misinformation. The recent historical and epidemiological reality described below raises serious questions about the effectiveness of the measles vaccine, the belief in "herd immunity," and the fantasy of 100% vaccine protection from measles. In the case of Disneyland, as elsewhere in the world, the 90–94% vaccination rate needed according to the theory of herd immunity was far exceeded.

The theory of "herd immunity" holds that immunity will occur for an entire group if 90–94% of its members have been vaccinated; but in the United States we are seeing measles outbreaks occurring in schools where the vaccination rate is over 98%—significantly higher than the 90–94% projection needed for "herd immunity." One measles outbreak occurred in an American school where 100% of the children had been vaccinated.[21] When measles occur where vaccination rates are 98–100%, we can't credibly blame the unvaccinated, and the herd-immunity theory can't explain measles outbreaks in completely vaccinated populations.

In 1984, measles occurred in a New Mexico junior high school in which 98% of the cases were recently vaccinated children.[22] Another 1984 breakout of measles occurred in an Illinois high school in which 100% of the cases occurred in vaccinated students.[23] There are at least fifteen other clearly documented examples of failed herd immunity.[24] The chart below is taken from Neil Z. Miller's book *Vaccine Safety Manual* (New Atlantean Press, 2008); it illustrates the epidemiological evidence of measles outbreaks in vaccinated populations, and dispels the 100%-protection fantasy.

Outbreaks of Measles
in Vaccinated Populations

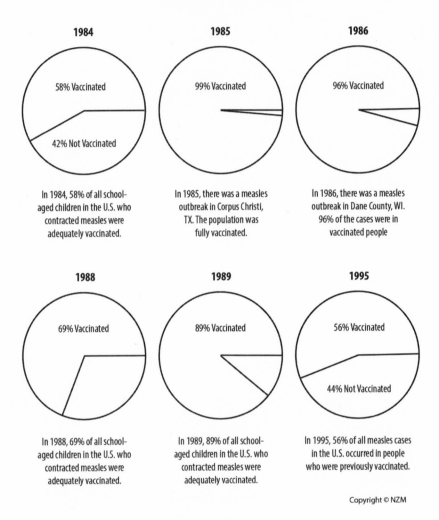

1984

58% Vaccinated

42% Not Vaccinated

In 1984, 58% of all school-aged children in the U.S. who contracted measles were adequately vaccinated.

1985

99% Vaccinated

In 1985, there was a measles outbreak in Corpus Christi, TX. The population was fully vaccinated.

1986

96% Vaccinated

In 1986, there was a measles outbreak in Dane County, WI. 96% of the cases were in vaccinated people

1988

69% Vaccinated

In 1988, 69% of all school-aged children in the U.S. who contracted measles were adequately vaccinated.

1989

89% Vaccinated

In 1989, 89% of all school-aged children in the U.S. who contracted measles were adequately vaccinated.

1995

56% Vaccinated

44% Not Vaccinated

In 1995, 56% of all measles cases in the U.S. occurred in people who were previously vaccinated.

Copyright © NZM

Source: *New England Journal of Medicine* 1987;316:771-74.
Journal of the American Medical Association 1990;263-71. Several CDS *MMWRs*.

As we look at the data, there is obviously a strong suggestion that the measles vaccine is not very effective, and that the idea of 100% protection from measles on a mass scale is a delusion. That fear-based notion, unfortunately, is part of what is driving the push for mandatory vaccinations, even though the hard epidemiological data upholds neither the theory of herd immunity nor the effectiveness of the measles vaccine. With the factual evidence in mind, the serious and significant risks of measles vaccination are a much more relevant consideration, from a risk/benefit perspective.

The next inconvenient epidemiological truth is that from 1915 to 1958, before the measles vaccine was introduced, the rate of deaths from measles had already declined naturally, through improved hygiene and plumbing, by nearly 98%. The rate has not dropped significantly further since the advent of measles vaccinations in 1958.

The death rate from measles had already declined by 97.7% at least 3 years before the first measles vaccination. The incidence of measles did decrease when the vaccine was introduced for a period of time, so it did appear to have some immediate effect for a limited period of time. The hardcore data, however, refutes the claim that the measles vaccine was the factor that largely eradicated measles.[25]

These "unexpected" measles outbreaks discrediting the herd-immunity theory are also happening in China, as noted above, where vaccination compliance is among the highest in the world, and in other countries. The rates of measles, mumps, and rubella vaccinations are reported to be higher than 99% in the Zhejiang province, but the incidence of measles, mumps, and rubella there is still high, and actually increasing.[26]

In France, the MMR vaccination rate was 96.8% in children under eleven years of age in 2008; yet from 2008–2011 there were 20,000 cases of measles. According to Dr. James Howenstine, measles outbreaks have occurred in schools with vaccination rates above 98% in all parts of the U.S. as well as China, including areas that had no cases of measles for years.[27] These facts are forcing us to look at some embarrassing truths about the theory of herd immunity, which epidemiological evidence does not support, as well as the overall effectiveness of the vaccine itself. A

THE MEASLES DEATH RATE WAS DECREASED ON ITS OWN *BEFORE* THE VACCINE WAS INTRODUCED

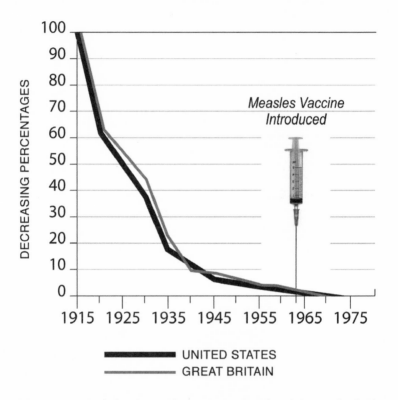

From 1915 to 1958, *before* the measles vaccine was introduced, the measles death rate in the United States and Great Britain had already declined on its own by 98 percent. Source: *International Mortality Statistics* 1981:182-83.

vaccine that may work for some people is clearly not guaranteed to work for all of them.

Considering the relative failure of measles vaccine as illustrated by the data, it is well past the time to consider other causes for worldwide measles outbreaks. One possible reason is the established fact that vaccinated children are carriers of the measles virus for at least two weeks after vaccination. Dr. William Atkinson, a senior epidemiologist with the

CDC, admitted that "measles transmission has clearly been documented among vaccinated persons."[28] Supporting this observation is data from the Amish, who are a basically unvaccinated community. They reported not a single case of measles from 1970–1987, while their vaccinated neighbors suffered cycles of epidemics every 2–3 years. The strange extrapolation of this is that measles may be more common in vaccinated populations. In addition, there are multiple strains of measles virus, as with the flu, which may also explain the proven ineffectiveness of the measles vaccines.

As we look at the larger picture of vaccines, and this apparently paradoxical situation in which diseases are breaking out in groups that are 97–100% vaccinated against those very diseases, there is a clear need to ask questions and try to understand the disconnect between the failed theory and the hardcore data. It is important to note that, in scientific circles, when a theory is not substantiated by scientific data, the theory needs to be discarded regardless of the politics, fear, or economics of the situation.

As mentioned above, people vaccinated with live measles viruses are proven carriers of the disease for at least two weeks after vaccination. This phenomenon may explain how the spread of measles infection may be caused by the MMR vaccination itself. Although this may not be the only explanation, it is amazing that so-called medical leaders in the world of pediatrics are still promoting the disproven herd-immunity theory by trying to shame, blame, and castigate parents who choose not to vaccinate their children. They do this in the face of actual data suggesting that, in highly vaccinated populations, it is actually the vaccinated who may be the disease carriers.

We suggest that parents of unvaccinated children keep their children away from children who have been vaccinated with live viruses for at least two weeks. It does not make sense that politicians and medical "authorities" who are calling for forced vaccinations have repeatedly ignored epidemiological evidence that vaccinated children represent the vast majority of those getting the measles in highly vaccinated populations, whether from the vaccines themselves or from infecting each other. It is also possible that vaccination weakens their immune systems, making them more susceptible to infections. The phenomenon of immune suppression by vaccines[29] was documented as early as 1981, and reconfirmed in 1992.

The reality of vaccinated individuals becoming active carriers of the disease was documented as far back as 1995 in a *Journal of Clinical Microbiology* article titled "Detection of Measles Virus RNA in Urine Specimens from Vaccine Recipients."[30] The study described in this article was conducted by professionals working at the CDC, and funded by the World Health Organization and the National Vaccine Program. It showed that the MMR vaccine led to measles infection in many of the children who received vaccinations. The live virus was found in the urine samples of newly vaccinated fifteen-month-old children as well as adults, using a technique called PCR testing to distinguish between wild and vaccine viruses. The vaccine-measles-virus RNA was detected in ten of twelve children, for a period of at least two weeks following vaccination and as early as one day afterward. This tells us that vaccinated children are indeed likely carriers of the measles virus.

PCR testing is acknowledged in the scientific community as a sensitive and specific way to distinguish between vaccine-strain measles and wild measles. We mention this because of the Disneyland outbreak, in which, as of April, 2015, 147 people were diagnosed with measles, and from which medical professionals immediately spread fear-based generalizations and assumptions without checking this key information. Since most of the people with measles had been vaccinated, it raises the question of whether it was transmitted by vaccinated or unvaccinated children. It would have been a perfect occasion for PCR testing to immediately distinguish whether wild measles or the vaccine virus was causing the measles—this would have established whether vaccinated or nonvaccinated children were the carriers. Any reasonable physician without a political agenda should have known to do this.

Instead, there was a hysterical mob response against nonvaccinated children and their parents, along with a propharmaceutical endorsement. Without data from PCR testing, there is nothing we can say except that the media and the health officials used it as a political opportunity. The only relevant question here is why they chose not to do immediate PCR testing.

Several months later, some data became available from at least nine of these cases, surprisingly opening a new and very significant possible cause for the Disneyland measles outbreak. In those nine people tested, the Disneyland outbreak was found to have been caused by a strain of measles called genotype B3, which is different from the only measles vaccine used in the U.S., called genotype A. The genotype B3 virus caused a measles outbreak in the Philippines in 2014,[31] and was found in more than fourteen countries and six U.S. states in the six months prior to the Disneyland outbreak.

It is important to note that there are twenty-three recognized genotypes of measles, of which type A is only one. The problem, as with flu-vaccine mutations and the high percentage of failure with the flu vaccine, is that the measles vaccines only work against type-A measles [32] and not against the other twenty-two genotypes. This is another possible explanation why, even with 97–100% vaccination rates in China, South Korea, France, and other U.S. communities, the occurrence of measles is increasing. In this case, with nine cases out of nine testing positive for the B3 measles virus, the leading reason for why the outbreak occurred, and also for why vaccinated people are getting measles, is that these are caused by a different strain of measles than the one addressed by the vaccines—not because of unvaccinated persons or a failure of herd immunity.

It is worth asking why people are not questioning the effectiveness of the measles vaccine. If the vaccine actually worked, and if the concept of herd immunity were true, there should be no hysteria; everyone would feel safe. Perhaps this medical overreaction reveals that people intuitively know about the (lack of) effectiveness of the measles vaccine and the very questionable theory of herd immunity.

The above evidence does not exclude the possibility that the forty-two other Disneyland measles cases may have caught the disease from a recently vaccinated person, as evidence does support the possibility of vaccinated persons transmitting infection. One example of this, selected from a variety of cases in which vaccinated persons transmitted measles to others, was a recent report of a person who was vaccinated twice in

New York City. He became infected with measles, and then spread it to secondary contacts, both of whom were also vaccinated twice.

This raises very interesting questions about vaccines, and the point that vaccination does not ensure immunization. The double failure of this MMR vaccine case challenges the pseudoscientific claim that when there's a measles outbreak, nonvaccinated or minimally vaccinated people are the "guilty ones." The vaccinated ones actually could have been the carriers in China, France, South Korea, and in communities in the United States where 96% to 100% of the people were vaccinated, as well as in this specific case in New York City.

The fact is that there are increasing outbreaks of measles worldwide, even in the 99% vaccinated populations. That is the issue that needs to be addressed: The data indicates that the problem may be a failure of the vaccine itself rather than a failure to use it.

What can we do to give our children real and safe protection? As we look at the general health of children and young adults, we see weak and vulnerable immune systems; we see them eating junk food, white flour, and white sugar, and living other components of an unhealthy lifestyle. It may be useful, in the face of infectious-disease outbreaks, to focus on building our children's immune systems by following a healthy organic diet, eliminating white sugar, white flour, grains with gluten and glia-din (a component of gluten), pesticides and herbicides, meat, and dairy, and instead following a diet high in organic, mineral-rich, plant-source nutrition supplemented with vitamin C, vitamin D, zinc, and vitamin A.

Vitamin A is highly specific and successful for ameliorating serious measles outcomes, hospitalizations, and deaths. Available but limited research shows that taking 200,000 IU of vitamin A for approximately three days and 100,000 IU for another week can significantly ameliorate serious effects. We additionally strongly suggest an herbal combination called Mega Defense preventively (at least one capsule twice a day for children, double that amount for adults, and triple that amount during a measles infection). These basic Chinese herbs include such key players as *Agaricus blazei* (*hime*-matsutake mushroom), *Lentinula edodes* (shiitake mushroom), *Grifola frondosa* (maitake, or hen-of-the-woods mushroom), reishi *(ling zhi)* mushroom, *Cordyceps sinesis* (caterpillar mushroom), amla berry extract, *Trametes versicolor* (turkey tail mushroom), *Pleurotus eryngii* (king trumpet mushroom), *Hericium erinaceus* (lion's mane mushroom), *Ocimum tenuiflorum,* also known as *Ocimum sanctum* (holy basil), and ginger, in the proper ratios for optimal function.

Building the immune system is safer than risking serious adverse effects. Since 2005 there have been no deaths in the United States from measles of the wild variety, yet there have been at least 108 deaths in a ten-year span, according to VAERS (the CDC's Vaccine Adverse Event Reporting System), from the MMR vaccine, sixty-eight of these in children under three years of age.[33] Other data suggest as many as 120 deaths from the MMR vaccine since 2005.

A survey of 635 children in the Netherlands in 2004[34] found German measles and whooping cough to be twice as common in unvaccinated children as vaccinated. However, throat inflammations, ear infections, rheumatologic problems, seizures, and febrile convulsions happened in the vaccinated at a much higher rate. There was also an increase in overall depletion of the immune system, and disordered neurological systems, in vaccinated children. There were eight times more aggressive behavior episodes in vaccinated children, and more sleep disorders. Thirty-three percent of vaccinated children required tonsillectomies, compared with 7.3% in the unvaccinated. When we look at the whole picture, it is hard to avoid the significant question of risks versus benefits.

The measles vaccine has a long list of serious adverse reactions that affect nearly every organ and body system—blood, lymph, cardiovascular, immune, nervous, respiratory, and sensory. Severe adverse reactions include encephalitis, the lethal subacute sclerosing panencephalitis, Guillain-Barré syndrome, convulsions, ataxia, multiform arrhythmia, deafness, and more.[35] Live-virus measles vaccines may also be associated with Crohn's disease (chronic inflammation of the bowel).[36] In 1995 *The Lancet* reported thirteen times more Crohn's disease and ulcerative colitis in people vaccinated for measles.[37] These serious, debilitating, and/or life-threatening clinical and scientific findings significantly contradict claims that vaccines are safe.

In addition to these documented serious adverse reactions, there is the disputed question of the possible link between the MMR vaccination and autism. Although the CDC maintains that there is no such link, their position is challenged by over 165 independent studies demonstrating that the mercury-based preservative thimerosal in this vaccine, as well as other vaccine components such as human DNA and aluminum, are in fact associated with autism.[38]

On September 23, 2014, an Italian court in Milan awarded compensation to a boy for vaccine-induced autism. The court ruled, based on scientific evidence presented, that a vaccine against six diseases caused the boy's brain damage and autism. The presiding judge, Nicola Di Leo, considered in his decision a previously unpublished, 1,271-page GlaxoSmithKline report providing ample evidence of adverse effects from the vaccine.[39] Amazingly enough, it included five known resulting cases of autism during the vaccine's clinical trials.

The Italian court's decision is important because it confirmed a vaccine-autism link. The court's decisions found that both the MMR and a hexavalent thimerosal and aluminum-containing vaccine can trigger autism. This is the second of two autism cases that have been judicially decided in Italy as caused by vaccines. Other cases in the UK, as well as many more in Italy, have further confirmed the vaccine-autism link regardless of the denials of pro-vaccine doctors and other vaccine promoters. Dr. William Thompson's unedited research at the CDC in 2004 showed an occurrence of autism approximately 336% that of the general population, in Afro-American children who received the MMR vaccination.

THE MYTH THAT VACCINES ELIMINATE DISEASE

When did the trend in infectious disease diminish? A CDC fact sheet cites vaccination programs in the U.S. as the main cause for reducing and eliminating many diseases. However, it does not mention the fact that there was a dramatic drop in disease, associated mainly with improved public health hygiene, that began at the turn of the twentieth century. In these graphs, one can see that most vaccines were not introduced until the last 4% of that reduction was already occurring.

MEASLES VACCINATION

THE FIRST MEASLES VACCINE WAS INTRODUCED IN 1963.

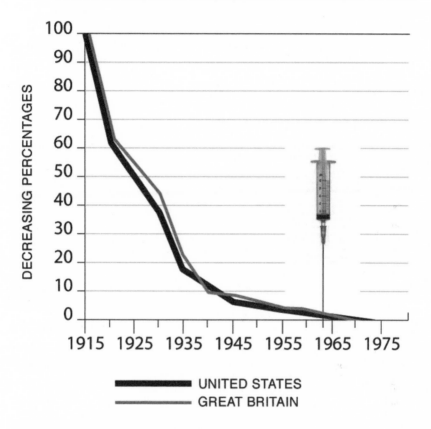

Graph showing the decrease in deaths from measles, leading up to the introduction of the measles vaccine in 1963. Graph created by Jared Krikorian from Figure 31 in *Vaccine Safety Manual* by Neil Z. Miller, with permission from the author.

PERTUSSIS VACCINATION

THE FIRST PERTUSSIS VACCINE WAS INTRODUCED IN 1927.

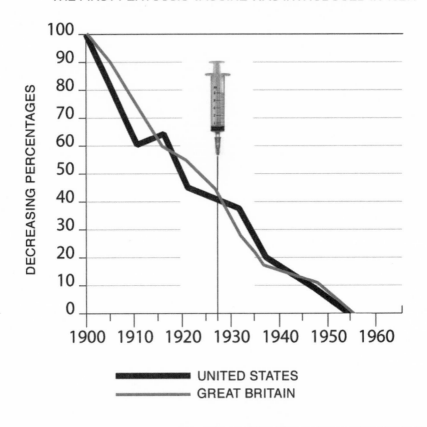

UNITED STATES
GREAT BRITAIN

Graph showing the decrease in deaths from pertussis, leading up to the introduction of the pertussis vaccine in 1927. Graph created by Jared Krikorian from Figure 25 in *Vaccine Safety Manual* by Neil Z. Miller, with permission from the author.

POLIO VACCINATION

THE FIRST POLIO VACCINE WAS INTRODUCED IN 1952.
THE ORAL POLIO VACCINE WAS INTRODUCED IN 1962.

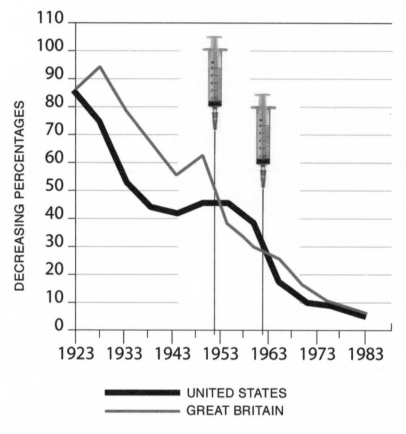

UNITED STATES
GREAT BRITAIN

Graph showing the decrease in deaths from polio, leading up to the introduction of polio vaccines in 1952 and 1962. Graph created by Jared Krikorian from Figure 10 in *Vaccine Safety Manual* by Neil Z. Miller, with permission from the author.

The National Bureau for Economic Research makes the point that mortality rates declined steadily and rapidly throughout the twentieth century. David Francis summarizes this fact: "Except for a ten-year period between 1955 and 1965, when the mortality rate was essentially flat, mortality rates have declined at a relatively constant rate of 1–2% yearly since 1900." [40]

If vaccines are responsible for this drop in disease, we should have seen mortality rates drop sharply in the latter half of the century as more vaccines were introduced. The report also mentions that by the mid-twentieth century a decline in death by infectious diseases was also assisted by the introduction of medical measures such as antibiotics, which have been especially helpful for the elderly as well as for young children.

Twenty-five percent of the reduction in child mortality in the U.S. occurred before World War II, and nearly ninety percent of the decline in child mortality from infectious disease occurred before 1940. Neither antibiotics nor vaccines were readily available before this time, nullifying the idea that vaccines and antibiotics were primarily responsible for the decline.

It is possible that these statistics reflect something very different from antibiotics or vaccines. Most analysts agree that major declines in child mortality in the first third of the twentieth century can be credited to public-health improvements in water treatment, food safety, solid-waste disposal, housing, and education about hygienic practices. Dr. Harris Coulter, an expert on the pertussis vaccine and author of *A Shot in the Dark,* states that the incidence of infectious disease began dropping around 1930, and that after World War II it continued to drop with further improvements in hygiene. The epidemiological data therefore refutes claims that vaccines are the main cause for reducing or eliminating acute diseases in the twentieth century.

The overall statistics suggest that vaccines have decreased infectious-disease occurrence by perhaps 2–4%. But since all of these diseases have been dramatically dropping since the turn of the twentieth century, before the introduction of vaccinations, even this 2–4% may be part of the same general trend. The vaccines emerged only at the very end of that dramatic drop. Vaccines do seem to help to a limited extent—but we must also consider the alarming collateral damage.

The Ethical Problem of Mandatory Vaccination

The argument of having to vaccinate one's children "for the good of the state" is scientifically questionable given what we have shared here. This argument is further compromised by the fact, for example, that the measles vaccine used in the United States is specifically effective for type A measles, and doesn't protect against the B3 or twenty-one other measles-virus genotypes, or from the documented transmission of the live virus by vaccinated children.

This new measles vaccine information resembles the pattern of failure associated with the flu vaccine—especially in children less than five years old, and in the elderly, where it has no proven efficacy. Desiring mandatory vaccination is therefore neither a scientifically based nor an ethical position of the state. It is, however, a common argument in totalitarian societies that "This is for the good of the collective."

According to the Nuremberg Code, medical ethics dictate that no one should be forced to undergo a medical treatment without informed consent to that treatment. This is especially important considering the apparently increasing lack of effectiveness of vaccination in populations even with vaccination rates as high as 97–100%. It brings to mind the forced sterilizations of the 1920s and '30s, the Tuskegee medical experiments that intentionally infected black prison inmates with syphilis, and the Nazi medicine that included involuntary euthanasia, experimentation, and sterilization—all "for the good of the state."

It is important that we protect ourselves against this sort of abuse of power. The push to vaccinate for the overall "collective good" has unfortunately already been abused, and continues to be. For example, the *Guardian* (September 26, 2000) reported the use of a virulent measles vaccine (Edmonson B vaccine) by a geneticist studying the indigenous Yanomami people of Venezuela. His measles vaccination "killed hundreds and thousands of indigenous people", "for the good of science."

According to Professor Terry Turner of Cornell University, "In its scale, ramifications, and sheer criminality and corruption, it is unparalleled in the history of anthropology."[41]

Is the state entitled to control our children's lives, and put our children at risk? Using the measles vaccine as an example of this medical-legal issue, we have grave doubts about the efficacy of the measles vaccination to protect our children, and documented evidence of its potential harm. Further complicating the decision is that safety tests are not done by the FDA, and have never been done. Almost every vaccine insert says, "not tested for adverse health effects." In terms of ethics and parental responsibility, there is a clear conflict of interest between governmental and/or pharmaceutical interests and parents who choose not to vaccinate their children for the well-being of those children and their overall quality of life into adulthood. The idea of mandatory vaccinations makes a mockery of the right of informed consent.

The definition of informed consent is to be fully informed without the intervention of force, fraud, deceit, duress, or other ulterior forms of constraint or coercion. But there is so much disinformation about measles-vaccine safety, effectiveness, and "herd immunity" that fully informed consent is not easily attained. Parents have to take real time to do research and become informed.

It is unethical, immoral, and contrary to the Nuremberg Code to force vaccination without consent. Vaccination is a medical treatment with risks that include death. It is utterly antithetical to all medical ethics to mandate that risk for others.

Given the complexity of the topic, the public controversy, and the fear-based statements, along with the actual scientific epidemiological data, the illusory and questionable "good of the collective" is a hard argument to make. Forced vaccinations may in time also be seen as causing a global weakening of the collective health, considering long-term studies about the other mental, chronic disease, and immune-weakening effects of vaccination, in addition to the short-term and acute problems associated with them.

Vaccination is a medical treatment that falls under the protection of informed consent. Informed consent is a basic human right, and is a parent's right in both ethics and law. Vaccinations are not harmless. About 2,000 severe reactions are reported each year (estimated to be 1–10% of the actual total by former FDA director Dr. David Kessler), resulting in prolonged hospitalization, permanent disability, and/or death. Over three billion dollars have been paid as settlements to victims of vaccine reactions. But no one has died of wild measles since 2005. Measles is not the bubonic plague, or ebola. Knowing the epidemiological facts, the risks versus the benefits of vaccination, and the possible causes of the Disneyland measles outbreak (most likely unrelated to unvaccinated children) will not incline us to forfeit our right to informed consent.

To help put it in perspective, the chance of being killed or injured by the measles vaccine, as previously mentioned, is actually greater than being killed or injured by wild measles itself. And if we move towards living with generally good health habits and eating a good diet, we will even further significantly decrease our children's susceptibility to all of these relatively harmless diseases.

Deciding for Ourselves: Informed Consent

Excess fear, public agency pressure, and social criticism are forcing children to submit to vaccinations against better parental judgment. Uninformed, uneducated school administrators, legal authorities, and pediatricians put pressure on parents. But this is not aligned with the medical or ethical meaning of informed consent which, according to the Nuremberg Code, is a decision without the intervention of force, deceit, duress, or other forms of coercion. The bottom line is that informed consent cannot happen if one is not properly informed.

In order to develop a truly informed consent, if they are to consent to vaccination, thoughtful parents need to do a serious risk/benefit analysis now that we have some knowledge of the real risks versus the potential benefits. We also need to regain perspective on the level of risks that these childhood diseases—which have been fading out since the early 1900s—actually pose. As we gain perspective and calm our media-stoked fears, we will be able to make thoughtful decisions. We will be able to optimize the long-term health and well-being of our children based on real science rather than on fear and manipulated studies from an allopathic medical community that appears to have lost perspective for a variety of reasons.

As concerned parents and grandparents with an instinctual, God-given duty to protect and optimize the health of our children and grandchildren—for their survival and the very survival of the species—it is important that we do all we can to educate ourselves and to listen to informed people guided by love and science.

INFORMED CONSENT REQUIRES
FULL SCIENTIFIC DISCLOSURE

Our primary focus in this chapter is to raise awareness among parents and grandparents of the potential vaccination risks, which have both short- and long-term, life-changing consequences. This information is generally insufficiently revealed by doctors, so that fully informed consent by parents is not possible. This crucial information is also often entirely missing from ads that promote vaccines. We parents and grandparents have a moral obligation, responsibility, and right to protect our children from harm, no matter what the economics, politics, or fear-based social pressures may be. This is similar to right-to-know issues about labeling GMOs, as is done in sixty-four other countries.

In order to make an informed decision about childhood vaccinations, one needs to know what the actual data is on both the upside and the downside of the issue. In the past few decades, we have seen a notable decline in communicable diseases such as polio, the plague, diphtheria, small pox, scarlet fever, measles, and whooping cough, while other serious diseases such as cancer, type 1 and type 2 diabetes, autoimmune disorders, and autism are skyrocketing.

Is the reduction of certain diseases a result of vaccination use? Even more disturbing is the possibility that we are putting ourselves at high risk for other serious chronic threats and health debilitation through the very practice of vaccination. According to a recent Internet article entitled "10 Reasons Why Flu Shots are More Dangerous than the Flu," we see that "a systematic review of 51 studies involving 260,000 children age 6–23 months found no evidence that the flu vaccine is any more effective than a placebo."[42] Researchers tell us:

> Medical journals have published thousands of articles revealing that injecting vaccines can actually lead to serious health problems including harmful immunological responses and a host of other infections. This further increases the body's susceptibility to the disease that the vaccine was supposed to protect against.[43]

Here in the United States, as mentioned above, we are also now seeing measles outbreaks occurring in schools where the vaccination rate is over 98%. One measles outbreak occurred in a school where 100% of the children had been vaccinated. Where measles occur in a population vaccinated at rates of 98–100%, we can't blame the unvaccinated, or use herd-immunity theory to explain it. By contrast, we see that there was a 97% decline in measles in London before the measles vaccine was instituted.[44]

INFORMED CONSENT REQUIRES KNOWLEDGE OF ACUTE ADVERSE EFFECTS

Another downside to vaccines includes a host of acute side effects. According to the CDC, the side effects of routine childhood vaccinations include: soreness, redness, swelling (at the injection site), fever (sometimes over 102°), nausea, vomiting, fatigue, poor appetite, diarrhea, abdominal pain, muscular and joint pain, swelling of glands, fainting, nonstop crying, temporary low platelet count, rash, hives, seizures, long-term seizures, loss of consciousness, permanent brain damage, coma, deafness, and illness resembling Guillain-Barré syndrome (GBS).[45] Another of many examples of acute or chronic post vaccination reactions is that those who received MMR vaccine are at greater risk for ITP (idiopathic thrombocytopenic purpura).[46] ITP is a serious autoimmune bleeding disorder, one of many documented autoimmune disorders that appear to increase with vaccinations. One study showed that children were six times more likely to develop ITP in the six weeks immediately following

MMR vaccination. True informed consent involves awareness of these potential trade-offs.

When we look at the well-documented acute adverse reactions, and at the chronic diseases that may result from vaccinations, we see that there are real life-crippling or -ending dangers, including Guillain-Barré syndrome, paralysis, seizures, unconsciousness, convulsions, swelling, chest pains, heart irregularity, kidney failure, vision problems, difficulty breathing, rashes, persistent vomiting, miscarriages, menstrual irregularities, reproductive-system complications, genital warts, vaginal lesions, and many levels of chronic disease, including asthma, atopic dermatitis, allergies, and ADHD, as well as death. While the CDC assures us that serious side effects are rare, the fact remains that the U.S. government has paid out over $2 billion to compensate families whose children have been seriously injured or have died as a result of vaccination.[47] To win such cases, the evidence must leave no shadow of a doubt. Vaccinations, according to these U.S. courts, are not safe.

The estimate by David Kessler, former commissioner of the FDA, as reported in the 1993 *Journal of the American Medical Association,* is that the documented cases of serious adverse vaccine side effects represent less than 1% of the actual occurrences, and by some estimates as high as 10%. In other words, what is reported to the CDC may be only one tenth—perhaps one hundredth—of what is actually happening.

INFORMED CONSENT REQUIRES KNOWLEDGE
OF LONG-TERM ADVERSE EFFECTS

Chronic diseases' link to vaccines must also be considered. Increased rates of cancer, for instance, are emerging in association with certain vaccinations. In 2002, the major British medical journal *Lancet* reported that a SV40-virus-contaminated polio vaccine was responsible for up to half of the 55,000 non-Hodgkins lymphoma patients that were occurring each year.[48] The SV40 virus has been found in a variety of cancers including lung, brain, bone, and lymphatic cancers. Data indicates that the SV40 virus causes malignancy. It has now been identified in 43% of cases of non-Hodgkins lymphoma,[49] and 36% of brain tumors.[50]

Jonas Salk's insights that vaccinations may cause the disease they are meant to protect against may have come from the unintentional results of his own experiments with the polio vaccine. According to the CDC, the last case of wild polio that was non-vaccine-associated occurred in 1979. From 1980 to 1999, there were no cases of wild polio. However, there were at least 144 cases of polio associated with the live vaccine during this period. There were also outbreaks of polio in the Dominican Republic and Haiti in 2002, which were also traced back to the polio vaccine.

In Nigeria, there was a serious outbreak of polio related to polio vaccination. Nigeria also has had a significant occurrence of autism. Thousands of children died after the polio vaccine was introduced in Uganda. In Zimbabwe, infant mortality tripled between 1990 and 2010, which is when most vaccines were added to the national vaccine schedule. In Australia, Archie Kalokerinos, MD, has pointed out in his book *Every Second Child*[51] that half of all vaccinated Aboriginal children died within days of being vaccinated. Many of these children in underdeveloped areas have extremely weak immune systems, and are simply unable to tolerate the immune stress of vaccination.

The epidemiological case studies of the polio vaccine are important in understanding the possible chronic effects of vaccinations, including infection with the disease itself. As previously mentioned, Dr. Jonas Salk himself, who created the killed-virus vaccine used in the 1950s, testified in 1976 that the live-virus vaccine that was used almost exclusively in the U.S. between 1960 and 2000 was "the principal, if not the sole, cause of all reported cases of polio in the U.S. since 1961."[52] Dr. Salk pointed out that the virus remained in the throat for one to two weeks, and in the feces for up to two months. Vaccine recipients themselves are at risk, and could also act as carriers of the disease to others, as long as fecal excretion of the virus continued.[53]

It is no accident that in 1992 the CDC published an admission that the live-virus vaccine had become the dominant cause of polio in the United States.[54] The CDC figures showed that every case of polio in the U.S. since 1979 was caused by the oral polio vaccine.[55] This strengthens the point that vaccinated children can indeed act as carriers of the live virus they have been vaccinated with. Vaccines cannot be considered safe.

The polio vaccine, as mentioned, has also been associated with a variety of cancers, including brain tumors and leukemia, some of its serious cross-generational, long-term chronic adverse effects. A study of 59,000 women birthed from mothers who had received the Salk vaccine between 1959 and 1965 revealed brain tumors occurring at a rate thirteen times that of women whose mothers did not receive the polio shot.[56] [57]

In April 2001, sixty-two papers from thirty laboratories around the world reported that the SV40 virus was in the tissue of tumors.[58] Dr. David Oshinsky, in his book *Polio: An American Story,* points out that both Jonas Salk and Albert Sabin, who developed Salk and Sabin vaccines, knew that the early vaccines were contaminated with a number of viruses, to which over 100 million people have now been exposed.[59] They knew this because Dr. Bernice Eddy, a microbiologist at the National Institutes of Health, proved that the SV40 virus was present in both killed and live polio vaccines, and caused cancer, particularly of the brain and nervous system.[60]

Adverse Effects of Vaccination

PHYSICAL ADVERSE EFFECTS

Perhaps more important in the parental decision-making process is the newer information that vaccinations are being linked to modern-day chronic illnesses such as type 1 and type 2 diabetes, developmental disorders, Asperger's syndrome and spectrum autism, brain tumors, leukemia, asthma, Crohn's disease, intestinal disorders, impulsive violence, and allergies. All of these were rare in children before the introduction of vaccinations.[61] Vaccinations have also been associated with increased incidence of ADD and ADHD.[62]

To establish clear evidence about the adverse results of vaccinations, a study that compares the health status of vaccinated versus unvaccinated people is called for. It is shocking to say that such an obvious study has never been undertaken by the CDC or any other agency of the U.S.

government in the last fifty years, even though the number of vaccinations have accelerated yearly.

Fortunately, other countries have done such studies. These studies comparing vaccinated and unvaccinated children reveal that a number of acute reactions may arise; but perhaps more significant and serious from a parent's point of view are the chronic long-term effects. A German study released in September 2011 compared approximately 8,000 unvaccinated and vaccinated children from 0–19 years in age. They found that the vaccinated children had two to five times more chronic diseases and disorders than the unvaccinated children.[63] This is highly significant information for a parent who wants to develop a truly informed consent.

Presently, about half the children in the U.S. suffer from some chronic disease, and 21% are developmentally disabled.[64] One in six children is seriously developmentally disabled. This cannot all be blamed on vaccinations, of course, but the evidence suggests that they play a significant synergistic role. The Salzburger Study, an ongoing survey on 1,004 unvaccinated children at the time of this publication, has found that 0% had asthma, compared to 8–12% of the vaccinated child population. They found that atopic dermatitis occurred in 1.2% of unvaccinated children, compared to 10–20% in the vaccinated population. Allergies were found in 3% of unvaccinated children, versus 25% in the vaccinated population. ADHD was in 0.79% of the unvaccinated children, versus 5–10% in the vaccinated population.[65] These chronic disease sequelae suggest another level of vaccine disabilities associated in particular with immune, autoimmune, and neurological chronic debilitation.

A 1992 New Zealand survey studied 254 children, of whom 133 were vaccinated and 121 were unvaccinated. Fifteen percent of the vaccinated children developed asthma, while only 3% of unvaccinated children developed asthma. Thirty-two percent of vaccinated children developed eczema and allergic reactions, while only 13% of unvaccinated children developed eczema and allergic reactions. Twenty percent of vaccinated children had chronic otitis, while only 7% of unvaccinated children had chronic otitis. Eight percent of vaccinated children had recurrent tonsillitis, while only 2% of unvaccinated children had recurrent tonsillitis.

Seven percent of vaccinated children experienced shortness of breath or sudden infant death syndrome (SIDS), compared to 2% of unvaccinated children. There was an eightfold difference in hyperactivity between vaccinated (8%) and unvaccinated children (1%).[66]

The results from these international studies speak clearly for themselves: Vaccinations are distinctly associated with at least some increase in chronic disease, particularly with immune, neurological, and central nervous system-based dysfunction and disease. Newer research also indicates that vaccines appear to weaken the immune system.

In 1977, a Russian study found that adults exposed to methylmercury or ethylmercury suffered brain damage years later.[67] Thimerosal, a mercury-based preservative used in vaccines and other products, was also found to create tubular necrosis in the kidneys, and nervous-system injury including coma and death.[68] As a result of these findings, Russia banned thimerosal from children's vaccines in 1980.[69] Denmark, Austria, Japan, Great Britain, and the Scandinavian countries have also banned the preservative. Presently they have taken thimerosal out of most U.S. vaccines with the exception of the flu vaccination, which they are still recommending for pregnant women and children. Each vaccination contains 25 micrograms of mercury per 0.5 mL (half-milliliter) dose. If these are given yearly, mercury will accumulate in the body to far beyond the acceptable level of toxicity, at least 25 times higher than "acceptable, safe" levels.

There are additional serious complications with vaccines, including death and Guillain-Barré syndrome, an autoimmune demyelinating syndrome that occurs in both children and adults. John Hopkins School of Medicine scientist Dr. Peter Doshi, in the *BMJ* (*British Medical Journal*), has strongly warned against the flu vaccine, saying that the only randomized trial of influenza vaccine done in older people found no decrease in deaths among those vaccinated. Doshi states, in an article entitled "Influenza: marketing vaccines by marketing disease":

> Few people realize that even the ideal influenza vaccine, matched perfectly to circulating strains of wild influenza and capable of

stopping all influenza viruses, can only deal with a small part of the "flu" problem…. Every year, hundreds of thousands of respiratory specimens are tested across the U.S. Of those tested, on average 16% are found to be influenza-positive…. It's no wonder so many people feel that "flu shots" don't work: for most flus, they can't.[70]

Dr. Doshi also points out that according to an Australian study, one in 110 children under the age of five had convulsions following vaccinations for the H1N1 influenza in 2009.[71] Another study found that the H1N1 vaccine was associated with increasing cases of narcolepsy among adolescents.[72] A 2014 study published in *Euro Surveillance* linked a fourteen-fold increase in narcolepsy with the H1N1 flu vaccine.[73] Narcolepsy is an incurable brain disorder theorized to be caused by autoimmune destruction of the brain cells responsible for maintaining wakefulness. A high percentage (90%) of these narcolepsy cases were flu-vaccinated children and adolescents.

Dr. Russell Blaylock, a well-known retired neurosurgeon, states that the H1N1 flu vaccine is completely worthless, and that the government knows it. Blaylock points out that the government recommends flu shots for the elderly to avoid secondary pneumonia, hospitalizations, and death. However, a study by the Cochrane Group, which studied hundreds of thousands of people, found that it offered zero protection for the specific things for which it is prescribed in the general community.[74] Another study found the flu shot to be perhaps 9% effective.[75]

Of particular concern, however, is the downside of the flu vaccine. As Dr. Blaylock points out, not only do children under five years of age receive no protection from it, they are still subject to the risk of serious adverse effects. Blaylock writes, "The government says that every baby over the age of six months should have the vaccine, and they know that it contains a dose of mercury that is toxic for the brain…. [and that] studies show that the flu vaccine has zero effectiveness in children under five."[76]

Dr. Blaylock further states that while flu vaccines don't prevent the flu, they do increase the odds of getting it, because the thimerosal in the vaccines acts as an immune suppressant. This immune suppression lasts for several weeks after the shot is administered, making people more susceptible to catching the flu. While the vaccine itself doesn't necessarily give them the flu, the temporarily suppressed immune system makes them vulnerable. Blaylock states, "The vast number of people who get the flu vaccine aren't going to get any benefit, but they get all the risks and complications."[77] In raising alive and conscious children, the same high risk/low benefit mechanisms are at play, as well as with the elderly.

Unfortunately, the relatively new "science" of virus and vaccination information does not offer a lot of definitive answers—with several exceptions. One is the very well-established and significantly documented association of both acute and chronic adverse effects with vaccinations, dismissed and denied by pro-vaccine allopathic doctors and pharmaceutical companies; when we examine the international data as we have just done, the ironic question arises as to who are the actual "vaccine deniers." Another is the established fact that recently vaccinated people are active carriers and transmitters of the disease who have been shown to infect both the unvaccinated and the vaccinated for a period of at least two weeks. And, finally, the myth of herd immunity is being exposed.

Except in these few areas, information that we need in order to make truly informed consent is missing due to a lack of research in the emerging field of vaccine and viral science. Specifically, we are missing information that could lead to an understanding of the negative ramifications of mass vaccination versus its short-term efficacy (fewer infections initially). Vaccine opponents may be surprised to hear us mention "short-term efficacy," but the statistics do show an initial "honeymoon" period of significant decrease in acute viral infection by measles, mumps, and pertussis. In other words, what some of the pro-vaccine allopathic doctors claim did indeed seem true for a period of time when vaccines were first instituted, during which there was a measurable drop in these infectious diseases.

The vaccines appear to create some level of short-term epidemiological remission, but this eventually gives way to a long-term resurgence in a stronger variety of the disease. For example, once the measles vaccine was properly developed around 1981, the number of reported measles cases did indeed drop initially. This honeymoon period ended in the mid- to late '80s, when thousands of cases of measles reemerged in the United States. The same pattern happened with chicken pox and pertussis. The reemergence of measles also occurred in China, with a 300% increase in the number of measles cases between 2012 and 2013. China, despite its 99% measles-vaccine compliance rate, had over 100,000 reported cases of measles, 50,000 of them confirmed.

What is going on? If full-population vaccination is supposed to work to prevent the disease, why is it getting worse, with infections among the vaccinated tripling even with essentially no unvaccinated children to blame? Vaccine viral science is significantly more complicated and less understood than the simplistic view of vaccine proponents. As evidenced by the recent measles outbreaks in China, South Korea, France, and the U.S., we have passed the "honeymoon" period in which the vaccines appear to be efficacious. The vaccine officials refer to this earlier period as a reason for continuing to do the same ineffective and possibly disastrous approach. We may be moving into a possibly pro-epidemic ecological phase of more virulent viruses generating epidemics that the newer and "improved" vaccines cannot stop, much like the "superbugs" that even newer antibiotics cannot treat.

One of the reasons for these vaccine failures is that the short-term efficacy of the vaccines essentially eliminated the natural wild virus. The wild-virus-infected people received more continual exposure to it throughout their lifetimes, which acted as a natural booster for their immunity. In other words, for immunity to be sustained there needs to be some wild virus circulating to induce immunity naturally.

Studies show that a reduction in the circulation of the natural chicken pox virus (due to the temporary efficacy of high vaccination rates) has actually been a causal factor in the epidemic increase of herpes zoster, which causes painful shingles in adults over fifty. In the past, adults relied on natural boosts to their immune system whenever they went out in public, which protected them against the varicella virus and ultimately shingles. The natural chickenpox virus circulating in the environment had provided natural antibodies that acted as booster shots for adults.

Although efficacious for children for a short time in reducing chicken pox, the vaccine has been associated with the increased outbreak of shingles in adults. Our society made a choice, in effect, to avoid chicken pox in children at an age when they can best handle it, at the expense of herpes zoster risk for adults. We have altered the ecology, and are experiencing the consequences. Vaccine recommendations now include herpes zoster shots for adults, in an attempt to undo this adverse effect.

The vaccination issue is far more complicated than the vaccination itself. Virus ecology needs to be part of this discussion if we are to address the entire vaccine issue intelligently. The basic ecology of viruses is that they mutate, becoming more virulent in order to cope with and overcome the vaccine. This is the way nature works. We see this in genetically modified plants that have become five times more resistant to glyphosates. We see this in bacteria that are becoming antibiotic-resistant, with virulent "superbugs" becoming the scourge of hospitals everywhere. We see this with antibiotic-resistant tuberculosis beginning to be a worldwide threat. These new antibiotic-resistant strains are often life-threatening.

Unfortunately, this is only part of the complicated story. The temporary partial efficacy of vaccines is enough that mothers no longer have natural antibodies against measles, and therefore fail to give their children protection against wild measles. Here, as before, the mothers had antibodies they had developed from the natural measles and shared with their babies through their breast milk and colostrum, protecting the babies for up to two years.

Research is beginning to indicate that, as the measles virus mutates, it has become more virulent for infants, teens, and elderly people rather than being confined, as in the past, to kindergarten through preteen ages. Grade-school years are when children can best defend against the disease. Short-term efficacy of a vaccine initially decreases the number of cases in this age group, but cases are now increasing in older children and adults as the virus mutates; over time, the number of infections among grade-school children has also increased.

Further complicating this concern is that the virus becomes more virulent in people who are vaccinated, as it mutates to survive the vaccine environment. This provides further danger for the unvaccinated, because the mutated wild or vaccine-associated measles virus can affect them more readily than vaccinated persons. It is important to note, as previously mentioned, that measles infection is presently seen mostly among the vaccinated, even in up to 99%-vaccinated populations such as China and certain U.S. states.

The idea of the initial quiescence and later activation of the virus over the years is not a new idea. The vaccine failures being reported as more and more children and adults contract measles were actually predicted by medical researchers. For example, Dr. David Levy in 1984 stated that the outbreaks were to be expected.[78] More recently, Dr. Heffernan in 2009 made predictions based on sophisticated mathematical computer analysis, in which he said:

> We predict that after a long disease-free period the introduction of infection will lead to far larger epidemics than that predicted by standard models…. Large-scale epidemics can arise, with the first substantial epidemic not arising until 52 years after the vaccination program has begun.[79]

For measles, that fifty-two-year period ends in 2015.

An additional consideration, as we see with the mutating flu virus and the resulting mass failure of flu vaccination, is that the measles virus does mutate, although not as fast as the flu virus. The same vaccine that may work for a five-year-old will be less effective for people at other ages at other times over the following years. The measles virus does mutate, although not as fast as with the flu. There is also genetic variation to consider. Research by Dr. Gregory Poland of the Mayo Clinic, editor-in-chief of the journal *Vaccine* as of 2015, is exploring the fallacy of the "one vaccine fits all" theory as it relates to the fact that we're all genetically different.[80]

This theory is not working effectively, as evidenced by Dr. Thompson's study, showing that African-American children experienced 3.36 times more autism in response to the MMR vaccination. He suggests that we develop a new measles vaccine to better fit variations in racial and ethnogenetic populations. The vaccines may also need to be different according to diet and vitamin A sufficiency, as these also affect our cellular immune status, the key defense mechanism against the measles virus. From this perspective we can see why there is a significant number of vaccine failures. We may even raise the question of not "who is immune?" but rather, "who is susceptible?"—which may not be the same question as who is or is not vaccinated.

In his research Dr. Poland shows that persons taking vitamin A, an important supplement for measles prevention and treatment, actually upgrade the epigenetic profile of their immune function. This brings us back to the debate from the 1800s between Louis Pasteur (founder of the "germ theory" on which allopathic medicine and vaccine theory are based) and Dr. Antoine Béchamp and Dr. Claude Bernard, who posited, "The microbe is nothing, while the terrain is everything." Their teaching was that fortifying the biological "terrain" is the key to protection against disease. This way of approaching disease is called pleomorphic medicine, as distinct from allopathic medicine. One's general health becomes the most important aspect of protection against viral illnesses and their effects. Many holistic physicians emphasize this approach.

Neil Z. Miller, who cites the link between measles vaccinations and cancer, highlights another serious ecological consideration.[81] The wild measles virus has been found to have oncolytic (anticancer) properties. Children who contract natural wild virus measles appear to be significantly protected against cancer later in life. Measles infections have even been found to create tumor remissions. This is well documented in the medical literature. In this context, children vaccinated against measles are being deprived of this oncolytic protection for their lifetime.

Several studies highlight the link between natural measles infections and cancer prevention. For example, Albonico et al. found that adults who had had childhood measles appeared to be protected against genital, prostate, skin, and lung cancer.[82] This protection was also found to a lesser extent with rubella. Montella et al. found that those who contracted wild measles had significantly less risk of developing leukemia.[83] Alexander et al. found that measles during childhood was associated with a 50% reduced risk of Hodgkin's disease in adults.[84] Glaser et al. found that after measles, mumps, and rubella in childhood, there is a reduced risk of lymph cancer.[85] Gilham et al. found that infants with the least exposure to common infections had the greatest risk of developing childhood leukemia.[86] Urayama et al. found that exposure to infections appears to be protective against leukemia.[87]

The point is that not only measles, but also other infectious diseases early in life, seem to protect against cancers later in life. This is a most interesting finding. Furthermore, children who are not the firstborn have fewer cancers than their older siblings, apparently due to more exposure to more illnesses. Children who attend daycare early are protected against cancers for the same reasons.

There is a major trade-off here. Babies and children who are unvaccinated and who become naturally infected with measles decrease their chances of cancer in adulthood. The vaccinated, on the other hand, have increased cancer rates. It's not for us to say which trade-off a parent may want, but it is important for parents to know there is a trade-off—this is true informed consent.

MENTAL AND BEHAVIORAL ADVERSE EFFECTS ASSOCIATED WITH VACCINATION

Eight million people in the United States suffer from severe clinical depression. About forty million adults in the U.S. suffer from moderate depression, and evidence indicates that vaccines may be contributing to this depression epidemic.

Vaccines cause the release of inflammatory cytokines that lower serotonin secretion. Serotonin has an antidepressant affect on the brain, and a deficiency of serotonin may increase the risk of glutamate, an excitotoxin that overactivates and destroys brain cells, and appears in spinal fluid and blood plasma. This is the same glutamate found in hydrolyzed soy protein and MSG (monosodium glutamate).

There's a great deal of research demonstrating and connecting chronic low-level brain inflammation created by child vaccinations with both elevated brain glutamine levels and depression. Many animal studies show that vaccinations increase inflammatory cytokines.

Children may also suffer from postvaccine encephalitis, either sub-clinical or clinical. Our children are exposed to a staggering amount of brain toxins in general. In July of 2005, the Environmental Working Group released a study of chemical exposure in newborns. They identified 287 chemicals in umbilical cords. Of these, 180 were carcinogens, and 217 were toxic to the brain and nervous system. About 208 were associated with birth defects.[88] These toxins tend to work synergistically with each other, maximizing toxicity when vaccines are later given. Infants have an immature immune system for the first several years of life, but vaccinations typically begin from day one to two months of age, and are given all given at once, which is potentially overwhelming. These vaccinations contain approximately sixty-six viral antigens, and a dozen different chemicals.

By the time a child is five years old and weighs about forty pounds, they will typically have received thirty-five injections. (Some estimate up to sixty-eight injections.) These will contain at least 110 weakened pathogens, and fifty-nine chemicals. If all recommended shots are administered, the child will have been injected with stray viral DNA and at least four types of animal tissues including pig and aborted human fetal tissue. These ingredients are all listed on the inserts, so it isn't a secret if one reads the fine print.

According to the U.S. Surgeon General, approximately twenty percent of American children and adolescents suffer from a mental disorder so significant that it interferes with their day-to-day life.[89] Is this a surprise, given how they start life? Typical diagnoses of these children and adolescents include behavior disorders, ADHD, hyperactivity, learning disabilities, a spectrum of speech delay, comprehension issues, and mood disorders that can include depression, bipolar disorder, anxiety, autism, and autism-spectrum diagnoses. An Oregon study of 900 boys showed that vaccinated boys had a 155% greater chance of having a neurological disorder, such as ADHD or autism, than the unvaccinated boys.[90]

The CDC estimates that over 5.4 million children ages four to seventeen have been diagnosed with ADHD, according to 2007 data.[91] This represents about one in ten children, and the numbers are increasing each year. Many of these children are medicated with Ritalin, which further disrupts normal brain function and development. Ritalin has been shown to delay or stunt growth, as it suppresses the release of growth hormone. Ritalin and similar drugs have also been implicated in increased susceptibility to drug addiction, especially to cocaine, in the teen and older years. Ritalin mimics a slow-acting cocaine.

Another behavioral disorder is oppositional defiant disorder (ODD), which typically manifests around age eight. Symptoms include frequent loss of temper, excessive arguing with adults, defying requests, refusing to follow rules, deliberately annoying others, and blaming others for mistakes and behavior. As of 2008, ODD was the most common reason for kids being referred to mental-health professionals. Most of these patients are boys, and they often end up on psychotropic drugs. Unfortunately, these allopathic treatments are neither orthomolecular or an organic, live-food diet, but antidepressants, mood-stabilizers, antipsychotics, and sedatives.

Clinical experience in holistic and orthomolecular psychiatry finds that many of these imbalances can be corrected through good nutrition and supplements. A recent sixty-nine-month study identified a total of 484 drugs given to children and teens and associated with 780,169 adverse reactions including violence and aggressive behavior.[92] Unfortunately, these drugs were also associated with 387 homicides, 404 physical assaults, 27 cases of physical abuse, 896 homicidal ideation reports, and 223 cases of violence-related symptoms.

Drugs used in an attempt to treat ODD include eleven antidepressants such as SSRIs (selective serotonin uptake inhibitors, including Lexapro, Paxil, and Zoloft), six sedative hypnotics (including Xanax and Klonopin, which may interact adversely with Zoloft), three drugs given for ADHD (including Ritalin and Concerta), and several antipsychotics (Seroquel, Zyprexa, and Risperdal). All these: vaccinations, pesticides, herbicides, heavy metals such as mercury, and psychotropic drugs cause inflammation, and synergistically react to significantly disorder our children's brains and nervous systems. We cannot of course blame all these symptoms on vaccines, but they are part of a complex synergy of toxic disruptive forces on our children's brains and bodies that we of course want to minimize if possible.

The pertussis vaccine, perhaps the second oldest after the smallpox vaccine, has been found to have profound effects on the development of the brains of children, and was the first to be implicated in the growth of autism-spectrum statistics and permanent changes in behavior, personality, intelligence, and emotional stability. These changes were noted from 1939 until the mid-1980s. One of the elephants in the living room is the association of vaccines with violence in America. The brain swells in a postvaccine inflammation which, according to Dr. Blaylock, is unfortunately more common than we would like to believe. When the brain swells, the mind may get confused, agitated, and hostile, and kids may act out.

Brain inflammation has both acute and chronic effects. A variety of brain and nervous system disorders can happen in response to vaccines, such as subacute sclerosis, encephalitis, brachial plexitis, postvaccine encephalitis, transverse myelitis, and peripheral neuropathies. Serious, chronic, long-term vaccine side effects that have been reported include neurological damage, encephalitis, transverse myelitis, peripheral nerve damage, autism, seizures, mental retardation, language delays, behavioral problems, and multiple sclerosis. That means, if we vaccinate our children, we're unintentionally exposing them to a risk of any of these potentially debilitating effects.

Dr. William Howard Hay, a New York doctor, author, lecturer, and founder of The East Aurora Sun and Diet Sanatorium, who developed a system of food combining, summarizes his clinical experience:

> It is now thirty years that I have been confining myself to the treatment of chronic diseases. During those thirty years I have run against so many histories of little children who had never seen a sick day until they were vaccinated and who, in the several years that have followed, have never seen a well day since. I couldn't put my finger on the disease they have. They just weren't strong. Their resistance

was gone. They were perfectly well before they were vaccinated. They have never been well since.[93]

Brain swelling and toxicity from vaccines reduce people's ability to think, learn, and function in childhood and even as adults. Vaccines activate the brain's own immune system, intimately connected to the body's immune system and made up of protective scavenger cells called microglia. Once this system is activated, the astrocytes, another part of the brain's immune system, move around the brain like amoebas, secreting toxic amounts of inflammatory chemicals called cytokines. Two forms of these excitotoxins are glutamate and quinolinic acid, which put the brain into the chronically inflamed and swollen state we have been discussing.

When the brain is inflamed, it swells, and people feel sick. They might feel that they have the flu. They have trouble sleeping restfully. They suffer from headaches. The high-pitched cries a baby may emit soon after vaccinations, known as encephalitic crying, is also a symptom of this brain inflammation (encephalitis). If a baby is crying this way after a vaccination, its brain is swollen and inflamed. Vomiting, loss of consciousness, seizures, and irritability are also signs of an inflamed brain. Vaccines can increase the rate of seizures threefold.

Brain inflammation is more likely to happen when multiple vaccinations are received all at once. The resultant overactivation of the body's immune system leads to overactivation of the microglial cells and release of excitotoxins that may lead to seizures. Enough research has been done that neurologists see this mechanism of postvaccine brain swelling as fact rather than theory.

The human brain develops slowly. Although most brain development is accomplished in the first two years, the brain continues to develop as late as age twenty-seven. Vaccinations may disrupt this critical growth process and delay or block the unfolding brain functions. Symptoms of this disruption may manifest as impaired thinking, concentration, attention, behavior, and/or language development. Additionally, there are toxic metals in vaccinations—particularly heavy metals such as mercury and aluminum, and animal proteins—particularly gelatin, hydrolyzed protein, MSG, and unknown factors such as the FC30 virus. All of these inflame the brain, overstimulate its immune reaction, and lead to loss and disruption of brain function. This is not theory; it is a proven fact in the scientific literature.

These viruses affect the whole brain. The first round of vaccinations may prime the microglia to chronically secrete inflammatory cytokines and excitotoxins; additional vaccinations and infections may greatly aggravate the immuno-excitotoxic region of a child's brain, and this again can cause mental, developmental, and behavioral problems, all of which are currently rampant in our society. Before the 1970s, this was not the case.

The neuroscience behind all this is very clear. As more critical research challenges the unsubstantiated claims of "safety" and "efficacy" of vaccinations, those are considered more and more imaginary among holistic and homeopathic physicians as well as in a growing number of allopathic physicians. There is also a growing number of parents who have done their research and are concluding that vaccines are neither safe nor effective.

For all of these reasons, one should be very careful about allowing a pediatrician or public health professional to give multiple vaccinations as if there is no risk. No studies exist showing that infants are unaffected by a synergistic toxicity from the eight vaccines recommended in the U.S. schedule at ages two, four, and six months. There is, however, evidence that the more vaccines babies receive at one time, the more likely they will be hospitalized and/or die.[94]

We also have concerns about vaccines containing bacteria, viruses, viral fragments, and mycoplasma (a type of antibiotic-resistant bacteria), which can reside in the brain for a lifetime, causing chronic brain swelling and ultimately accelerating brain degeneration. This may be why we are seeing such an increase in Alzheimer's disease—it may start in our children with vaccinations, as part of a synergy of toxins. What we do with our children in terms of vaccinations and nutritional patterns will be with them for the rest of their lives, and can be positive or negative. For the informed parent and grandparent, there is reasonable concern that vaccines given early in life may affect brain and immune function for a lifetime. They may also make one susceptible to chronic diseases such as heart disease, autoimmune diseases, diabetes, and a variety of cancers.

It is interesting to note that this only applies to vaccine viruses. Wild viruses, such as measles, do not remain in the system after the infection if there is good cell-mediated, natural immunity.

Some vaccinations, besides increasing cancer rates, increase the rates of multiple sclerosis. It was found that people receiving a complete series of hepatitis B vaccines experience a 300% higher risk of developing MS compared to the unvaccinated public.[95] To further complicate the issue, low-virulence viruses that are attenuated or "killed" can be converted over a lifetime by free radicals into a potential for stronger viral effects.

In addition to the nervous system and mental complications that vaccines potentiate in our children, there is the issue of the SV40 virus, a polio-vaccine contaminant, has been distinctly linked to brain tumors, mesotheliomas, and osteosarcomas, medulloblastomas, ependymomas, and choroid plexus papillomas.[96] Most people infected with the SV40 virus in the polio vaccine have also passed this virus on to their children.

More and more informed physicians are beginning to comment on the real danger of vaccination:

> The vaccines are not working, and they are dangerous... We should be working with nature (Lendon Smith, MD, "The Children's Doctor," American obstetrician and gynecologist, pediatrician, author, and television personality).

THE AUTISM-VACCINE CONNECTION

Another tragic potential downside to vaccinations appears to be autism, which is still considered a debatable long-term adverse effect. A number of independent studies reveal the epidemiological correlations of vaccine schedules and autism. This, of course, is hotly contested by the CDC. A study on monkeys shows notable behavioral changes and development differences in vaccinated monkeys, compared to monkeys who were not vaccinated. (While this information has been given here to inform parents, it does not mean that the authors of this book support animal testing.) These changes include significant neurodevelopmental deficits, increase in gastrointestinal-tissue gene expression, and inflammation.[97]

These are all classic symptoms experienced by children with autism.

The association between autism and the MMR and pertussis vaccines is another area of much disagreement. The existence of autism was initially identified in 1943. People at first believed it to be a psychological problem caused by poor parenting. It was soon linked to the pertussis vaccine. Over time, many researchers, notably Dr. Andrew Wakefield, also implicated the MMR vaccine. In 1998, Wakefield published a landmark study linking MMR vaccination to autism.[98] This preliminary study of twelve patients was heavily attacked, and his paper was withdrawn. This active discrediting of Dr. Wakefield is now used as "scientific evidence" to support claims that there is no connection between autism and vaccinations.

Studies by F. Edward Yazbak also showed a direct correlation between MMR and autism, especially when given to mothers during pregnancy.[99] Adding to this debate, Dr. Walter Shilling published independent research suggesting that children who receive all the recommended vaccines "are approximately fourteen times more likely to become learning disabled, and eight times more likely to become autistic as compared to children who have not been vaccinated."[100] Dr. Mark Geier has published several studies linking autism with thimerosal in vaccines. These studies are all thoroughly reviewed in Neil Miller's book *Vaccine Safety Manual for Concerned Families and Health Practitioners*.[101]

The following graphs were taken from that book, and designed by Jared Krikorian with permission from the author. They clearly illustrate the epidemiological research for both the MMR vaccine and vaccines in general.

Also linked to the autism/brain-disruption spectrum of disorders are hyperactivity and brain dysfunction. Although vaccines appear to play the major—or least an associatively significant—role in causing autism, the disease has many other potential causal factors, including a particularly negative association with a variety of environmental toxicity factors. The data also clearly implicates a time-and-number association between autism and the number of vaccinations given, as well as the introduction of the MMR vaccines. We don't necessarily believe vaccinations are the

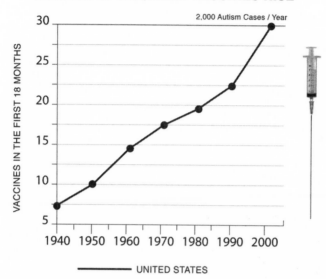

AUTISM CASES INCREASE AS THE NUMBER OF REQUIRED VACCINES RISE

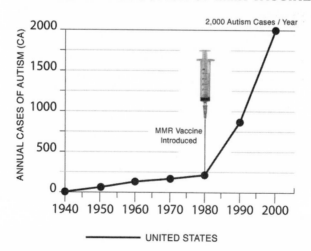

AUTISM CASES SOAR IN RELATIONSHIP TO THE INTRODUCTION OF MMR VACCINE

Graphs showing increase of autism rates correlative with intensification of vaccine schedules between 1940 and 2000. Graphs created by Jared Krikorian from Figure 52 in the *Vaccine Safety Manual* by Neil Z. Miller, with permission from the author.

sole cause of these debilitating effects on the nervous system and brain, but they seem to be a major factor that requires consideration.

While the pandemic rates of autism continue to rise among the vaccinated population, it is useful to point out that autism did not apparently occur before the 1940s—before pertussis, DPT, or MMR vaccinations became common. By the 1970s, the incidence of autism was one in 10,000. Now it is one in 68, and one in 42 among boys, according to the CDC. There are no cases of autism among the Amish, who have never vaccinated their children.

According to the late Mayer Eisenstein, MD, of Homefirst Medical Services in Chicago: "We have about 30,000 or 35,000 children that we've taken care of for years, and I don't think we have a single case of autism in children delivered by us who never received vaccines.... We do have a sample. The numbers are too large not to see it." Such strong epidemiological statements are hard to explain away through coincidence.

While numerous parents of autistic children have linked the disorder to their children's vaccinations, not all have been lucky enough to prove it in court. However, the vaccine-autism connection has been made in Italy, and was also reported by *The New York Times, Medical News Today*, and CNN, where Johns Hopkins neurologist Dr. Jon Poling and his wife Terry Poling, RN won U.S. government compensation for the vaccination-induced autism of their young daughter Hannah. In 2012, the court in Rimini, Italy also ruled that the MMR vaccine was responsible for the autism of one-year-old Valentine Bocca, who had an immediate reaction to the vaccination at the age of fifteen months.

According to the UK newspaper *The Independent*, about 100 similar cases are now being examined by Italian lawyers, and more cases may appear in court. Additionally, laboratories in England, Ireland, and Japan have found evidence of MMR vaccine viruses in the intestinal tracts of autistic children, but not in normal children in control groups.

In reviewing this overall correlative evidence, there does indeed seem to be an association between vaccines and autism. The evidence is incriminating, but it may be years before it is unquestionably definitive. Initially the evidence was only about the pertussis vaccine in the mid-1940s, and now it is also implicating the MMR vaccine. We therefore return to the sage advice of Maimonides, who taught that we should not wait for evidence of danger to be definitive before taking action to avoid it.

FALSIFICATION OF RESEARCH ON VACCINES AND AUTISM

Although the CDC maintains its position that there is no connection between thimerosal and autism, this position is challenged by over 165 independent studies demonstrating that this mercury-based vaccine preservative is in fact associated with autism.

Another challenge was revealed at the CDC conference "Scientific Review of Vaccine Safety Datalink Information," held in June 2000 at the Simpsonwood Methodist retreat and conference center in Norcross, Georgia. At this conference, data was presented from the Vaccine Safety Datalink examining a potential connection between thimerosal in vaccines and neurological problems such as autism in the children who received them. During the conference, Dr. Thomas Verstraeten of the CDC shared unpublished data that found a 7.6-fold increased risk of autism from exposure to thimerosal during infancy.[102]

Dr. Verstraeten's report was not well-received by the vaccine companies. It has been claimed that he was told to "clean up" his report. He tried to do this in a later paper, which was then exposed as manipulated misinformation by Dr. Brian Hooker.

An article by Dr. Hooker et al. titled "Methodological Issues and Evidence of Malfeasance in Research Purporting to Show Thimerosal in Vaccines Is Safe,"[103] reviewed six studies, on the basis of which the CDC had claimed there was no connection, and found, upon careful review, that these studies had severe "methodological difficulties," partly explaining the disparate findings in them. There is obviously a question of credibility here. According to the evidence that Dr. Hooker revealed, Dr. Verstraeten of the CDC appeared to have reworked that data until he was able to statistically do away with the mercury-autism connection.

Dr. Hooker states that Dr. Verstraeten included an additional piece of data from a very questionable source. He also failed to include any written data in his paper to support his later conclusion that there was no link between mercury and autism.[104] Verstraeten used records from four HMOs showing that infants exposed to twenty-five or more micrograms of mercury in vaccines at the age of one month were 7.6 times more likely to have an autism diagnosis than those not exposed to mercury vaccines. In the same abstract, Verstraeten reported the risk of neurodevelopmental disorders after vaccination as 1.8 times greater, the risk of speech disorders as 2.1 times greater, and of nonorganic sleep disorder as five times greater. All relative risks were statistically significant.[105]

Verstraeten's analysis in 2003, however, excluded more than 50% of all autism cases from a particular HMO (Harvard Pilgrim). The point is not to present an exposé, but to emphasize how difficult it is to get trustworthy data. All of this information can help us as parents to make informed, intelligent, and wise decisions.

Thimerosal also appears to be a risk factor for tics,[106 107] speech delay, language delay, and attention deficit disorder (ADD).[108 109 110 111] Hooker's paper titled "Methodological Issues and Evidence of Malfeasance in Research Purporting to Show Thimerosal in Vaccines Is Safe" concludes by stating:

> Considering that there are many studies conducted by independent researchers that show a relationship between thimerosal and neuro-developmental disorders, the results of the six studies examined in this review, particularly those showing the protective effects of thimerosal, should bring into question the validity of the methodology used in the studies.[112]

The significance of this is larger than the issues of mercury, autism, and neurodevelopmental disorders. We now have two pieces of evidence that warn us about our ability to trust the CDC regarding their vaccine research. According to Hooker's article, "five of the publications examined in this review were directly commissioned by the CDC, raising the possible issue of conflict of interests or research bias, since vaccine promotion is a central mission of the CDC."

Another CDC scandal emerged in 2014 around a 2004 CDC study in which the data clearly showed that African-American children three years old and younger developed autism at a rate that was 336% of the general population after receiving the MMR vaccination. Responses of various races to various vaccines do appear to differ. The CDC data apparently was altered to remove evidence of association between MMR vaccination and autism, according to a public admission by Dr. William Thompson, a senior CDC researcher. This purposeful disinformation was revealed in 2014 by Dr. Thompson himself, who was part of the original study. He confessed, in a moment of conscience, that they had in fact changed the data to make it appear that there was no association.

The significance of this revelation is only now becoming clear. The chief CDC investigator, Frank DeStefano, denied that any of this was the case; however, after the actual data was released and examined, it was clearly seen that the rate of autism in African-American boys who received the MMR was indeed approximately 3.36 times as much as for other races.

This purposeful disinformation has massive implications. Based on this study that denied any connection between the MMR vaccination and autism, there followed ninety-one studies and over 300 articles influenced by its conclusions. The implications here are that physicians in the public-health field, as a result of this purposely altered data, felt assured in their belief that there was no connection between MMR vaccinations and autism; they therefore disregarded statements by Dr. Wakefield and everyone else connecting vaccinations with autism.

In effect, parents, grandparents, sincere pediatricians and family physicians, and researchers, because of this falsification, were denied critical decision-making information. Dr. Brian Hooker reevaluated the data and provided this new information in the scientific journal *Translational Neurodegeneration*. In the wake of Hooker's revelations, Dr. William Thompson admitted to omitting the relevant data in the 2004 study, thereby admitting the falsity of its conclusion that there was no connection between MMR vaccination and autism. Unfortunately, Hooker's paper was "suddenly withdrawn." (This has also happened with GMO studies unfavorable to GMO promotion.)

Also in 2014, in the court case United States vs. Merck and Company, two former Merck scientists claimed that Merck "fraudulently misled the government and omitted, concealed, and adulterated material information regarding the efficacy of its mumps vaccine in violation of the FCA (False Claims Act)." The court documents of the two whistle-blowers showed that Merck "failed to disclose that its mumps vaccine was not as effective as Merck represented, ... manipulated testing methodology (and) ... falsified test data."

These critical data distortions are part of what may be a serious disinformation trend that has undermined the credibility of claims by the CDC, other government agencies, and pharmaceutical-company research. After the revelations at the Simpsonwood Conference and about the falsified CDC 2004 study, can we trust the CDC, the FDA, or any other agency that is heavily funded by pharmaceutical companies? Can we trust the vaccine developers, after hearing from the Merck whistle-blowers? Whom can we trust, and where do we go from here? Does this put the onus on responsible parents to become specialized in studying scientific papers? The more informed parents and general public are, the less likely they are to ostracize thoughtful parents who choose not to vaccinate their children based on scientific evidence.

INCREASED VACCINATIONS LINKED WITH INCREASED INFANT HOSPITALIZATION AND DEATH RATES

We are not pleased to point out that the epidemiological data indicates that the higher the number of vaccinations, the higher the infant mortality and hospitalization in the first year of life. The U.S. gives the most vaccinations—and has the highest rate of infant mortality and hospitalizations in year one—of the top thirty-four industrialized nations.

An important and elegant epidemiological study published in October 2012 by Gary S. Goldman and Neil Z. Miller in *Human and Experimental Toxicology* should get our attention. The study was titled "Relative trends in hospitalizations and mortality among infants by the number of vaccine doses and age, based on the Vaccine Adverse Event Reporting System (VAERS), 1990–2010."[113] Goldman and Miller discovered a clear linear correlation in the thirty-four industrial nations between the number of vaccine dosages and the rates of hospitalization and death at the

MEAN INFANT MORTALITY RATES /
MEAN NUMBER OF VACCINE DOSES
BASED ON STATISTICS OF TOP 34 NATIONS-
UNITED STATES HAS HIGHEST NUMBER OF VACCINE DOSES AND HIGHEST IMR.

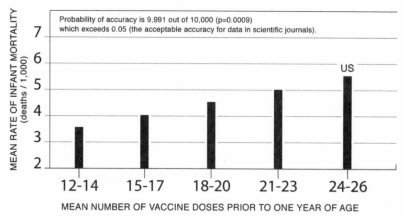

Graph created by Jared Krikorian with permission from Neil Miller, based upon research presented in Goldman and Miller's study "Relative trends in hospitalizations and mortality among infants by the number of vaccine doses and age, based on the Vaccine Adverse Event Reporting System (VAERS), 1990–2010," published in *Human and Experimental Toxicology*.

end of one year. They analyzed literature between 1990 and 2010, and the records of 38,801 hospitalized or deceased infants. The country with the most infant hospitalizations and deaths in the first year of life—the United States—also had the most vaccinations. In no uncertain terms, the facts from the morgue and in the hospital show that the more vaccinations given to a nation's infants, the more hospitalizations and infant deaths occur in that nation. This correlation is accurate to a probability of .0009—significantly better than that considered acceptable (.05) for scientific papers.

Heated opinions and personal agendas are trivial compared to the weight of statistical fact. Parents must ask: Is vaccination a risk I want to take? King Solomon is credited with saying, "The wise understand the implications of their actions." Regardless of the prejudices of the "experts," the facts derived from these correlations speak for themselves. This is not unlike the research conducted on heights, weights, and BMI in children on vegan diets, which shows that vegan children have above-average heights and weights. A picture is worth a thousand words, especially if it is science-based. After studying graphs illustrating the research, it is easy to agree with Dr. J. Anthony Morris (former Chief Vaccine Control Officer and Research Virologist for the U.S. FDA) when he said, "There is a great deal of evidence to prove that immunization of children does more harm than good."

Other doctors, based on their clinical experience and the scientific data, have similar opinions. Dr. Robert Mendelsohn, for instance, said,

> The greatest threat of childhood disease lies in the dangerous and ineffective efforts made to prevent them through mass immunization.... There is no convincing scientific evidence that mass inoculations can be credited with eliminating any childhood disease (Robert Mendelsohn, MD, pediatrician, student of Dr. Benjamin Spock, and author of How to Raise a Healthy Child in Spite of Your Doctor).

VACCINATIONS MAY BE LETHAL

Unfortunately, the vaccination story becomes even more tragic, as vaccines have been linked to a number of deaths. In June 2002 there was a congressional hearing regarding vaccines containing thimerosal that had been tested on meningitis patients and resulted in 100% fatality. According to *Judicial Watch*, twenty-six children died after receiving the HPV (human papilloma virus) vaccine between September 1, 2010 and September 15, 2011.[114] *Judicial Watch* reports that the total number of U.S. deaths from the HPV vaccine is over 100 as of 2015.[115]

In the book *Every Second Child*, we read the firsthand account by world-renowned Dr. Archie Kalokerinos about the vaccination of Aboriginal children, half of whom died shortly after receiving vaccinations. Recent deaths of children in India due to vaccinations have made headlines as well. Union Health Ministry information obtained under the Right to Inform Act shows 111 reported deaths of Indian children in

2008, 116 in 2009, and 128 in 2010 due to adverse effects following immunization (AEAI). And the vaccination-induced death count for Indian children has continued to rise.[116]

Some Indian villages have discontinued vaccination programs after the deaths of four children due to measles vaccinations. In all four cases, the children under two years old were reported to have fainted soon after inoculations; they went into seizure and were not able to receive emergency care in time to save their lives. According to the *American Chronicle,* India also suspended the use of the Gardasil HPV vaccine after the deaths of four Indian girls and injuries to 120 Indian girls after receiving this vaccine.[117]

Sudden infant death syndrome (SIDS) has grown from 1953 (at 2.5 deaths per 1,000 live births) to 1992 (eighteen deaths per 1,000 live births). That's a sevenfold increase, and the numbers continue to grow. The peak incidence of SIDS is between ages two and four months, which is precisely the age when many vaccines are given. Eighty-five percent of SIDS occurs in the first six months of infancy. Neil Miller's book *Vaccine Safety Manual* points out that 70% of SIDS cases have been shown to follow pertussis vaccinations within three weeks.[118] An uncomfortable association is emerging between SIDS and the timing of vaccinations; it is fiercely denied by vaccination advocates, but that denial is getting harder and harder to uphold.

The film *Vaccine Nation* by Gary Null, PhD documented the tragic case of Alan Yurko, whose infant son died as a result of a reaction to vaccinations and subsequent iatrogenic complications in the hospital. When the problem was misdiagnosed as shaken baby syndrome (SBS), the grieving father was sentenced to life in prison. Fortunately, however, with the support of medical experts and vaccination-safety advocates, he was released from charges and freed from prison (after serving over six years of time).

Upon Alan Yurko's release, he made the following public statement:

> I would never plead guilty to harming or abusing my son. However,
> I do take responsibility for the fact that as a parent I could have

and should have taken a stronger role in his healthcare. I could have stopped his vaccinations. I could have been more inquiring and demanding about his care in the hospital, and I could have researched the health and science issues thoroughly. I did not do any of these things, and therefore I cannot escape the fact that I have some culpable negligence in his death.

What parent wants to go through this?

Yurko went on to say,

> I did not shake, abuse, or hurt my son, and did not plead guilty to any such thing. I pled no-contest to manslaughter in hopes that people would see the message and parents would take more responsibility and active roles where these matters are concerned.[119]

How could a violent reaction to vaccinations be misdiagnosed as shaken baby syndrome? According to Dr. Archie Kalokerinos, pathologies found by autopsy in many SIDS cases include intracranial and retinal hemorrhages, and bone changes caused by infections and toxins, which can be mistaken for trauma fractures. Dr. Kalokerinos further says:

> If the vitamin C status of an infant is borderline, the administration of a vaccine, particularly (but not only) pertussis vaccine, can result in endotoxaemia, which results in a severe reaction to the vaccine, a tremendous increase in the need for vitamin C, and the precipitation of some of the signs and/or symptoms of acute scurvy.[120]

The onset may be so rapid that the classical signs of scurvy may be absent. Sudden death, unconsciousness, shock, or spontaneous bruising and hemorrhaging may occur, which can be wrongly attributed to shaken baby syndrome rather than vaccinations. Medical experts including Dr. Kalokerinos are now suspecting that vaccinations are a key factor in SIDS. Other physicians feel the same way; for example, "The evidence for indicting immunizations for SIDS is circumstantial, but compelling," says William Campbell Douglass, MD, twice honored as the National Health Federation's "Doctor of the Year."[121]

A particularly important study challenging unsubstantiated pro-vaccine "safety" claims was conducted in Guinea-Bissau. It observed

15,000 mothers between 1990 and 1996, and found that the death rate in children injected with DPT (diphtheria, tetanus, and whooping cough vaccine) was twice as high as that in unvaccinated children. The unvaccinated children had a death rate from diphtheria, tetanus, and whooping cough of 4.7%, while the vaccinated children had a death rate of 10.5% from the very diseases against which they had been vaccinated.[122]

Several questions begin to haunt us: What to do? Why is there a controversy surrounding vaccinations? Why do so many parents and doctors who have studied the material contend that vaccines are unsafe? Is an informed risk/benefit analysis or discussion available from the vaccine advocates? Why do so many others believe vaccines are necessary? The Centers for Disease Control is obviously very pro-vaccine—where is the legitimate scientific basis for such a strongly held position? These questions should have been answered by now.

With the perspective provided above, you may begin to notice that the actual scientific data does not support the pro-vaccine position.

Contaminants in Vaccines

CONTAMINATION WITH VIRUSES

Not only do some standard vaccines contain the live virus of the diseases we are attempting to prevent, we are also seeing a problem with accidental viral contamination of vaccines as well. Because various vaccines include animal tissue such as African green monkey kidney cells, bovine (cow) serum, chicken-embryo cells, pig tissue, aborted human fetal tissue and DNA, Chinese hamster ovary cells, dog kidney cells, and mouse brain cells, there is potentially dangerous residual DNA and RNA contamination in the vaccines.

It is clear from the above that vaccines are not a vegan product. Depending on various levels of interpretation, vaccinations may be against religious law for orthodox Jewish people and/or Muslims because of the use of pig tissue, though some say this technically only applies to oral vaccines. Various chicken viruses have been found in the Rimavex measles vaccine. *Acanthamoeba* (sometimes called a brain-eating amoeba), as well as simian (monkey) cytomegalovirus have also been found in the polio vaccine.[123] Bird-cancer viruses and pestivirus (a virus causing abortion and diarrhea in cows) were found in the MMR (measles/mumps/rubella) vaccine, and duck, dog, and rabbit viruses have been found in the rubella vaccine. Avian (bird) leucosis virus has been found in flu vaccines as well.

The implications of this cross-species viral and DNA contamination need to be much more seriously researched and considered.

CONTAMINATION WITH HUMAN DNA

In addition to the use of animal DNA, twenty-four common vaccines are grown on aborted human fetuses. For some people, aborted fetus and human DNA may bring up religious and/or moral as well as health issues.

The issue of human tissue and human DNA in vaccines is not one that is understood clearly. Moreover, most parents are not informed that human DNA is in a vaccine so that they can choose a vaccine compatible with their conscience. Interestingly enough, the use of aborted fetal cells in producing these vaccines began in the mid- to late 1970s. The vaccine companies, with no evidence at all, decided that using aborted human fetal cells would result in more efficient vaccine production. There was very little discussion at the FDA level of the potential adverse health consequences of using human DNA.

More questions arise; for instance, should parents and grandparents know that their children are receiving DNA from aborted human fetuses in their vaccinations? Presently there are no laws that required drug manufacturers to inform the public of this. What are the health consequences of adding human DNA to these vaccines—could this have the potential to trigger autoimmune responses, or other unknown potential problems? Does the human DNA in vaccines have the potential to become incorporated into our own DNA, through a well-documented process call homologous recombination (when a DNA sequence is pushed out and replaced by foreign DNA, which can occur during cell division or DNA repair)? Do we want our children getting someone else's DNA, when no one knows with any certainty how it could affect who they are, physically, emotionally, mentally, and spiritually? How might human DNA-contaminated vaccines contribute to human diseases? Is it acceptable that our child's genes become contaminated with those of an unknown aborted fetus through this process of homologous recombination?

It doesn't take much imagination to picture the consequences of DNA from an aborted fetus that may have lower brain capacity, for instance, potentially affecting our own child's developing brain. Please keep in mind that these thought-provoking considerations are unresearched, and theoretical—but scientifically based—possibilities. They are not proven facts, but they absolutely need to be addressed before injecting human DNA into our children.

Human DNA is recognized as a powerful immune stimulant, able to activate body and brain inflammation and/or autoimmune diseases such as type 1 diabetes, multiple sclerosis, and lupus, as well as allergies, asthma, hyperactivity, and autism. There is indeed an increase in autoimmune diseases in those who are vaccinated. The worldwide rate of type 1 diabetes, depending on the country and study, is between 50 and 150% higher in vaccinated children.[124]

Additionally, an increasing amount of worldwide evidence points to a link between child vaccines and autism, particularly in association with the MMR vaccine. It is not clear why, but the use of human aborted fetal DNA may be a factor. Aborted fetal cells containing human DNA have been used since 1983 in the MMR vaccine. It is more than an interesting coincidence that the increase in autism, began to rise in 1983 as well. Aborted-fetal-tissue use in the MMR vaccine was introduced in the UK about ten years later, and again coincided with a spike in autism levels there.

This epidemiological evidence establishes some level of association, and adds weight to the rarely discussed link between MMR vaccination and autism as well as autoimmune diseases. Unfortunately, no well-designed studies, retrospective or prospective, have ever examined this. Because of the epidemiological suggestion of this link, it may be useful to ask your physician if his or her recommended vaccines contain aborted-human DNA.[125]

It is important to note that some mandatory kindergarten-entry vaccines, including MMR and chicken pox, are only available in the U.S. with aborted fetal DNA. The human DNA cell lines used are MRC-5 and YI-38, which are derived from aborted human fetal tissue. According to Dr. Theresa Deisher, "Not only are the human fetal contaminated vaccines associated with autistic disorder throughout the world, but also with epidemic childhood leukemia and lymphomas."

There are obvious health, moral, philosophical, and religious reasons some people want to know if DNA from aborted human fetuses is indeed being injected into their children. In an article called "Finally the Truth," a study was highlighted that showed a rise in autism cases where vaccines made with aborted human baby cells had been used. The study reported that "increases in autism rates were directly linked to the introduction of human aborted DNA vaccines."[126]

At three points in time between 1987 and 2002, when human DNA developed from an aborted human cell line called WID8 was added to vaccines, or increased in the vaccine schedule, there was a correlative increase in autism.[127] This increase in autism following the addition of human fetal cell DNA three separate times presents a significant warning: Parents who choose to vaccinate their children need to check what is in the vaccines.

CONTAMINATION WITH HEAVY METALS
AND OTHER TOXINS

Unfortunately, these human DNA and cross-species viruses and tissues are not the end of the list of potentially harmful substances found in vaccines that could be associated with autism, ADHD, and a variety of chronic inflammatory diseases. According to the Centers for Disease Control (CDC), other ingredients include thimerosal (mercury), MSG, aluminum, antibiotics, formaldehyde, and a wide variety of lesser-known toxic adjuvants and substances. The scientific literature has ample evidence of the body and brain toxicity caused by these substances.

In essence, if your local doctors strongly recommend vaccines, they are suggesting, without saying it explicitly, "I hope you don't mind, but to get a stronger response we added a few extra ingredients, including MSG, aluminum, formaldehyde, neomycin, sorbitol, chick-embryo cell culture, WI-38 human lung fibroblasts, sucrose, bovine calf serum, recombinant human albumin, hydrolyzed gelatin, MRC-5 cells, Medium 199, Minimum Essential Medium, sodium phosphate dibasic, sodium bicarbonate, potassium phosphate monobasic, potassium chloride, potassium phosphate dibasic, potential unknown viruses, and aborted-tissue human DNA."

Ways to Proactively Minimize Childhood Disease

Scientific research is strongly suggesting that vaccinations have the potential for highly dangerous acute and chronic adverse effects, at a much higher frequency than some of us as parents are comfortable with. How then do we proactively prevent childhood diseases, and serious harm from those diseases?

Some epidemiological common sense helps provide clarity. First of all, we see that the historical drop in epidemics of communicable diseases coincided with a time of substantial improvements to public sanitation and hygienic awareness. As we now know, having clean, drinkable water is absolutely essential for disease prevention.

Working to provide clean drinking water to countries most at risk for communicable disease could be our number-one strategy for helping the world's children who still lack this basic necessity of life. The Tree of Life Foundation, for instance, an international humanitarian, educational, and religious 501(c)(3) not-for-profit organization headquartered in Arizona, is creating new wells and providing purified drinking water in Mexico, Ethiopia, Nigeria, Cameroon, and Ghana.

We also now know that supporting the human immune system with proper nutrition is highly effective for disease prevention, and ameliorates a disease already contracted. An example of this is the dramatic positive effect of vitamin A for measles. When we trust and support the innate intelligence of the body with high-mineral, organic, vegan, living, low-to moderate-glycemic foods (sugar suppresses the immune system and inflames the brain), we see a dramatic decrease in sickness and acute viral diseases.

This profound and exciting strategy equips our wondrously designed bodies to do their job of protecting us from infectious disease, or minimizing their negative effects. The key is to build the health of our children's bodies with good organic nutrition, to eliminate white sugar and white flour, junk food, gluten and gliadin grains, chicken, fish, beef, and dairy, to add positive thoughts, and to minimize chronic stress. Certain basic supplements are also very supportive, since topsoils are so depleted that most food grown today is deficient in minerals and vitamins.

The work of Thomas E. Levy, MD, JD gives us additional confidence in the immune-boosting power of vitamin C. "Amazingly," says Dr. Levy, "vitamin C has already been documented in the medical literature to have readily and consistently cured both acute polio and acute hepatitis, two viral diseases still considered by modern medicine to be incurable." Because "many viral infectious diseases have been cured and can continue to be cured by the proper administration of vitamin C," Levy suggests that "the vaccinations for these treatable infectious diseases are completely unnecessary when one has the access to proper treatment with vitamin C."[128]

As previously noted, vitamin D3 is also a highly effective preventative measure for the flu and for most infectious diseases, as is vitamin A. Vitamin A is especially powerful for ameliorating the serious effects of measles. We also recommend prevention and treatment with a Chinese herbal combination for immune-system support called Mega Defense, or other combinations of Chinese herbs as previously outlined. We further recommend an essential-oil formulation called Immortal Immune, available in a nebulizer for children seven and younger. These are simple and powerful prevention strategies as well as complementary treatments.

As supplemental support for a vibrant family lifestyle, there are also homeopathic "immunizations" that are both safe and effective for strengthening immunity to various childhood diseases. There was an epidemic of diphtheria in Buenos Aires, Argentina, for example, in which half of the city received homeopathic immunizations and the other half received conventional vaccines. Although neither was 100% effective, those who received the homeopathic immunization had a substantially higher rate of protection against the disease than those who received the conventional vaccinations.

There was also an "unplanned" study in Petaluma, California during an outbreak of pertussis. Of the children who were conventionally vaccinated, a high percentage became infected. None of the children who received homeopathic immunity treatments became ill. According to the late Julian Winston, author of the book *The Faces of Homoeopathy* and codirector of Wellington College of Homeopathy:

> The Journal of the American Institute for Homeopathy (May 1921) had a long article about the use of homeopathy in the flu epidemic. Dr. T.A. McCann from Dayton, Ohio reported that 24,000 cases of flu treated allopathically had a mortality rate of 28.2%, while 26,000 cases of flu treated homeopathically had a mortality rate of 1.05%. This last figure was supported by Dean W.A. Pearson of Philadelphia (Hahnemann College) who collected 26,795 cases of flu treated with homeopathy with the above result.[129]

The point is that there are valid, noninvasive, and much safer and healthier ways than vaccination to prevent acute infectious diseases. The ramifications of acute and chronic adverse reactions to vaccination are becoming alarming to a growing number of parents. There are close to six million autistic children in the U.S. today; in 1990 there were practically none. The number of children with allergies has doubled over the last decade or so. Over 100 American girls have died from receiving the HPV vaccine. And no true double-blind studies have ever been done on vaccinations in the U.S. to test the validity of vaccine theory. We need to ask why such studies have not been done.

A Biblical Perspective

In Rabbi Gabriel's religious tradition, Moshe ben Maimon (known as Maimonides, or "Rambam"), the world-famous twelfth-century sage, rabbi, and chief physician to Saladin, sultan of Egypt, in his *Codification of Jewish Law,* gave the following wise advice to parents and people in general:

> If any impediment has the potential of danger to life, it is a mitzvah (good deed) to remove it, and protect oneself from it, and to be extremely vigilant concerning it, as is written (in Deuteronomy 4:9 and 4:15): "Watch over yourself, and be careful concerning your life soul." And if one fails to remove such hazardous obstacles that can endanger oneself or others, they violate this positive commandment and also the negative commandment, "You shall not enable situations that can spill blood [i.e., endanger life]" (for instance, see Deuteronomy 22:8). Many things did the sages forbid to us because they were dangerous to our well-being. Anyone who transgresses these prohibitions and says: "I am willing to endanger myself, and how is it my business if in so doing I also endanger others?" or "I don't care about any of this," is deserving of severe beatings (Mishneh Torah, Hilchot Ro'tzeach U'Shemirat Nefesh 11:4–16).

Maimonides then goes on to list prohibited foods and drinks, forbidden not because of any violation of *kashrut* (kosher) laws but because of their possible danger to health. Vaccines are prohibited substances in both of these contexts, and thus fall into the forbidden category. In the next series of laws in the same section (12:1–5), Maimonides extends the prohibition to include food and drink items that may contain poisonous elements from their preparation process or their ingredients, such as poisons from venomous creatures who may have bitten into it or drunk from it. Ingesting such foods, even though they may be kosher, is strictly forbidden because of the possibility of danger to one's health and possibly life.

A more recent *halakhic* (Jewish law) authority, the late Rabbi Moshe Feinstein, applied these rulings even to situations where we are not 100% sure about the danger of something, but have a suspicion. For instance, we may not be absolutely certain that a venomous snake had drunk from a basin of water, but we are still forbidden from drinking it if it was left uncovered in a snake-infested region "because of danger to life" (Igrot Moshe, *Orach Chaim* 2, no. 100). This sage advice from the twelfth century, repeated in the twentieth century, applies today, and may provide a good gauge for health issues we face today including vaccination. This is "sage" advice from great and holy sages, given for our benefit and without any political or economic ulterior motive except for the protection of our and our children's health, well-being, and expanded consciousness.

The question that we ask ourselves as grandparents and parents is, "Am I willing to take the lifelong responsibility of vaccinating my children, and the risk that they will possibly develop lifelong debilitation as a result of that decision, or have an increased risk of cancer as an adult.... Could I live with that? Is it worth a lifetime of guilt and the potential chronic debilitation or death of my child?" And/or: "Am I willing to risk not vaccinating, which may either increase (as when infected by the vaccination itself, such as with polio) or decrease the risk of contracting an acute infectious disease?"

These are tough but heartfelt questions that we need to ask if we are committed to raising alive and conscious children, and developing and maintaining our responsibility of informed consent.

Moving Out of Polarity

With such a complex, emotional, media-driven, and socially laden issue, the answer of what to do isn't easy. It is easier simply to look at the science-based epidemiological hard facts. Each parent needs to do this in a deep way, evaluating their sensitivities and fears (imagined or real) as to which risk is greater.

The difficult news is that a hard look at the scientific data at this point does not give us an overwhelmingly definitive answer acceptable to parents and medical authorities. As mentioned before, it took thirty years for general acceptance of the fact that smoking causes lung cancer. But possibly, in time, enough data will be revealed about the long-term health damage associated with vaccinations, and their apparent lack of effectiveness, that the decision will become undeniably clear.

There is an interesting teaching that the heat of an argument is inversely related to the knowledge of the participants. It is important that parental and medical communities such as those concerned about measles vaccine decrease the violence of their rhetoric and increase their actual knowledge—and maintain personal compassion for each other in struggling with this rather difficult question.

Despite the fierceness of the debate, there is common ground for pro- and anti-vaccine parents—they both want their children to be protected and to thrive. The unnecessary rhetorical violence aimed at nonvaccinating parents, who may have a significantly higher level of education than those who choose to vaccinate (at least ten studies have made this point[130]), is a dangerous form of "mobocracy." This chapter is not written to give answers but to encourage you to make a thoughtful decision, weighing the risks and benefits as well as the idea of the theoretical "collective good" as part of the consideration.

The most basic point of all is that the danger of vaccination is not yet clearly understood. It took thirty years to prove that smoking causes cancer. As already noted, there are significant potential risks with the MMR and pertussis vaccines, as well as others, and there appear to be questionable benefits—certainly not the 100% protection fantasy many parents and doctors would prefer to believe. With minimal scientific knowledge and searching-out of true evidence, however, a parent will find clear pros and cons as to what types of risks to take in regards to their children.

Parents who choose not to vaccinate based on the scientific evidence showing both the dangers and the ineffectiveness, for example, of the measles vaccine will find no compelling evidence that their children pose a risk to vaccinated children. For those who trust in the authorities, there is enough social pressure supporting their choice to vaccinate. Rather than upsetting parents into fear and panic, it would be helpful to get evidence-based clarity rather than the unfortunate and clearly unethical efforts to suppress or even alter the data, as has been documented by the Thompson study. To claim a scientific "consensus" in favor of vaccination, or that the "science" surrounding vaccinations is a "finished book," as the media is trying to do, is a wild distortion of the scientific data available.

Time and again throughout history, the "consensus science" has been, in many cases, proven wrong. A classic example of this was the case of Dr. Ignaz Semmelweis (1818–65). Dr. Semmelweis pointed out that doctors who would perform autopsies and then examined pregnant women without washing their hands increased mortality tenfold from "childbed fever" (uterine infection). Although simple hygiene is commonsense today, it was rejected in his times as "not aligned with the medical consensus."

We simply cannot thoroughly understand the toxic synergies among vaccines, psychotropic medications, and environmental toxins. What we do know, at this point in history, is that it is very difficult to raise healthy children in such a toxic stew. The best that we as parents and grandparents can do is to minimize their exposure to all these toxic forces—and to remain vigilant, without becoming obsessive.

Summary

We as parents and grandparents are legitimately tasked with making a choice of fully informed trade-offs. First, there was clear evidence that vaccines can have a short-term efficacy, at least at the beginning of the vaccine usage, which can decrease the incidence of acute disease such as measles, mumps, rubella, and pertussis in the short term. We conscious parents need to ask the question: Is this approach effective for our overall, long-term health and well-being? As noted above, many acute and chronic diseases have been documented as resulting from vaccinations.

Second, we understand now that natural viruses, particularly measles, rubella, and mumps, have oncolytic effects that protect against a variety of cancers in adulthood. Third, virulent mutations have already been documented in measles, chickenpox, and pertussis viruses, and may evolve into serious epidemic problems similar to those caused by antibiotic-resistant bacteria that cause so much concern in hospitals.

Fourth, will the short-term decrease in infectious viral disease be offset by long-term virulent epidemics of viral infections, as theoretically predicted by several doctors?

A problem we all face is that there is not yet enough good scientific information about viruses and vaccinations for anyone to make fully informed decisions, so we simply need to do the best we can. In time, the information will unfold, and we will have the answers we are seeking.

In this context, we have choices as conscious parents. We can choose to build up the cellular immunity in our children and ourselves by eating a healthy diet, as discussed in this book, paying attention to our mental and physical health habits, and taking proper dietary supplementation to boost immunity, including vitamin A, vitamin D, adequate zinc, and vitamin C to upgrade our epigenetic (beyond the immediate influence of genetics) program to protect us against diseases. Although no approach guarantees 100% protection, this approach to building and maintaining a strong biological terrain, if we are willing, offers a viable regenerative solution—and healthier children.

If we choose a diet high in white flour, white sugar, junk food, pesticides and herbicides, without proper nutritional support, we will decrease our epigenetic cellular immunity, and our children will become more susceptible to viral infections. Data is clear about this in developing countries: Children who are malnourished and without supplementation are considerably more susceptible to infectious diseases such as measles, and suffer far more serious sequalae from these infections. Such people in the short term may potentially benefit from vaccinations, buying them time to ultimately build up their cellular immunity.

These are difficult decisions. Up to this point in history, the choice remains ours.

There is one final consideration.... A thoughtful vaccine choice can actually go beyond the medical/biological risk/benefit trade-off question. In a larger, more conscious context, it is also a lifestyle choice, and a worldview choice. Disease throughout history, until the emergence of allopathic medicine, was understood as activated by an imbalance in relationship with both natural and cosmic laws. At this deeper level of considering the vaccine question, we may be inspired to ask: Do we choose to live in a way that enhances our biological terrain—a holistic way of life that brings us into body-mind-spirit harmony with all of creation and the cosmos, that enhances the web of life for all of creation, and that elevates our souls?

CHAPTER 10

Maximizing Aliveness by Minimizing Toxic Synergy

Vaccines are only one part of a tremendous and complex synergy of toxic disruptive forces affecting our children's brains and bodies. As responsible parents and protectors, it is important for us to address all the issues of raising a healthy child. This quest can become obsessive, but it makes sense for us to minimize this toxic synergy in any areas where we have some control.

Gluten

The question of gluten in the diet speaks to a major issue facing our children's brains and mental health as well as their physical health. This question must be addressed, though freeing ourselves from gluten does create some initial inconvenience.

What is gluten? It is a glue-like protein composite that holds everything together in foods such as bread, pizza dough, and baked goods in general. Gluten is not a single molecule, but a combination of two groups of proteins, glutenins and gliadins. Gliadins contain twelve smaller antigenic proteins. All twelve of these, plus the glutenin, have the potential to cause inflammation throughout the body, particularly in the brain.

Gluten-free grains include buckwheat, corn, rice, amaranth, millet, quinoa, sorghum, oats (if properly milled), and teff. Pure oats are gluten-free, but because they often are milled in gluten-contaminated situations, they often do contain gluten.

Glutenin and gliadin are found in wheat, barley, rye, spelt, Kamut®, couscous, triticale, bulgur, and semolina. Gluten components are also found in other grains and products including durum, *seitan,* farro, emmer, graham, malt, and einkorn. Some ingredients containing gluten include brown-rice syrup, caramel coloring if it is made from barley, dextrin, hydrolyzed malt extract, hydrolyzed protein, maltodextrin, modified food starch, natural flavoring, soy protein, and texturized vegetable protein (TVP). Gluten and gliadin are also often hidden in processed foods as additives to give them bulk. Some hidden sources include soup mixes, sauces, soy sauce, candies, salad dressings, frozen meatballs, cold cuts, low-fat foods, and no-fat foods. These are just a few examples that illustrate how widespread glutens are in our food supply.

In most people's minds, gluten is associated with celiac disease, although celiac disease actually represents only a small part of the larger problem of gluten sensitivity. Celiac disease, also known as "sprue," is an extreme gluten sensitivity involving a specific allergic reaction in the small intestine. The number of people that have celiac disease may be as high as three percent. However, nearly twenty-five percent of the American population may have a genetic tendency toward celiac disease, especially those with northern European ancestry.

Celiac disease is better understood as a symptom of a larger issue called gluten sensitivity. There seems to be a wide genetic spectrum of gluten sensitivity. Some feel as much as thirty to fifty percent of the population may have some degree of gluten sensitivity. When people have an inflammatory reaction to gluten, commonly referred to as gluten sensitivity, it may lead to inflammation in any organ of the body, with or without the small intestine's involvement.

The brain is most at risk from gluten sensitivity. When people are gluten-sensitive, the immune system responds to gluten by sending out inflammatory substances called cytokines. These can damage the tissue they are trying to help, such as worsening "leaky gut" in the small intestine, or inflammation in the brain. As with vaccines, brain inflammation causes a number of symptoms. We see these, in worst-case scenarios, as elevated cytokines in Alzheimer's disease, Parkinson's disease, multiple sclerosis, and autism. Some doctors feel that ninety-nine percent of people whose immune systems react negatively to gluten are unaware of their reaction because it occurs subtly and may become more active elsewhere in the body, often as a neurological disease. Brain inflammations can occur without any gastrointestinal problems such as celiac disease.

While the idea of celiac disease may be new to some people, it was first diagnosed in the first century AD by Aretaeus of Cappadocia, a famous Greek physician. In the seventeenth century, people began to refer to the ailment as "sprue," or chronic diarrhea. No one knew what caused it until the 1940s, when Dr. Kirel Dickel connected it with consumption of wheat flour. In 1952, doctors made the link between celiac disease and gluten. But as early as 1937, the Archives of Internal Medicine published a study from the Mayo Clinic pointing to the neurological component of celiac disease.[1] They didn't understand that the inflammation didn't need to occur with celiac disease, but they began to establish the connection.

In 2006, the Mayo Clinic published in the *Archives of Neurology and Psychiatry* a report linking celiac disease with cognitive impairments.[2] These included ataxia, neuropathies, numbness, weakness, pain, amnesia, confusion, and personality changes. Other symptoms of celiac disease include myoclonus (muscle spasms) and epilepsies. These symptoms typically reverse in three to six months with a gluten-free diet, and sometimes right away. Suddenly people began to see this as an issue distinct from nutritional deficiencies.

The percentage of people impacted by gluten sensitivity is much higher than originally suspected. A 2009 article from New Zealand titled "The Gluten Syndrome: A Neurological Disease,"[3] represented a further refinement in our scientific understanding. It described a study that furthered shifted focus away from the small intestine and onto gluten sensitivity as "interference with the body's neuronetwork," saying that "gluten is linked to neurological harm in patients both with and without evidence of celiac disease."[4] It is becoming clear that the brain and the nervous system seem to be the prime site for inflammation from gluten sensitivity, potentially resulting in chronic neurological and brain damage. Brain disorders from gluten sensitivity may include schizophrenia, depression, bipolar disorder, autism, and ADHD.

The gluten reaction can be quite powerful. At an orthomolecular psychiatric training in the 1980s, Dr. Gabriel saw a person receive an injection of wheat extract and begin hallucinating within fifteen seconds. Research is also showing that people with celiac disease have increased free-radical damage in their fat, protein, and DNA. These people can even lose their antioxidant support through lowered levels of glutathione, the main anti-inflammatory support factor, as well as lower levels of vitamin E, retinol, and vitamin C in the blood. Gluten reaction wears away at the system.

Gluten sensitivity increases the production of inflammatory cytokines, which are major players in causing brain inflammation resulting in neuro-degenerative conditions. That is why this is so important for our children to avoid gluten, or to be checked for gluten sensitivity. The question arises: We've been eating wheat for 10,000 years, so why are we having this problem now? The answer is: The original grain is genetically different than what we have hybridized into being. Today's grains contain up to forty times the gluten of the original grains—and the higher concentration of gluten makes a significant difference in its ability to cause inflammation.

Also connected with gluten sensitivity is the obesity epidemic, because fat is our "inflammation organ." The fatter a person is, the more cytokines they produce, which worsen inflammation. Gluten sensitivity makes a person crave what they are allergic to, namely, wheat and other gluten grains that make us gain weight. Symptoms of gluten sensitivity in children include ADHD, Tourette syndrome, anxiety, loss of balance, autism, ataxia, immune disorders including diabetes, Hashimoto's thyroiditis, rheumatoid arthritis, brain fog, cancer, chest pain, chronic illness, dairy intolerance (wheat and dairy intolerance seem to go together), delayed growth, depression, digestive disturbances such as gas, bloating, and diarrhea, hives, rashes, irritable bowel syndrome, migraine headaches, nausea, and sugar cravings.

Gluten makes us crave sugar, and those two work synergistically to both inflame tissues and cause mental and physical symptoms.

The brain doesn't work as well when its tissues are inflamed, and there is a higher rate of emotional volatility, outbursts, and poor functioning, including ADHD. The treatment for ADHD is often medication, and in some schools in the United States as many as twenty-five percent of students are receiving legally prescribed mind/brain-altering drugs. The side effects of these prescription drugs can lead to long-term neurological developmental problems. As of March 13, 2014, according to the CDC, nearly one in five high school boys in the U.S., and about 11% of school-age children had been diagnosed with ADHD. This is a 53% rise in ADHD in the last decade. About two-thirds of these children are receiving Adderall or Ritalin.[5]

Anxiety is another potential reaction in gliadin/gluten sensitivity, and the use of anti-anxiety drugs increased 45% in females and 37% in males between 2001 and 2010. Research shows that depression and anxiety are often high in children with gluten sensitivity. Many children are being placed on antidepressants and antipsychotics as young as four and five years old. Before we put our children on drugs, what if we simply took them off all gluten foods for three to six months? Cytokines produced in a gluten reaction block neurotransmitters, including serotonin, recognized as one of the most important of the brain's own antidepressant neurotransmitters.

We estimate that up to ninety percent of children with ADHD could be helped with a gluten-free diet, as well as high amounts of DHA and a whole, organic, vegan diet with no white sugar. This will make a difference in the long run. By keeping children off drugs, we are much more likely to optimize normal brain development. New research has emerged indicating that some drugs used to treat ADHD have created permanent Tourette syndrome.[6] This began to be documented in the 1980s.

An interesting piece of research was done in 2006. It was a "before-and-after" story of people with ADHD that went gluten-free for six months. The ADHD symptoms were measured using a behavioral scale called the Conner Scale Hypescheme. They found that the ability of the children to pay close attention to details increased by 36%; their ability to sustain attention increased by 12%; their ability to finish a project increased by 30%; and their tendency to be easily distracted diminished by 46%. The overall symptomology of the people in the study decreased by 27% when gluten was eliminated from their diet for six months.

Autism represents a complex synergy of causative factors including vaccines, environmental toxins, and reactions to additives and coloring, Gluten is yet another factor contributing to the entire autism spectrum. Research suggests that children put on a gluten-free diet had some improvement in their autism symptoms. The data isn't overwhelming, but there does seem to be a connection between autism and celiac disease—namely, brain inflammation. We can think about celiac disease as inflammation of the small intestine, and autism as inflammation of the brain, and they tend to overlap. If we can reduce the cause of the inflammation in both cases by taking away the gluten, then it is reasonable to assume that relief from gluten sensitivity is the cause.

A 1999 study in the United Kingdom observed a significant improvement in twenty-two autistic children placed on a gluten-free diet for five months. They also noted that when the children were put back on gluten, there was a rapid degeneration.[7] It takes at least three months to see the results of a gluten-free diet.

Research supports the idea that inflammation affects both the brain and the small intestine, showing an overlap between celiac disease and depression. Two 1998 studies found that a third of those with celiac disease also had depression.[8][9] In a 2007 study, Swedish researchers evaluated 14,000 celiac patients against control patients.[10] They found that 80% more patients with celiac disease had depression than in the control group; and those who were depressed had a 230% higher likelihood of having celiac disease. In 2011, another study from Sweden found that risk of suicide amongst those with celiac disease was higher by 55%.[11] An Italian study showed that those with celiac disease had a 270% higher risk of depression.[12] Another study found depression in about 52% of gluten-sensitive individuals.[13]

Brain inflammation is associated with depression, and it is associated with gluten sensitivity. It is important for us to consider protecting our children against these. Gluten-sensitivity tests are available and can provide a measure of clarity. However, a good start may be to simply take your children off gluten and watch what happens.

There is recent evidence that gluten sensitivity may be genetically passed on. The children of gluten-sensitive mothers are nearly 50% more likely to develop schizophrenia later in life. If you happen to be a mother who is gluten-sensitive, the obvious thing to do is to help your child begin life without gluten. Gestation conditions may affect a child's entire lifetime. A prenatal dietary sensitivity may cause the development of schizophrenia up to twenty-five years later.[14]

Headaches are another common symptom of gluten sensitivity. Headaches immobilize children and adults alike. As many as forty-five million people suffer from chronic headaches. If your child suffers from chronic headaches, it is well worth trying a gluten-free diet. One well-documented study showed that chronic headaches occurred in 56% of gluten-sensitive people, and 30% of those with celiac disease. A group of Italian researchers conducted a gluten-free experiment on eighty-eight children with celiac and chronic headaches, and found that 77% of them experienced significant improvement and relief from headaches on a gluten-free diet. Twenty-seven percent of the children became headache-free when they stayed on the gluten-free diet. They found that 5% of those with headaches who were not previously diagnosed with celiac disease were found to have the disease.

What happens in childhood follows us into adulthood. Research shows that children who suffer from migraines have a 50–75% chance of becoming adults with migraines. Childhood migraines constitute the third leading cause of absences from school.[15] These are things to consider; the solutions are simple, and do not require medications. Adult drugs used for headaches on children are often ineffective and often have side effects.

Obesity is also connected with headaches because of the direct correlation between fat and cytokines. A 2006 study examined 30,000 people and found that 28% more of the obese had chronic daily headaches than those with a healthy BMI. Those who were morbidly obese had a 74% higher occurrence of daily headaches. A Norway study of 5,847 adolescents with headaches found that the children who were overweight were 40% more likely to suffer from headaches.[16] All this points at reducing sources of inflammation—which is caused or worsened by both obesity and gluten sensitivity.

In looking at brain inflammation, neurobiological symptomology, and neurological development from a variety of angles and causes, we see that gluten sensitivity completes a synergistic picture of inflammation in our children's brains. There are things we can do to avoid this. A gluten-free diet is not simple, but if the whole family can do it, this may be best because of the genetic transmission of gluten sensitivity; the whole family can then benefit from it.

The health of parents also affects the health of the kids. When we eat organic, noninflammatory vegan foods and minimize all sources of inflammation in the household, our children are bound to have healthier, more loving, happier, and better-functioning brains, minds, social interactions, and relationships, and more functional, alive, and conscious lives.

Marijuana: Toxicity to the Brain

Although the authors are in favor of decriminalizing marijuana, and are aware of good research suggesting that it may be useful in certain cases as a cancer therapy and to many people suffering from chronic pain, this does not mean that it is a totally innocuous herbal substance.

From a holistic perspective, although good for ameliorating some pain and cancers, the research shows that marijuana has highly undesirable effects on our children's brains and minds. It shows that smoking marijuana affects brain development in teenagers by altering the neuronal connections in the brain "at a time when the brain should be at a clear state of mind in accumulating memory and data and good experiences that will lay a good foundation for the future" (Reuben Baler, National Institute of Drug Abuse).[17]

There is a correlation between adolescent pot smoking and an increase in imbalanced relationships and exacerbated intimacy difficulties later in life, irrespective of social upbringing, personal hardships, or other potential challenges. In other words, research shows that regularly smoking marijuana as a teenager affects the brain in a way that impacts intimacy capacity and relationship capacity in general. Marijuana affects the brain in the immediacy, over the long run, and during adulthood, even after stopping the use of marijuana.[18] And marijuana use affects people in terms of addiction as well as cognitive development.[19]

In Dr. Gabriel's observation of this phenomenon as a family therapist since 1973, he has seen that if one member of the family is smoking marijuana, there is a block in the communication and intimacy amongst family members, because they are working on different planes. Marijuana smoking can be seen as a way of subtly undermining the intimacy process. Although those who are smoking may believe they are more "in touch," others who are not smoking have a much different experience of the interpersonal communication and emotional interplay.

Marijuana also affects social and work-related willpower. For example, the *Washington Post* reports that teenagers who smoke marijuana daily are 60% less likely to complete high school.[20] In Colorado, where pot has been legalized, there has been an increase in marijuana use by teens, which is manifesting in increased marijuana-related suspensions, expulsions, and emergency room visits (up 57%). It is common knowledge amongst psychiatrists working with drug addiction that higher doses of marijuana can cause temporary psychotic reactions in some people, including hallucinations and paranoia. CNN cites seven studies that have found this to be the case.

Teenagers with family histories of schizophrenia are also at a higher risk of developing schizophrenia after using marijuana. These observations certainly support those of Dr. Gabriel, who has had a number of patients who became psychotic every time they smoked marijuana. These people were otherwise able to function in the world. Their treatment was to help them break their addiction to marijuana, so that they wouldn't need to smoke and/or become psychotic each time they smoked.

Research on long-term use of marijuana (twenty or more years) in Jamaica, as far back as the 1970s, showed that chronic users suffered significant brain-cell loss.[21] Since marijuana has become legalized in Colorado, traffic fatalities among drivers testing positive for marijuana has increased 100%, with the majority of DUI arrests involving marijuana. Twenty-five to 40% were for marijuana alone.

Furthermore, according to a White House statement on the public consequences of marijuana legalization, marijuana is the second leading substance for which people receive drug treatment, and is a major cause of visits to the emergency room. The *Washington Post* also notes a significant (57%) increase in marijuana-related visits to the emergency room. Not only does research show an increase in traffic fatalities, but the *British Medical Journal* reports that marijuana users who drove within three hours of smoking doubled their risk of an accident. According to the CDC, cannabis users have a 4.8-fold risk of heart attack during the first hour after smoking.

The main point here, however, is that teenage and child brains are still undergoing neurodevelopmental processes that appear to be disrupted and delayed, at least temporarily and perhaps permanently, by smoking marijuana. Although the subject requires more research, this significant statement was made by the National Institute on Drug Abuse.

For all of these reasons, we don't recommend any use of marijuana by teenagers or young adults, as there is ample information to suggest that the neurodevelopmental and cognitive processes are indeed, to some extent, blocked, delayed, and/or otherwise disrupted by marijuana use. It is hard to be fully alive and conscious when one's brain and neurodevelopmental function are disrupted.

Fluoride: Toxicity to the Brain and Body

To support parents further in protecting their children from toxins, we must also discuss fluoride, a known neurotoxin that damages the brain, delays and disrupts neurodevelopment, and has been associated with lowered IQ.

In 2012, researchers from the Harvard School of Public Health published a review of fluoride's effects on the brains of children. They felt that the results supported the "possibility of the adverse effects of fluoride exposure on children's neurodevelopment."[22] Basically, they found that children with a higher exposure to fluoride had lower IQs than those exposed to less fluoride. Twenty-six of the twenty-seven studies they reviewed indicated a connection a relationship between lower IQ and increased fluoride intake. These studies were based on research from all over the world, including China, India, Iran, and Mexico, over twenty years.

A study published in 2010 in the *Journal of Hazardous Materials* also documented an association between lower IQ and fluoride intake.[23] Researchers measured fluoride content in urine samples and compared those results to the children's IQs. They found a direct correlation between increased fluoride levels in urine and lower IQ. They also noted that a rise in fluoride levels from .3 ppm to 3 ppm was associated with a five-point IQ drop.

The justification that putting fluoride in water will protect teeth has been completely debunked. According to the WHO, there is no discernible difference between tooth decay in developed countries that fluoridate their water and those that do not. The decline of tooth decay in the U.S. in the last sixty years has been falsely attributed to fluoridated water. In reality, as with vaccinations, the decline of tooth decay occurred in all developing countries, including those that do not fluoridate their water. This strongly suggests there is no valid reason to add fluoride to municipal water supplies.

Some dentists place a fluoride coating on teeth. We do not recommend this practice because of the potential neurodevelopmental dangers from fluoride wearing off the teeth and being ingested. Fluoride not only lowers IQ but also effects emotional function, making people more emotionally imbalanced, fearful, and submissive, while decreasing willpower and fertility. This is why the Nazis used fluoride in the water in their concentration camps. Besides the U.S., only seven other countries in the world now fluoridate their water; in Europe, only Ireland fluoridates its water. Fluoride coating applied to teeth may possibly strengthen tooth enamel, but this is a layer approximately six nanograms thick—so small that it wears off during the simple act of chewing.

Beyond fluoride's neurodevelopmental dangers, according to L. Valdez-Jiménez et al., fluoride induces degenerative changes, to the brain's physical structure and biochemistry that affect neurological and mental development.[24] Fluoride also negatively affects cognitive processes such as learning and memory.

New evidence suggests that fluoride activates calcification in the pineal gland, which is important for melatonin secretion and also for proper timing of menses. Fluoride causes the onset of menses at an earlier age, which is also associated with an increased risk of breast cancer. Spiritually, the pineal gland is considered to be the seat of the soul, and it is contraevolutionary to have this special organ become calcified with calcium fluoride.

Because so many people in the U.S. are deficient in iodine, a competing halogen to flouride, we strongly recommend iodine as a way of flushing fluoride out of the pineal gland and key organs that accumulate fluoride, such as the thyroid. Various iodine and kelp supplements (5 tablets daily) have been successful for this. The most effective supplement, and easiest for children of all ages, as it is a liquid, is a liquid iodine preparation called Illumodine. The iodine in this preparation is already broken down from I_2 to I-, the active form of iodine in thyroxine (a thyroid hormone).

Today, because of the Fukushima disaster, 28% of babies born on the American West Coast as far north as Alaska, and 44% of babies in Fukushima, are born with a congenital hypothyroid condition. Ninety-four percent of Americans are deficient in iodine, and so are prone to accumulate radioactive I-131. The best defense for ourselves and our children is supplementation with some other form of iodine to protect us from absorbing I-131.

Research has also associated fluoridation exposure with acceleration of the aging process.[25] This is because fluoride disrupts metabolic enzyme production, acting as a poison that increases the rate of aging through metabolic disruption.[26] Fluoride has also been associated with increased cancer rates[27] and Alzheimer's disease rates.[28] Fluoride has been shown to increase the bioavailability of aluminum, which may account for its Alzheimer's-promoting effect. Drinking fluoridated water allows aluminum to be transported more easily across the blood/brain barrier, to be deposited in the brain. The combination of fluoride and aluminum has been shown to cause the same changes in brain tissue as those found in Alzheimer's patients.

Fluoride impairs the body's antioxidant system. Fluoride has also been associated with depression, emotional volatility, and bipolar diseases. It disrupts the circadian rhythm because it disrupts pineal gland function. As a metabolic poison, fluoride deactivates sixty-two different enzymes, and inhibits more than 100. Unfortunately, over forty percent of American teenagers show visible signs of fluoride overexposure, with the demonstrable emergence of dental fluorosis as mottling of the teeth. Fluoride exposure is also associated with hardening of the arteries, and there appears to be a significant correlation between a history of cardiovascular disease and the amount of fluoride in the arteries.

Fluoride is more toxic than lead, and increases the amount of lead that is absorbed into the system. Fluoride disrupts the endocrine system, creating hypothyroidism through competitive inhibition (forcing iodine out of the thyroid gland). It also increases the occurrence of hip fractures in the elderly because it makes the bones brittle. Epidemiological research shows that the number of hip fractures amongst the elderly is particularly high in those communities with fluoridated water.

On November 9, 2006, even the American Dental Association issued an alert advising patients to avoid using fluoridated water in reconstituted infant formula.

Fluoride stands out as a particularly neurotoxic mineral that all our children are potential exposed to. It has no proven benefits, and doesn't seem to be associated with a decline in tooth decay.

Although it is said that .7 to 1.2 ppm of fluoride is safe in the water, we do not believe there is any safe level, because fluoride accumulates in the body. That cumulative effect disrupts the synthesis of collagen, and breaks down the collagen in bone, tendon, muscle, skin, cartilage, lungs, kidneys, and trachea. Fluoride depletes energy reserves and the ability of white blood cells to destroy foreign agents through phagocytosis. It stimulates granular formation and oxygen consumption in white blood cells, but it inhibits that process when white blood cells are challenged by a foreign agent in the blood. This means that it also weakens the immune system. It has also been associated with autoimmune diseases, and inhibiting antibody formation in the blood.

In summary, fluoride increases lead and aluminum absorption and brain damage, lowers IQ and lowers thyroid function, contributes to genetic damage and accelerates aging, disrupts the synthesis of collagen, increases rates of arthritis and most cancer, particularly osteosarcoma, creates hyperactivity and/or lethargy, creates emotional volatility, fear, and weakened willpower, aggravates dementia, disrupts the immune system, creates muscular disorders, inhibits the creation of antibodies, increases infertility, and damages sperm. Fluoride is a general systemic toxin.

Many municipalities routinely fluoridate public drinking water supplies. If the water in your area is fluoridated you have two choices of action: Use distilled water and activate it, as described in the "Living Water" section of *Spiritual Nutrition* (page 384); or use reverse-osmosis filtered water.

Since ninety-six percent of the population is deficient in iodine,[29] and since iodine is so important for thyroid, brain, and endocrine functions, and for metabolic support against fluoride toxicity, everyone can benefit from a certain amount of iodine supplementation. The best thing we as parents can do is to make sure our children do not drink fluoridated water or soft drinks, most of which contain fluoridated water.

EMFs and Our Children's Brains

There is not much information on the topic of electromagnetic exposure to make our knowledge definitive. If there is a potential danger, however, should we not act preventatively?

Present epidemiological studies strongly correlate low-frequency, nonionizing electromagnetic radiation exposure (EMFs) with an increased incidence of cancer. This not only includes low-frequency, nonionizing electromagnetic radiation from cell phones and WiFi, but also extremely low-frequency, nonionizing electromagnetic radiation from power lines and cell phone towers. A large number of epidemiological studies are beginning to demonstrate a correlation between exposure to EMF radiation and the incidence of certain cancers in large populations.

In 2009, the *Journal of Clinical Oncology* published a review of twenty-three epidemiological studies of the link between cell phone use and cancer.[30] Ten of the twenty-three studies found a significant association between phone use and tumor risk. Another fifteen studies investigating cell-phone use over the course of ten or more years also found a significant association with tumor risk, especially for brain tumors.[31]

A 2007 review of sixteen studies showed that all sixteen found an increased occurrence of brain tumors known as glioma and acoustic neuroma. These are tumors that grow on the nerves associated with hearing and balance, located on the sides of the face where cell-phone users typically placed their phones. The studies found that the potential for tumor growth on the same side of the head where the cell phone was placed had increased 240% (the average from the sixteen studies combined). Some of the studies showed a risk higher than 240%. One study associated increased incidence of acoustic neuroma with cell-phone use of at least ten years, with a 90% increased risk of auditory nerve cancer and a 390% greater occurrence on the side where the cell phone was used. The study showed little difference with cell-phone use of less than ten years, the implication being that long-term use may be a key determinant of outcome.

Children are much more sensitive to shorter exposures. Another study done in 2009 by Dr. Lennart Hardell reported that those who began using cell phones before age twenty had a 520% increased risk of developing gliomas,[32] and this occurred after only one year of use. In 2008, Dr. Siegal Sadetzki and her colleagues published results in the *American Journal of Epidemiology* associating heavy cell-phone use (over twenty-two hours per month) with a 50% higher likelihood of cancer of the parotid gland (one of the salivary glands). Dr. Sadetzki found a much higher occurrence on the side where people placed their cell phone. Her research enforced the link between the use of cell phones and the occurrence of cancer. She concludes, "This unique population has given us an indication that cell-phone use is associated with cancer."[33] [34]

A review of deaths between 1970 and 2006 in the Israeli National Cancer Registry found that "the total number of parotid-gland cancers in Israel increased fourfold between 1970 and 2006." In other salivary-gland cancers, there was no change at all. We are getting clear indications that cell phones are carcinogenic in adults, and are particularly carcinogenic in children.

The cell phone and WiFi industries are fighting these findings, just as the tobacco companies did with cigarette research. They are even funding studies that support their position that cell phones, WiFi, and cell phone towers don't contribute to cancer. This is the same pattern we have seen with vaccines, cigarettes, and GMOs, where profit motives attempt to influence science itself.

The effects of EMFs involve a variety of physiological functions, but we are choosing to focus on cancer since it represents the most serious of those problems.

Studies indicate a relation between cancer and proximity to cell towers. Cell-tower radiation is equivalent to secondhand smoke. The closer you are, the higher your cancer risk, especially if you live in the building where the transmission occurs. This is common in Israel. There also is a notorious tower in England known as the Tower of Doom, referring to a pair towers owned by Vodafone and Orange (a UK mobile operator), erected atop an apartment building. After they were installed in 1994, the people living in the apartments noted an increased incidence of health ailments including cancer, specifically breast and uterine cancer. Five of eight apartments' occupants became ill. The cancer rate on the building's top floors was ten times higher than the national average. So it appears that proximity to cell towers also carries risk.

The question of long-term effect is relevant here. Many of these results were not apparent until after ten years of exposure. One study compared cancer cases occurring within 400 meters of towers to others farther away. After ten years, those living near the transmitters had over three times the rate of cancer than those living at a distance.[35]

These studies have been somewhat duplicated in Brazil, where they found the greatest number of cancers among those living nearest the cell towers. Research in New Zealand by Dr. Neil Cherry, an environmental scientist, associated health risks with television and FM-radio broadcasting antennas (which also broadcast EMFs). This correlation was also found in San Francisco near the Sutro Tower broadcasting antennas. In a section of the population from 1937 to 1988, researchers discovered 123 cases of cancer among 50,686 children, and cancer rates were lower further from the tower. This is a large enough sampling to clearly demonstrate that children living closer to the towers did have a higher risk of cancer than those at a distance.

This has also been demonstrated with FM-radio transmitters. The Karolinska Institutet in Sweden did a study from 2002 to 2008 and found a carcinogenic association in proximity to FM-transmitting towers. Melanoma was particularly common, and the rate of melanoma increased with the rate of exposure to FM frequencies. They concluded that melanoma risk is associated with FM broadcasting. As with cell phones, the rate of cancer was twice as likely under exposure to FM or TV towers over time.

The research of Dr. Sam Milham correlated increases in death rates with the onset of electrification via power-line exposure. His research findings supported the fact that childhood leukemia, with a peak incidence in children three to four years old, correlates with levels of exposure. Even the World Health Organization, since 2002, is now including EMFs among possible causes of childhood leukemia.

This is not a new finding; the danger to children has been recognized as far back as 1979. Nancy Wertheimer and Ed Leeper found a correlation between EMF exposure from power lines and childhood leukemia. They noted that even very low levels of EMF radiation seemed associated with leukemia in children. Children's bodies are in a state of rapid growth, which means that they undergo a more rapid pace of cell division; thus the DNA of children is more vulnerable to errors that may occur during normal protein synthesis. Any damaged DNA is therefore likely to pass into the cells during cell division as well as replication, creating disruption. Additionally, the bone in children's skulls is thinner, providing less shielding than in adults.

At the University of Helsinki in Finland, researchers demonstrated that children are susceptible to more subtle effects on brain function, showing a greater decrease in cognitive function in children from cell-phone radiation exposure in the range of 902 megahertz. They found decreases in auditory memory and cognitive processing.[36] In short, the findings in all this research show that the same cell phone, held in the same position for the same length of time, does more harm to children than to adults.

In the Stewart Report, published in 2000 by an independent group of experts on mobile phones at the request of England's Ministry for Public Health, deduced:

> (C)hildren may be more vulnerable because of their nervous system, the greater absorption of energy in the tissues of the head, and a longer lifetime of exposure.... We believe the widespread use of cell phones by children for nonessential phone calls should be discouraged. The mobile-phone industry should refrain from promoting the use of mobile phones by children.[37]

But no studies have been done on children to determine safe levels of exposure. The standards set for adults are being applied to children without considering their heightened vulnerability.

Baby monitors are another potential difficulty, utilizing radio waves and presenting a similar danger. Other research shows that the average exposure to WiFi radiation by the time children graduate high school is equivalent to 12,960 hours of exposure.

Recent studies are also connecting cell-phone usage with sleep problems among teens. One of these, conducted by Gaby Badre, MD, PhD, showed that teens with high cell-phone exposure reported greater restlessness, fatigue, stress, difficulty falling and staying asleep, and consumption of "energy drinks" than teens with lower cell-phone exposure.[38]

Another study, sponsored by the Mobile Manufactures Forum and conducted by scientists from Karolinska Institutet and Uppsala Universitet in Sweden and Wayne State University in Michigan, also linked radiation from mobile phones with symptoms of insomnia, confusion, chronic headaches, and depression (affecting adults as well as teens).[39] Thankfully, we now have some radiation-protective devices that can be added to personal phones.

The general recommendation of experts is: *Adults should limit cellphone use, and children should have no cell-phone use.* This includes kids up to the age of twenty. They should also minimize exposure to WiFi networks. This is of course an interesting issue, because many places now offer free WiFi, including many schools that feel they are doing an academic service. These WiFi networks run all day long and, of course, so does their damaging impact. One solution is to simply return to using Ethernet technology.

Although these technologies represent advancement, the price is too high when we add up the increased medical bills, parental and childhood suffering, and increased mortality, simply for convenience. The problem is, as always, that we are not using intuition or foresight, so it will take many years and a lot of cancer to drive home the point. In the meantime, it is best for us to go by the principle that if it looks dangerous, maybe it is dangerous.

WiFi is set up for entire schools; "smart" electric meters are installed in schools; we are likely looking at significant future increases in brain cancer, salivary-gland cancer, and cancer in general. Although there is less specific research available on smart meters, the principles we have discussed, and some recent research, strongly suggest that they are and will be a major health risk.

For more information you may visit the following websites:

- www.magdahavas.com/category /electrosmog-exposure/schools/
- www.safeschool.ca
- www.citizensforsafetechnology.org
- www.wiredchild.org

One study indicated that if pregnant mothers are exposed to sixteen milligauss (mG) of magnetic exposure for even a short period, they are twice as likely to miscarry. It suggests that acute high exposure could even trigger a miscarriage. The risk of miscarriage increased for all participants in the study by at least eight percent. The risk was high for early miscarriages, at 220% of the norm; and it was particularly high for women with problems in prior pregnancies, at 400%.

EMF exposure also seems to be associated with increased occurrence of asthma. Research shows that children born to mothers with an average EMF exposure greater than or equal to 2 mG during pregnancy were 3.5 times as likely to develop asthma by age thirteen. The research showed the children's asthma risk increasing in a dose-related response, according to the mother's EMF exposure while pregnant. Every one-mG increase in the body of the pregnant mother was associated with a fifteen-percent increase in the child's risk of asthma.[40]

A correlation has also been noted between the rise in childhood obesity and exposure to EMFs.[41] We're looking at a global problem that has been thus far been minimally addressed. What we do know is that we need to protect our children. Not every technological change is for the best, particularly if one does not know how to use it in a safe way.

Global Radiation Toxicity

At the time of this writing, we are facing the class-7-level disaster of Fukushima, which is the most drastic category. It has resulted in acute planetary exposure to radiation. We are now seeing, for example, 300 times higher levels of radiation in the continental-U.S. milk supply, and 2,033% higher than permissible radiation levels in the Hawaiian milk supply. Reports of higher levels of radiation in general have also come from Los Angeles, San Francisco, Philadelphia, Niagara Falls, Denver, Detroit, Trenton, Oakridge, Cincinnati, Pittsburg, and Boise.

This event is considered to be 1,000 times worse than ever anticipated by nuclear-reactor builders. As we have seen with Chernobyl, also listed as level 7—where resulting deaths after twenty-five years are estimated at one million or more—this is a grave global issue that requires a proactive and protective response. But first we need to get a feeling for the degree of the danger. Radioactive cesium, for example, stays in our environment for thirty years. Children are especially susceptible to radiation poisoning because their cells are more rapidly dividing and growing than adults. Since Fukushima, 44% of babies in Japan and 28% on the North American West Coast are now born with congenital hypothyroidism as a result of I-131 (radioactive iodine) exposure.[42]

Research on children exposed to nuclear radiation after the disasters at Chernobyl, Fukushima, and Three Mile Island show a strong correlation between radiation exposure and increased incidence of type 1 and type 2 diabetes. Sixty percent of children twelve and under in the Fukushima area now have type 2 diabetes.[43] After Chernobyl, the rate of type 1 diabetes in children (under age fifteen) was at least doubled,[44] with the highest incidence occurring in the most contaminated local districts. From 1986 to 2002, there was a 100% increase in type 1 diabetes in children and adolescents in the Chernobyl region. Further research uncovered that in the regions surrounding Chernobyl there has been a significant increase in type 1 diabetes since the nuclear disaster 25 years ago—up to 200% more than before the Chernobyl event.[45] Workers who cleaned up after that event have higher insulin levels in their blood, which is a precursor warning of type 2 diabetes.[46]

After the Three Mile Island nuclear power plant accident, the rates of cancer and both type 1 and type 2 diabetes in the region were about doubled, and the rate of type 2 diabetes increased as residents aged. Survivors of the atomic bomb in Hiroshima also had an increased rate of type 2 diabetes thirty years or more after their radiation exposure.[47] Diabetes screening has been conducted on 64,000–113,000 atomic bomb survivors living in Hiroshima City since 1961. From 1971 to 1992, type 2 diabetes mellitus increased 2.7 times in males and 3.2 times in females.[48] We also see data indicating that children who undergo total body irradiation for cancer treatment may also develop a state of insulin resistance.[49]

The Pacific region and the island regions around Bimini showed the largest rise in fasting blood-glucose levels in the world between 1980 and 2008, and correspondingly the highest rates of diabetes prevalence in the world by 2008. This region was subjected to nuclear weapons testing from 1946–1958, and all residents there were exposed to acute and chronic radiation fallout.

We are also exposed to dangerous amounts of radiation when we are subjected to x-rays and CT scans (which expose patients to hundreds and sometimes thousands of times as much radiation as other x-rays and mammograms). The "naked body" scanners previously used by the U.S. Transportation Security Administration (TSA) in airports also exposed passengers to dangerous amounts of radiation, which concentrate in the skin and then spread throughout the body. A Los Alamos scientist has shown that TSA scanners "shred" human DNA.[50]

Because we are exposed to increased solar radiation when flying in an airplane, Dr. Gabriel recommends that women in their first trimester of pregnancy do not fly at all, in order to protect the fetus from radiation exposure. Dr. Stewart showed that women exposed to x-rays during pregnancy had offspring with double the average rate of leukemia. Giving pregnant women x-rays during the first trimester of pregnancy was associated with a twelve times higher rate of leukemia in the children.[51]

Thankfully, there are radiation-mitigation devices that can be placed onto personal cell phones, such as cell-phone discs by Tachyon Technologies, as well as nutritional supplements known to be effective for radiation protection. Our favorite of these supplements is Rad-Neutral, an odorless, flavorless, and safe product that has been shown to neutralize intracellular radiation for up to two years. (Both of these products are available at www.DrCousensOnlineStore.com.)

NCD-Zeolite (ten drops, four times a day) also helps to safely eliminate radiation from the body; after the Chernobyl disaster, children were given zeolite cookies to eat to decrease the negative effects of radiation.

Foods high in antioxidants are also beneficial, because radiation tends to oxidize the brain, promoting depression. We recommend eating as much sea vegetation as possible—but ideally not from the Pacific Ocean. Sea vegetables, particularly kelp, also help the body to eliminate radioactive minerals from the body.

When whole kelp is soaked in water for a few hours, quite a bit can be blended up as a thickener for soups and salad dressings without dominating the flavor of the food. Dried kelp powder, in contrast, can be fairly strong in flavor for children, even in small amounts. The Miso-Kelp-Dulse Broth recipe may also be helpful as a practical way to take sea vegetables daily.

Miso-Kelp-Dulse Broth (Phase 1)

1–2 tablespoons light miso

1–5 teaspoons kelp powder

1–5 teaspoons dulse flakes

½ teaspoon garlic powder

½ teaspoon onion powder

¼ teaspoon coconut oil (optional)

1½ cups warm (not boiled) structured or filtered water (see "Living Water," page 384)

If these foods are new to you, start with fewer sea veggies and work your way up to more. Simply stir ingredients together, and drink while still warm.

By following a plant-sourced lifestyle, we are lowering our families' risk of radiation toxicity. Flesh food on the average contains fifteen to thirty times more radiation than plant-sourced foods—with the exception of Pacific Ocean fish, which is much higher. This is true of all animals on the planet, including wild game and free-range farmed animals. During times of acute exposure, an alkaline, plant-sourced diet, antioxidants, and anti-radiation supplements are all essential.

Summary

As aware parents and grandparents, we now have some information to further protect our children and ourselves from toxic synergy. Every amount of protection, no matter how small, does make a difference. What we do matters, on multiple levels.

In looking at the few challenges we have listed, which affect our children's brains, nervous systems, endocrine systems, and organ systems, parents and grandparents may feel that the challenge of avoiding or eliminating the toxic dietary and environmental brew is overwhelming. In each subsection we have provided a few simple things that can reasonably be done, such as avoiding gluten and gliadin foods, and minimizing the use of cell phones for our children.

It is helpful to communicate with our children and grandchildren the power of positive thinking to create a diet and lifestyle with some of the unique supplementation we suggest, leaving our children filled with good feelings about their actions rather than fear. It is helpful to know that this positive lifestyle minimizes toxic synergy.

Keep in mind that our mental state also plays an important role in minimizing its effects. Research in Chernobyl, for example, showed that those who meditated experienced fewer toxic effects from the radiation exposure. Our focus, then, is on creating a lifestyle that naturally involves an optimistic approach to what we can do, versus being weighted down by the thought of all the toxins that the population of our planet is now exposed to.

CHAPTER 11

Supporting the Child's Spiritual Development

Every child you encounter is a Divine Appointment.

—Wess Stafford, President Emeritus
of Compassion International

The soul needs nourishment as well as the body.

—Rudolf Steiner

Every child is a spark of God. Our job as parents is to support them in becoming a flame of the Divine throughout their lives

—Rabbi Gabriel Cousens, MD

Spiritual Nutrition for Childhood

The secret of spiritual nutrition is to eat in such a way as to be a superconductor of the Divine.

—Rabbi Gabriel Cousens, MD

Beloved, I pray that you may prosper in all things and be in health, just as your soul prospers.

—3 John 1:2

Behold, I have given the grasses and herbs of the field, and the fruit of a seed-bearing tree. That shall be your food.

—Genesis 1:29, on the original food for the Adamic Race

The eating of meat extinguishes the seed of great compassion.

—The Buddha (Mahaparinirvana Sutra)

To avoid causing terror to living beings, let the disciple refrain from eating meat.... (T)he food of the wise is that which is consumed by the *sadhus* (holy men); it does not consist of meat.... There may be some foolish people in the future who will say that I permitted meat-eating and that I partook of meat myself, but ... meat-eating I have not permitted to anyone.... I do not permit, I will not permit, meat-eating in any form, in any manner, and in any place; it is unconditionally prohibited for all.

—The Buddha (in the Dhammapada)

Dear Father, hear and bless Thy beasts and singing birds; And guard with tenderness small things that have no words.

—Book of Prayers for Children (a Little Golden Book)

To create holiness in eating is to eat in a way that sanctifies and transforms the consciousness of the individual and affirms all of life.

—Rabbi Gabriel Cousens, MD

Much of the current treatment of animals in the live-stock trade makes the consumption of meat produced through such cruel conditions *halakhally* (by spiritual law) unacceptable as the product of illegitimate means.

—Rabbi David Rosen, Former Chief Rabbi of Ireland, and Director of the American Jewish Committee's Department of Interreligious Affairs and the Harriet and Robert Heilbrunn Institute for International Interreligious Affairs

The welfare of a soul can only be achieved after obtaining the well-being of the body.

—Moses Maimonides, in o'Hilchot De'ot

When the body aches, the soul too is weakened and one is unable to pray properly, even when clear of sin. So you must guard the health of the body carefully.

—Baal Shem Tov

The wolf will dwell with the lamb, and the leopard will lie down with the young goat.

—Isaiah 11:6

Because childhood is a time of spiritual sensitivity, the child benefits greatly when what we think, say, eat, and do is consistent with the great wisdom teachings that we follow within the home. Spirituality by example is the great teaching style that children understand, remember, and learn from.

By digging deeply to reconnect with our spiritual roots, whatever the tradition, we often bring to light precious gems that have been lost or cast off in the mad rush of a commercialized, amoral culture. When we were children, our spiritual training included recommendations to avoid cigarettes, alcohol, and illegal drugs, in order to honor the body as a holy temple of the Divine. And yet, because of widespread nutritional ignorance at the time, we faithfully bowed our heads over an alarming amount of sugary, fried, chemical-laden, and fast foods served around religious functions.

Our hearts were stirred by Bible stories, prayer, and devotional music—yet as young adults grow older, it is common to experience a conflict between spiritual heritage and the internal conviction to care about the environment, the humane treatment of animals, and the optimal nourishing of our living temples. This separation of "church and plate" is often reconciled when young adults come across Bible-based ecology books and other information casting light upon the ungodly practices of factory farming and lending spiritual support to people of faith who respond with veganism.

The Judeo-Christian scriptures are a treasure-trove of teachings on the protection of animals and of the Earth, as well as instruction for holistic health and vitality. For a more in-depth discussion of this, we highly recommend the Animal Humane Society's booklet entitled "The Bible's Teachings on Protecting Animals and Nature," available free of cost at www.humanesociety.org/assets/pdfs/faith/replenish-booklet-in-color.pdf.

As live-food educators, we are also encouraged by the work of Hallelujah Acres Lifestyle Centers to support modern-day Christians with living, plant-sourced nutrition, as well as the Tree of Life Center U.S., and Congregation Etz Chaim in Patagonia, AZ, which supports and empowers people of all traditions in successfully following Genesis 1:29. These efforts are helping families to integrate faith with holistic lifestyle choices, to help end the separation of "church and plate."

As discussed in *Conscious Eating*, the spiritual practice of nourishing the mind, body, and spirit with living foods is found at the heart of most of the world's wisdom traditions, including Hinduism, Buddhism, Taoism, Judaism, and Christianity. We see that the inner circle of the ancient Jewish Essenes, the rishis of ancient India, and the Taoists were also eating diets of primarily plant-based living foods. This is not so surprising because what is alive is what best supports us in our own aliveness. What is whole is what best supports our wholeness and holiness. Living foods, which literally hold light through photosynthesis, serve to support the alchemical process of attuning us with our light-bodies and our own unfolding enlightenment, and ultimately stimulating the inner light.

In *Creating Peace by Being Peace,* Rabbi Dr. Gabriel speaks of food as a "living field," referring to the work of Professor Fritz-Albert Popp, who was able to show that wild food has approximately twice the biophotons (energetic radiations) as organically farmed food, and that raw organic food has eighty-three times as much biophoton energy as junk food. Popp's work also revealed that healthy individuals have a higher cellular charge of biophotons than those who are unhealthy. He also found that the average junk-food eater had an average measure of 1,000 biophotons, whereas the average baby had an average of 43,000. A person with a fairly healthy, organic, cooked plant-based diet also has an average of 23,000 biophotons, while live-fooders showed a biophoton count of 83,000.

The more biophotons we have, the more our communication with the cosmos is enhanced; and so, the more biophotons we radiate, the more strongly we feel our connection with the cosmos and the Divine. This is one reason why we feel more "turned on" when we start eating live foods, and our awareness of the oneness of life is enhanced. Also, the more biophotons we have, the greater intracellular and intercellular communication we have, which means better intracellular and extracellular function.

By contrast, foods such as white sugar, white flour, and processed foods, which are stripped of nutrients and therefore fragmented from their wholeness, tend to aggravate human conditions of depletion, fragmentation, and alienation from our own wholeness. Choosing to eat meat and dairy products is choosing to take into our bodies the suffering and victim-consciousness of the animal. As the enlightened Swami Prakashananda Saraswati, one of Rabbi Dr. Gabriel's main spiritual teachers, said:

> Every animal that is slaughtered for human consumption brings the pain of death into your body. Think about it: The animal is killed with violence. That violence causes the animal to experience very intense pain as it dies. That pain remains in the meat even after you've prepared and cooked it. When you eat the meat, you eat pain.

That pain becomes lodged in your body, heart, and mind. The violence and pain that you consume will eat you also. It consumes you, so that you must experience the same pain in your life also.

In the Ayurvedic tradition of spiritual nutrition, foods are classified as being *sattvic, rajasic,* or *tamasic. Sattvic* foods are pure foods that support the cultivation of a quiet mind and stimulate the most spiritual energy; *rajasic* foods activate outward thinking and actions, which may be good for warriors or businessman/woman energy; and *tamasic* foods are analogous to junk food, white flour, white sugar, and processed foods, and drugs, transmitting vibrations of suffering, meanness of spirit, sloth, addiction, and criminal activity. The *tamasic* results of the SAD (standard American diet) are unmistakably evident in today's society.

A study of the world's spiritual traditions reveals that not only within the Torah or Biblical traditions but also in the Hindu, Taoist, and Sumerian traditions, there is a subtle reference to the "great galactic summer." This refers to preflood times of 6,000 years ago, when the Earth's climatic conditions were similar to that of a greenhouse, and therefore optimal for the plant-sourced living-foods lifestyle. This is a partial explanation of why the diet in Eden was 100% living food.

As Earth's climate slowly changed and vegetation was less plentiful, there was a slow change in the human diet for some. According to the famous archeologist Richard Leakey, a good case can be made that humans as far back as three million years ago had a 97% vegan diet, similar to that of chimpanzees. Certainly there have been times, such as the Ice Age, in which a meat-based diet was necessary for human survival.

Also, after the Biblical flood, Genesis 9:3 states: "Every moving thing that is alive shall be food for you; I give all to you, as I gave the green plant." This is because people who were not ready to go back to being immediately vegan were given the biblical dispensation to slowly transition away from meat-eating back to a Garden of Eden live-food vegan diet. This is according to many rabbis, including the first chief rabbi of Israel, Rav Abraham Isaac Kook, who was himself a vegetarian.

We are presently living in a time, however, when a return to our original plant-based diet is needed for physical planetary healing and for the spiritual development of Earth's inhabitants. As Rabbi Dr. Gabriel has said, "In each generation we are given the medicine for healing the generation. In our generation, live food veganism is the medicine for healing ourselves and the planet."

According to Torah tradition, there will be a time when even the predatory animals will be herbivores: "And to all the beasts of the Earth and all the birds in the sky and all the creatures that move along the ground—everything that has the breath of life in it—I give every green plant for food" (Genesis 1:30), and "The wolf and the lamb shall feed together, and the lion shall eat straw like the bullock" (Isaiah 65:25).

Retold as part of a scripture-based homeschool curriculum, modern-day animal stories can also help validate this potential for students. In the first (true) story, a rat snake in Tokyo surprised all of its zookeepers by becoming best friends with a hamster who was put into his cage for food. The second true story features a lion named Little Tyke, also living in captivity. Because his caregivers, Georges and Margaret Westbeau, believed that he would not survive without eating meat, they tried everything they could to make him accept it. Little Tyke, however, voluntarily remained an ovo-lacto-vegetarian for his entire life, feeding on grain, rice, milk, and eggs.[1]

This zoology textbook, widely used among homeschoolers, also encourages students to consider that, just because we've all been taught that sharp teeth are for tearing flesh, doesn't necessarily make it true. If we look inside the mouth of the panda bear, for example, we can see that its long, extremely sharp incisors and canines are ideal for eating bamboo. Dr. Gabriel and his wonderful wife Shanti visited a Buddhist sanctuary monastery in Thailand, where a large number of tigers were raised for their entire lifetimes on a vegan cuisine. Although some were on chains, people could pet them, and Rabbi Dr. Gabriel and Shanti even guided one on a leash for a walk. There was a waterfall and swim pond where humans and tigers (not on a chain) could be together. The reality of Genesis 1:30 seemed already true. A peaceful diet, including peaceful people and tigers, can bring peace.

Another book in which we've found prophetically peaceful cross-species stories is *Unlikely Friendships* by Jennifer S. Holland. While many of these stories include domesticated animals, such as a companionship between a rat and a cat, some of these remarkable friendships were observed even in the wild—a lioness who mothered a baby oryx, and a leopard who literally lay down beside a cow, who would groom her when she made her nightly visits.[2]

Every shamanic tradition acknowledges that when we eat animals, regardless of how they were raised, we are literally taking in the spirit of the animal. This is expressed in the Biblical teachings of a kosher diet. The original dietary recommendation of Genesis 1:29 is clearly plant-sourced: "… every seed-bearing plant that is upon the Earth, and every tree that has seed-bearing fruit, they shall be yours for food," as this is the most peace-promoting cuisine.

When people strayed from eating only plant-sourced foods, they were advised to at least eat only herbivorous animals, which are more peaceful than carnivores, and to strictly avoid the consumption of blood (seen as containing the spirit of the animal), as a practical starting point for returning to greater harmony by reducing the violence in the animal qualities being consumed. Kosher food guidelines were a way of helping the people transition back to the vegan cuisine of Garden Eden. The spiritual subtlety of vegan cuisine helps us bring a holiness and bloodless *ahimsa* to life, to separate us from our own lower nature and from the decay, disease, destruction, depletion, and degeneration associated with killing animals and bringing their death and blood into our bodies and lives.

Veganism is a brilliant approach for elevating human consciousness and avoiding the energy of death and degeneration associated with killing animals for food, which enters us when we eat their flesh and blood. Live-food organic veganism sanctifies the natural boundaries in nature between animal and humanity, which become blurred when we consume animal flesh. In this context, vaccinations composed of a variety of animal components such as pig, monkey, and cow parts represent a failure to separate species, and thus are a violation of the Divine order in creation.

By sanctifying the boundaries in nature, on the other hand, we uplift human consciousness and health. Killing animals to satisfy our lust is a degenerate behavior that does not support the regeneration and evolution of life and consciousness. Dominion, presented in the Bible as the role of humans on Earth, does not mean domination. We are put on Earth not to create degradation and death but, through aware, awake, and veganic dominion, to sanctify and upgrade the web of life on Planet Earth—and we can do this every time we sit down to eat. These are profound, three-times-a-day, compassion-and-peace teachings for our children, which they can receive at a level appropriate to their age.

Although people were given a temporary biblical dispensation, the eating of "kosher" meat is not the Judaic ideal. Israel has the second-highest percentage of vegetarians in the world (8.6% of the population). India is first, with 40%, and Europe and the U.S. have an estimated 3.3% vegetarian population. In the Torah tradition there are blessings for every food—except meat. In addition, at this time in history because of the "unkosher" practices of kosher meat-processing plants, there is arguably no truly kosher meat available, as in Biblical times. Not only do most animals suffer inhumane farming practices, but factory-farmed herbivores are now given processed feed that contains the ground-up flesh of other animals. As Rabbi Joseph Albo stated:

> Aside from the cruelty, anger, and fury in killing animals, and the fact that it lends human beings the bad trait of shedding blood for naught, eating the flesh even of select animals will yet give rise to a man of insensitive soul.[3]

As a holistic physician and rabbi, Dr. Gabriel has observed firsthand in thousands of people that plant-sourced living foods are the most powerful foods for enhancing the flow of the Divine feminine energy, known as the *shekhinah* in Hebrew, *kundalini* in Sanskrit, or Holy Spirit in Christianity. A natural flow of this energy within each person brings us a deeper perception of truth, reality, and universality.

In these ways, an 80% live-food vegan cuisine provides powerful support for enhancing spiritual life in our children.

Supporting the Spirit of the Child with Silence

In quiet listening we penetrate a depth of truth that can renew our souls. The subtleties of nature vibrate with ancient wisdom. If we are silent enough to hear the invitation, we are welcomed as humble participants into the most tender movements of creation.

—Shea Darian, in *Seven Times the Sun: Guiding Your Child Through the Rhythms of the Day*

The child, with unaffected innocence, will understand the message of silence.... Through the secret that silence holds, the child will seek out his spirit. As he stands closer to God or nature by virtue of his lesser years, he will recognize it and know it as part of himself.

—Elizabeth Caspari, friend and student of Dr. Maria Montessori, and cofounder of Caspari Montessori Institute

Mom, can I sit up in the tree and be quiet for awhile? It helps me to be present.

—Leah's daughter Quinn, at age eight

You have to meditate and play, both at once.

—the Dalai Lama (as quoted in the book Zen Baby)

You can get help from teachers, but you are going to learn a lot by yourself sitting alone in a room.

—Dr. Seuss

My son and daughter were regularly meditating in adult meditation groups since the age of three. At three years old, my daughter would awaken early with me and meditate in my lap every morning, for months at a time.... At ages five for my daughter and eight for my son, of their own choice and willpower, they successfully participated in an eight-hour-per-day adult meditation weekend intensive with Swami Muktananda in India. Children raised in a spiritually supportive environment without television are capable of much more than we usually expect of them.... Parents and children can communicate in the sweetness of their silence when they meditate together.

—Rabbi Gabriel Cousens, MD

When offering her little students candy as a reward for being quiet, Dr. Montessori observed that, once the children had tasted the deliciousness of silence, they refused her rewards of sweets. It was as if it spoiled the spiritual experience—and most of us would be worried about spoiling their dinners!

It has also been a great pleasure to observe children in their journey into silence. Whether it's just one minute of silent pause before a meal with preschool students, or an hour-long meditation with our children or grandchildren, it is a delight to see how the child is drawn to the experience when readiness is present. Once Leah was leading a group of preschool and kindergarten children on a nature walk, and they came upon a lovely place to sit. Leah invited the children to "make silence" with her as a group. Some opted to go back to the classroom with the teacher's aide, while others chose the experience of silence.

On subsequent nature walks, upon passing that same spot, a child would say fondly, "Remember when we made silence there?" Or they would even ask, "Can we make silence there again?" One little boy's experience with silence touched Leah's heart in particular, for he had explained to her that he wanted to calm his body down. When they started playing silence games together as a class, this extremely active boy's face lit up, and he asked to hold the silence together longer, as it appeared to be helping his hyperactive state. Not only that, but he also asked Leah to tell his mother about this stillness, so that he could do this with her and his older brother at home. Being on a spiritual path herself, his mother was very happy to hear this news.

In the book *Calm and Compassionate Children,* author and educator Susan Usha Dermond recommends calm and soothing music as a way to ease out of a lifestyle of high-media consumption of TV, radio, and video games, into one that includes silence. Dermond also points out that our children need plenty of outdoor time and physical activity in order to be able to be still during quieter times of the day.

The best way to teach meditation to our children is for them to see that we meditate. From infancy on, our children learn what to value in their lives by the values we demonstrate. When we weave meditation, prayer, and other spiritual practices into family life, they become just as natural as eating, sleeping, toileting, working, playing, storytelling, or anything else that initially takes repetitive practice.

For very young children who are relying on their absorbent minds rather than logic and verbal cognition—in other words, before the left- to right-brain crossover that generally happens around the age of three—the living example is enough, and no explanation of meditation is necessary. For older children who want to understand why we include silence in our day, the following exercise helps to illustrate this: Take a glass jar and fill about one quarter of it with dirt. Now add water to the jar until it is full. With your child, cap and shake the jar vigorously, and then set it down to watch what happens. Explain that the jar with swirling contents is like our active minds, and that when we sit in stillness our minds begin to calm down—just as the contents of the jar settle and allow the water to clear—until we feel settled and our minds become quiet and at peace.

In classic Montessori classrooms, lessons on observing silence are given to help develop stillness within children age three and older. The child is invited to these lessons, but is not forced, as children come into readiness for silence with their own individual timing. Practicing silence is introduced only after the child has received other lessons that support their coordination and movement control, many of which can be demonstrated with little verbal instruction. This is because an ability to control one's bodily movements is needed in order to be still.

As part of the spiritual fasting retreats at the Tree of Life Center U.S., not only do fasters meditate each day but they spend one day of their week in silence. This is an opportunity to be further supported in turning inward. Likewise, spending a portion of the day in silence with your child can also be rewarding, as long as the child wants to play along. You can pass notes when needed, if the child is old enough to read and write. The benefits of this exercise may include a more tranquil atmosphere; no nagging, lecturing, or scolding; a greater awareness of reactionary impulses, surrender, mystery, practice of intuitive communication skills; and quiet giggling.

Imagination

> The wild dream is the first step to reality. It is the direction-finder by which people locate higher goals and discern their highest selves.
>
> —Norman Cousins

> I want to draw a picture of a jewel to remind you of your heart. I think our hearts are really jewels. I imagine it that way. Are our hearts jewels? Do you think that too? ... Our hearts are a secret treasure, and we know where that treasure lies. We want the treasure, don't we?
>
> —Leah's daughter Quinn, at age five

While imagination is often associated with childhood fantasy, the ability to make a mental picture can also increase one's awareness of what we often call reality—three-dimensional, Earth-plane phenomena. Albert Einstein used to conduct what he termed "thought experiments." In one of these experiments, Einstein imagined riding sunbeams to the far reaches of the universe; upon finding himself returned, illogically, to the surface of the sun, he concluded that the Universe must indeed be curved, and that his previous logical training was incomplete. Einstein then rounded out this thought experiment—a right-brained exercise— with numbers, equations, and words, using his left brain, to arrive at the intuitive-scientific theory of relativity.

We also see the use of imagination in healing with visualization during prayer and other forms of guided imagery. In Brandon Bays' book *Journey for Kids*, we read the following example of a child seeing with his mind's eye to resolve a traumatized cellular memory stored in his ear:

> Six-year-old Oliver held up his "before" and "after" paintings, and the "after" looked just like a shell. A medical doctor attending the ... retreat gasped when he saw it. He asked if he could speak to the child, and went up to Oliver saying, "That's an anatomically correct picture of the cochlea in the ear—you can't have taken anatomy lessons at your age, can you?" Oliver: "I just went in here (pointing to his ear), and found this shell inside. It looked all gunky at first, but now it looks clean and shiny!" He had painted rays of light coming from the shell in the "after" picture.[4] What Journey facilitators have observed is that whether the image created by a child is anatomically accurate or is a metaphorical picture, the results are the same: profound healing occurs.

Inspiring visions and dreams also come to us through imagery, connecting us to our intuition. Observing the imaginative play of a child can be a profound experience as well. One morning when Leah was waking, her son Levi, who was four at the time, bounded into the room, threw a blanket over her head, and exclaimed, "Mama, you're a present!"

"Really?" Leah asked from underneath the blanket. "Who's going to open me?" Without a moment's hesitation, Levi answered, "You are. Because it's yours." This playful declaration moved Leah deeply, reminding her of the profound teaching: I will become what I already am. Levi's creative expression led his mother into the sacred reality of the journey to the self. While accurate observations about the Earth plane, astral plane, and other levels of awareness are all important, in the context of liberation we see that ultimately the Divine is the only true reality, existing prior to and shining in the Earth plane.

What are some ways to nurture creative imagination?

- As the parent, allow yourself to express creativity.
- Minimizing media intake is a precious gift, especially for the very young child.
- Tell uplifting stories.
- Pray or meditate together.
- Draw, color, or paint your mental pictures.
- Sing songs, or read poetry with rich and meaningful metaphors.
- Create artful and therapeutic puppet plays (see "Resources," page 485).

Is fantasy healthy? For the adult, the experience of fantasy fades as a natural part of identifying with the ego. For the child, however, who is still in the stage of ego-development, the authors feel that fantasy plays an important role. When the child is engaged in fantasy play, this is an etheric, dreamlike experience that we can appreciate as a healthy part of spiritual development.

Just as we need not interfere with the child's fantasy play, neither do children require us to inundate them with excessive materialism to nurture fantasy. Technology-based fantasy such as TV, movies, and video games is not generally recommended, as these actually limit the flow of fantasy.

Meaningful Work

Work that connects the child to life, and to the creative spark within, is what we are looking for in the environments we prepare for children. Activities with predictable and repetitive motions such as knitting, crocheting, embroidery, snapping peas, peeling almonds, or counting objects, tend to quiet the mind. Like devotional chanting and mantra repetition, these serve as preparation for meditation, which takes us beyond the mind. They also provide a gently grounding influence.

Wisdom Teachings

Bringing up a child in a Divine-focused tradition helps to guide them and provide avenues of spiritual expression. These traditions also tend to provide supportive community relationships, a sense of morality and ethics, opportunities to serve, and, most of all, support for one's relationship with the Divine.

Music

After silence, that which comes nearest to expressing the inexpressible is music.

—Aldous Huxley

Music is the mediator between spiritual and sensual life.

—Ludwig van Beethoven

Take a music bath once or twice a week for a few seasons. You will find it is to the soul what a water bath is to the body.

—Oliver Wendell Holmes

The musician hears the pulse of the divine will that flows through the world; he hears how this will expresses itself in tones.... The effects of music on the human soul are so direct, so powerful, so elemental.

—Rudolf Steiner, in his lecture
"The Inner Nature of Music and the Experience of Tone"

In our culture, music education for children is often limited to an appreciation of its mathematical aspects, music theory, a potential career option, or a means for "creative expression" regardless of the musical content. However, in the context of liberated culture, we see that music also has the potential to unify the human family and to help the child attune to higher vibrations. It is with a deeper understanding of music's role in childhood that the Association of North American Waldorf Music Educators (ANAWME) states, "Musical instruction is presented in such a way as to encourage musical living."[5]

Anita Wolberd of Caspari Montessori Institute tells the story to teachers in training of one of her kindergarteners, who had a somewhat troubled home situation. He came to school exclaiming that the song "Love Within" had come to him upon waking, and that they had to sing it together! The class had sung that song together in circle time, with the following words: "Love within, love without. Love is ever 'round about. Here at hand, near and far, love is always where we are."

Children will often use the tool of sacred song to center themselves. In *Creating Peace by Being Peace,* Rabbi Dr. Gabriel says, "The acts of listening, chanting, or playing sacred music empower the soul to perceive and release illusions of fear, pain, separation, and suffering, so that it experiences and remembers the reality of the love it already is."

Sacred sound has been a part of all historical times and cultures. Devotional music has been shared by the Essenes, Sufis, Native Americans, Gnostics, Hindus, and many other Divine-focused cultures. Music has the potential to bypass the ego and dance with the soul. Music moves us emotionally and subliminally, affecting our consciousness through two laws of physics known as sympathetic vibration and entrainment. This is why paying attention to the type of music in the child's environment is so important.

While music can deeply touch the child's soul and nurture their aliveness, certain types of music, conversely, can undermine the yearnings of their souls. As described in Rabbi Dr. Gabriel's book *Creating Peace by Being Peace,*

In 1993 Dr. Jonathan Klein published the results of his survey of 2,760 adolescents ranging from fourteen to sixteen years of age: "There is clearly an association between embracing heavy-metal music and risky behavior (smoking marijuana, cheating, stealing, drinking alcohol, and having sex)."

Various studies of music's effects on plants, as well as Dr. Masaru Emoto's water-crystal photos in the book *Hidden Messages in Water*, also reveal a dramatic distinction between the vibration of heavy-metal music and that of classical music, which was often dedicated to the Divine, or other devotional types of music.

Unfortunately, it is not just heavy metal that delivers undermining vibrations. As we've all likely noticed, much of today's pop music, including rock, rap, country, and heavy metal, inundates the child with messages that glamorize death-culture behavior, and encouragement of drug and alcohol use, materialism, sexism, and other forms of disrespectful sexuality. Our culture's most heavily marketed music for tweens and teens so often offers to the impressionable child celebrity role-models whose lyrics, music videos, and lifestyles clearly undermine holistic character and spiritual development.

Just as the least nutritious foods today—typical school-cafeteria fare, fast-food kid meals, sugary breakfast cereals, and chemical-laden processed lunchbox products—are considered to be "kid food," we also see that highly commercialized, spiritually depleted "ear-candy" is also assumed to be what children want or, by implication, feel they are worth. Rather than investing in "the best for the youngest," as Dr. Montessori recommended, the culture of death capitalizes on its most vulnerable citizens by hooking them on food and media products that are both highly addictive and cheap to produce. That is part of why we have emphasized the importance of healthy food and uplifting media for supporting the spiritual life of our children.

As the culture of life is revived, however, it is very fun to see that— just as the child will initiate healthy food choices when given the option and support—children are also very capable of experiencing the joy of spiritually uplifting music when immersed in this type of environment. In Leah's own childhood, she would often sing songs she had learned at church, many of them scripture verses, throughout her day and during long rides in the car. These were key spiritual experiences that followed her into her teen years, as she continued to select artists whose music was devoted to their relationship with the Divine. These songs were food for her soul, long before she was introduced to living nutrition. Participating in sacred song at the Tree of Life Center is always a special time for her and for her family.

In *Creating Peace by Being Peace,* Rabbi Dr. Gabriel says:

> Our music can either reflect the lowest emanations of a culture such as fear, hate, and murder, or those of peace, compassion, and love.... What do we choose to listen to, and what does the mass media, which usually reflects the culture of death, promote?
>
> As we create a world culture of peace, it is important to create a world music that shares the vibration of peace and love, and the process creates a sharing of the best of the different world cultures, which in turn creates respect for all the gifts of the different planetary world cultures. The real power of culture through music is the potential to spread the vibration of the joy of inner and outer peace through the subtle effect of music on the heart and mind.[6]

Its effect on the heart and mind gives music the potential to stimulate healing. Music therapy, for example, has been found to be helpful for physical needs such as pain management for cancer and leukemia patients, treating autism and headaches; for emotional and cognitive needs such as reducing depression and negativity, and aiding concentration, memory function, and spatial-temporal reasoning; and for social needs as well.[7] "Music therapy quite literally can soothe the soul," says pediatric oncologist Dr. Rob Goldsby.[8]

Sacred dance, which has been practiced since ancient times, also offers participants an avenue for transformation. As seen in the film *Dance of Liberation,* sacred dance is also being offered as a support for liberating the shining potential within teens. In Waldorf education, we see a musical art form called eurythmy that was designed to treat illness holistically through movement.

As parents, we have the beautiful options of music, song, and dance to uplift the home environment and to educate our children in the importance of these choices. What a blessing we have in music, to carry the energetic frequencies of love, joy, and peace in support of the child's mind, body, and spirit.

The Spirituality-Enhancing Power of Love

Perhaps the most powerful spiritual motivation, teaching, and evolutionary upliftment for children of any age is love. We have already discussed the importance of a child being and feeling love as powerful for building their self-esteem, but this discussion includes a more expanded approach.

A primary spiritual teaching of love and relationship for children is the parents' intimacy process. It starts before pregnancy, in the actual lovemaking. When there is true love, every cell is filled with love, including the sperm and ovum. This union, as love-into-oneness, is the ultimate love-merging on the physical plane, in which the two literally become one with each other and the Divine in order to start new life. In the womb, the baby feels the love of the mother for herself, and for it as a wanted baby.

Love is again amplified at birth, and throughout childhood, by the parents. This is the ideal, in which the child experiences love throughout childhood. We realize that not everyone is blessed with ideal inputs, and this may not happen every step of the way, in the context of the variety of ways a child may experience love and the variety of failed and successful relationships happening today. There are many adults who did not receive this love during childhood; but this can be remedied by a long-term intimate relationship and/or ultimately by experiencing the love of the Divine within.

When we experience the love spark of the Divine within, often as the result of meditation and prayer, we know directly that we are loved, and that we are love. Then we move from having a belief about "God-love" to the direct experience, sustained by faith, that we are loved. This direct experiential awareness empowers our faith in the Divine love reverberating within us, which leads us to the infinite love of the Divine that heals all our loveless wounds.

Parental intimacy enhances this high spiritual level in the family, as parents become an active, nonverbal role model of love and spiritual development for the children.

One of the fundamentals of understanding love is that love comes from within oneself rather than from someone else. Getting this understanding backwards is a not-so-subtle misunderstanding that usually leads to codependency, when we believe someone outside of us is the source of love. It is true that someone else can help you access and amplify that place of love within yourself, but they are not the source. Not acknowledging or consciously accessing the Divine source of love within is where people often get very confused in relationships.

Another level of relationship confusion is the politically correct term "unconditional love." Rabbi Dr. Gabriel Cousens, as a family therapist, consistently sees the contrary, where even healthy and successful people and relationships usually have a "bottom line." In other words, there is a healthy conditionality in relationships, and it needs to be respected and not idealistically ignored.

This dynamic can also be played out in parent/child relationships, both directly and as practice for future healthy relationships. It is important to be sensitive to this, because if these bottom lines get crossed there may be irreversible damage to the relationship. It is important that the children see their parents maintain dignity and self-respect in relationship. Even if a relationship ends, it is important that everyone should come out of the relationship loving themselves. Respected bottom lines are healthy because they maintain self-esteem, create a sense of safety, and help to avoid unnecessarily irreparable damage to a relationship, which can often occur when bottom lines are crossed.

It is productive to verbalize these (often suppressed) bottom lines in relationships among all family members, so that everyone knows where they stand. It may be confusing for parents and/or children if they have theoretical, "politically correct" beliefs that they "should" be unconditionally loving, and therefore "anything goes"—rather than setting healthy physical, psychosocial, and spiritual boundaries that honor and protect the love in a relationship. A healthy relationship benefits immensely from boundaries and clarifications. These create safety, which is essential for mature intimacy to develop. It is a powerful, beneficial teaching for a child's developing relationship skills to be involved in conscious discussions about these issues.

A healthy intimate relationship involves the physical aspect, the mental aspect, the emotional aspect, and the spiritual aspect. All of these have to be in line for a full, sacred and intimate relationship. Sacred relationship invokes the Divine in all levels of interaction, and includes commitment to elevating your partner and family member as well as yourself to the highest spiritual potential. This is an optimal interdependent, not codependent, relationship.

For a child to witness this sacred, intimate kind of relationship is a powerful spiritual teaching for building sacred relationships themselves. In an interdependent relationship, you are happy in the relationship but do not *need* the relationship. You are choosing the relationship because it is one that creates continuous spiritual elevation, but your survival or happiness does not depend on the other. Naturally, when two people partner there has to be a cooperative interdependence. A key part of relationship is the joy of working as a team. In the most successful, evolving sacred relationships, the Divine is also included as a partner. This is another aspect of the sacred relationship that a child can understand—that teamwork is in the context of interdependence, not codependence; of choice, not need.

Love is the language of relationship. The love-connecting fire of relationship opens up the door to intimacy. It is healthy for children to see and feel the love-fire and romance of their parents' relationship. It provides a powerful, Divine, love-intimacy experience for children to witness and feel in their family. It helps them understand the intimacy of couple and family as an evolving spiritual path that they share to some extent.

Intimacy can be talked out, and valued for the challenge that it creates for character and spiritual growth. Consciously teaching children about relationship intimacy is important for their life training. (It is of course important to put healthy boundaries around "adult" aspects of the relationship, such as the sexual aspects, which generally are not appropriate for them.)

Intimacy is an enduring aspect of relationship in which people are able to maintain an openhearted love and sense of safety. In order to have intimacy, you have to feel safe. Feeling safe is key to a healthy, happy childhood. Moments of intimacy are not the same thing as steady, safe, and ongoing romantic love that sustains through the ups and downs of whatever happens. It is a great spiritual teaching and experience for children to see in their parents and also to experience for themselves in the parent-child relationship, with appropriate parent-child boundaries. This takes mature parenting skill. This is why sacred relationships are both the oldest and the newest frontier.

One contributing factor in our societal breakdown is fear of intimacy. This fear is often a result of growing up in a dysfunctional family. In some segments of our society, fear is becoming stronger than the power of love. The challenging question that we are posing is: *Are you willing to allow the power of love to overcome your fear of intimacy?* The cosmic play in relationship is when love encourages us to overcome our fear of intimate relationship. This is a spiritually evolved setting for a child to witness and be inspired by.

When we look at the complexity of relationship, we can understand that a major spiritual purpose of relationship is to enhance one's spiritual development. There are other forms of relationship besides sacred, intimate relationships: There are, for instance, dharmic relationships, which may even involve raising children or sharing a life mission; and there are relationships where there is a healing of the rift between male and female energies. In Biblical teaching, the he-Adam and the she-Adam were one, before there was a split. Intimate relationship slowly brings them back together again. The cosmic teaching is that one becomes two, which become one flesh again.

The meaning of intimacy—the goal of sacred relationship—is as a spiritual path. Love of self, partner, and the Divine is the foundation of all sacred relationships, and in fact almost all relationships. The ability to love another transcends gender; it depends on experiencing the source of love within our own hearts, and experiencing and rejoicing in that in the other. This is far beyond sexual lust as a foundation of relationship.

Sacred intimate relationships in any form remain the great and challenging frontier of our society and times. The ability to love intimately is the eternal and final frontier. Are we up to the challenge? Through the intimate love and sacred relationship in our lives, we can inspire our children by allowing them to experience loving, intimate family and to witness healthy levels of parental intimacy, preparing them to take on the spiritual challenge of their own sacred intimate relationships, as children and also when they reach mature adulthood.

In a deep and heartfelt way, as parents and grandparents involved in conscious parenting, we find, through a variety of ways, the profound, sweet, and holy responsibility of supporting our children's spiritual unfolding. May we be blessed with beautifully honoring this sacred responsibility!

In this spirit, we end this chapter with a quote from the much-loved children's musician Raffi:

> We find these joys to be self-evident: That all children are created whole, endowed with innate intelligence, with dignity, and wonder, worthy of respect.
>
> The embodiment of life, liberty and happiness, children are original blessing, here to learn their own song. Every girl and boy is entitled to love, to dream and belong to a loving "village." And to pursue a life of purpose. We affirm our duty to nourish and nurture the young, to honor their caring ideals as the heart of being human. To recognize the early years as the foundation of life, and to cherish the contribution of young children to human evolution.
>
> We commit ourselves to peaceful ways, and vow to keep from harm or neglect these, our most vulnerable citizens. As guardians of their prosperity, we honor the bountiful Earth whose diversity sustains us. Thus we pledge our love for generations to come.[9]

CHAPTER 12

Recipes for Children

The Phase Chart of food lists below, as developed by Rabbi Dr. Gabriel for his book *Rainbow-Green Live Food Cuisine,* can be extremely helpful for parents in getting an idea of how much sugar is in their children's meals. Although sugar is attractive to children, it clearly isn't the best food for their general constitution. According to the classical Ayurvedic system, all children tend to be on the *kapha* side—plump and watery—and do best with bitter, pungent, astringent foods.

However, classical Ayurveda includes all the tastes—sweet, sour, salty, bitter, and pungent—all of which belong in a balanced diet and life. Unfortunately, the American diet focuses on the sweet. What parents and children become accustomed to eating has significant long-term negative ramifications for their long-term health and longevity.

The Phase Chart is a guideline for parents and grandparents to the amounts of fructose or glucose that occur in various foods. We have based our recipe section on this Phase system, so that we can better guide you in using recipes to balance children's constitutions with bitter and astringent foods and tastes. At the same time, the recipes provide enough sweetness to make children want to eat the foods. We also varied the colors, making the food an even more enriching, exciting journey for them.

The Low-Sugar Piece to the Food Puzzle

While a small percentage of the population does well with a high-fructose diet, this is certainly not the diet for the vast majority, and especially not for children. High blood-sugar levels, even from sugars in whole foods, completely interfere with the growth hormones of childhood development. This because a high-sugar diet raises insulin, which is a hormone that inhibits the human growth hormone.

Not surprisingly, a high-sugar diet also appears to increase tooth decay. If we look at how much fruit humans have eaten historically (except in the tropics), we had limited access to fruit sugar and glucose. This helps explain how excessive amounts of glucose and fructose, which indirectly raise insulin and diabetes rates, can lead to an unhealthful way of life for most people. Nature made fructose and glucose scarce, and humans made it plentiful.

High blood sugar in the body is also associated with an increased risk of heart disease and trace-mineral deficiencies, specifically of chromium, copper, calcium, vanadium, and magnesium; it is also implicated in emphysema, and the depletion and imbalance of neurotransmitters. When sugar intake is raised, neurotransmitter levels go down, and depression, anxiety, ADD, and ADHD go up.

High blood sugar has also been connected to type 2 diabetes, hypertension, hyperactivity, increased triglycerides, skin wrinkles, obesity, PMS, weakened immune system (by blocking access of vitamin C to the cells), alcoholism, asthma, arthritis, colitis, drowsiness and inactivity in children (when they hit the low after the sugar high), Alzheimer's disease, multiple sclerosis, weakened eyesight, varicose veins, and raised adrenaline in children. Additionally, all sugars feed candida and cancer cells, and contribute to hypoglycemia. We also see that type 2 diabetes greatly increased from 1992 to 2002, jumping from appearing in 4% to 24% of children in general, and up to 75% of children in African-American communities in Arkansas and Ohio.[1]

In the "Reversing Diabetes" program at the Tree of Life Center U.S., participants with type 2 diabetes are 97% successful in reducing insulin

dependency and even coming off insulin entirely, through a holistic program of spiritual fasting, supplement support, and adopting a moderately
low-glycemic, living-foods diet. The statistics revealed in *There is a Cure
for Diabetes* (revised edition) show 61% of the non-insulin-dependent
diabetics and 24% of the insulin-dependent diabetes were healed in three
weeks. A moderately low-glycemic "Phase 1" diet is the foundation of
this healing process. Phase 1 cuisine includes vegetables, leafy greens,
sprouts, nuts, seeds, and sea vegetables, altogether comprising 95–100%
live foods.

For day-to-day family life, we recommend a 25–45% moderately low-
carbohydrate, mineral-rich diet made up of at least 80% vegan, living
foods, with 25–45% of it raw plant-based fats, especially long-chain
omega-3s; and from 10–20% of it protein for children and perinatal
mothers, so that there is enough protein while childbearing, breastfeeding, and to support the children's growth.

Long-chain omega-3s and cholesterol are particularly important for
brain development. A safe amount of fructose (sugar from fruit) for most
people is around fifteen to twenty-five grams a day. This is the equivalent
of two bananas, two Medjool dates, one quarter-cup of raisins, or two
kiwis.[2] In addition to building a foundation for overall health, reducing
sugars helps to minimize emotional and energetic spikes and lows; as
sugar rises, much-needed neurotransmitters go down. Rather than pulling
calcium from the teeth, as sugars do, the chlorophyll in fresh leafy greens
cleans and strengthens the teeth and gums.

It is also interesting to note that babies who experience the bitter flavor
of dark-leafy greens, green juices, green powders, etc. via amniotic fluid
while in the womb (if mom is eating these) and while breastfeeding via
mother's milk, actually prefer the bitter flavor to sweet, once they start
on their own solid foods. According to Ayurvedic tradition, more bitter
foods are highly beneficial for the child because childhood is a more *kapha*
stage of life, and bitter, pungent, and astringent foods balance *kapha*. The
kapha stage of life is from infancy through puberty. It is the time when all
children's physiology is the most watery, and there is the highest tendency
to problems involving mucus, such as colds, flu, earaches, and tonsillitis.

The following Phase Chart (from *Rainbow Green Live-Food Cuisine*) lists foods with no-to-low sugar, and foods with moderate-to-high sugar content.

Phase Chart: The Sugar Content of Various Foods

PHASE 1 FOODS

These foods are recommended for an optimal healing diet generally, and specifically for type 1 or 2 diabetes.

Note: A Phase 1 salad with a small amount of Phase 1.5 fruits and vegetables is also considered to be Phase 1.

Foundation Vegetables

green juices and smoothies

leafy green vegetables

green sprouts

other veggies (unless noted)

Sea Vegetables

dulse

kelp

nori

sea lettuce

sea palm

Non-Sweet Fruits

cucumbers

lemons

limes

red bell peppers

tomatoes

Fats/Oils

almond oil

avocados

cacao beans (not for diabetics)

chia oil/seeds/powder

coconut oil

flax seeds

hemp oil/seeds/powder

olives/olive oil

pumpkin oil

sesame oil

other nuts and seeds

Superfoods and High-Protein Foods

blue-green algaes

chlorella

green powders

mangosteen extract

marine phytoplankton

noni extract

spirulina

wheatgrass juice

Fermented Foods

apple cider vinegar

cultured-seed "cheeze"*

cultured-seed "mylk"*

kimchi

sauerkraut

soy-free miso

Sprouted Legumes
(for moderate use; both of these
sprouts are good for diabetics)

lentil sprouts

mung bean sprouts

Sweeteners

erythritol

stevia

xylitol

Teas, Spices, and Herbs

all herbs and spices

caffeine-free herbal tea

white and green teas

Supplements

enzymes

garlic extract

herbs

ionic minerals

medicinal mushroom extracts

probiotics

silica

vitamin C

Pure Salt

raw Himalayan salt

raw scalar salt

PHASE 1.5 FOODS

A Phase 1.5 diet is for optimal maintenance and growth. It includes Phase 1 foods in the list above, plus the following additional foods.

Note: A small amount of Phase 2 fruits and vegetables in a salad is also considered Phase 1.5.

Vegetables
(raw or lightly cooked)

beets

carrots

parsnips

pumpkins

rutabagas

hard squash

hard squash

summer squash

sweet potatoes

yams

Fruits

blueberries

cherries

coconut meat/pulp/crème/flakes

cranberries (fresh, unsweetened)

grapefruit

green apples

kiwis

oranges

pomegranate

raspberries

strawberries

Grains

amaranth

buckwheat

millet

quinoa

rice

teff

Superfoods

bee pollen

goji berries

maca root

pomegranates

Condiments/Sweeteners

cacao oil/butter

carob (raw)

mesquite meal

Fermented Foods

coconut kefir

cultured coconut meat*

Juices

grapefruit juice (diluted
with an equal amount of water)

PHASE 2 FOODS (PARTY FOODS)

Note: A small amount of Phase 2 fruits and vegetables in a salad is considered Phase 1.5.

Vegetables (raw)

parsnips

pumpkins

rutabagas

Fruits

apples

blackberries

coconut water (diluted with other
    ingredients)

oranges (seeded)

peaches

pears

plums

Sweeteners

inulin

lucuma

yacon

Teas

black tea

Dried Fruits

dates

figs

raisins

Fruit/Carrot Juices

fresh, raw fruits or carrots,
 diluted with an equal amount
 of water

**High-Sugar Fruits
(for minimal use)**

apricots

bananas

cherimoyas

durians

figs

grapes

mangos

melons

papayas

persimmons

pineapples

raisins

rambutans

sapotes

tamarinds

FOODS TO AVOID

agave syrup (dark or light)

alcohol

animal products (flesh, dairy,
 eggs, low-quality honey)

bottled juices

brewer's yeast (except to
 activate breast milk in
 mothers having trouble
 starting lactation)

caffeinated drinks

corn

cottonseed

grains (except those listed)

heated, refined, or processed
 oils and margarines

nutritional yeast

peanuts

processed foods

soy sauce, *nama shoyu* (raw,
 unpasteurized soy sauce)
 and soy-based "liquid aminos"

sugar

tobacco

uncontrolled fermented foods

white potatoes

NATURAL LOW-SUGAR AND NO-SUGAR SWEETENERS

Note: Artificial sweeteners and chemical sweeteners such as NutraSweet (aspartame) are harmful to health, for reasons other than sugar content, as they are "excitotoxins." These overstimulate neural activity, and are associated with disorganization and inflammation of the brain, increased brain-cell death, and obesity.[1]

Stevia (Phase 1) is a green herb that is very sweet to the taste but does not raise blood-sugar levels. It can be homegrown and dried, or purchased in liquid (plain or flavored) or powdered form. It is the lowest-glycemic sweetener.

Cinnamon, cardamom, fennel, allspice, star anise, and vanilla-bean powder (Phase 1) are other culinary herbs that lend a gentler sweetness. These are especially delicious in teas and desserts.

Xylitol (Phase 1) is a granular or powdered sweetener derived from birch-tree bark. Xylitol can also come from corn and other vegetables, but these are not recommended because most modern corn has been genetically modified. Xylitol is a diabetic-friendly sweetener because it tastes sweet but does not raise blood sugar. It has also been found to prevent tooth decay. Xylitol can replace equal quantities of white sugar or other granular sweeteners in any recipe.

Erythritol (Phase 1) is a granular sweetener very similar to xylitol in appearance and usage. Like xylitol, it does not raise blood sugar, making it safe for diabetics. Some people find erythritol easier to digest than xylitol.

Carob powder (Phase 1.5) is often toasted but can also be purchased raw. Ground carob pod can reduce or replace cacao (raw chocolate) or sweeteners in dessert recipes. While cacao is high in beneficial antioxidants and magnesium, it is good to be aware that it has a stimulant effect, and stresses the adrenal glands. Chocolate is also commonly eliminated when treating childhood allergies and ADHD. Because of carob's high tannin content, which binds mucous membranes in the intestinal tract, it has also been used to treat diarrhea in young children and infants.

Mesquite powder (Phase 1.5) can be imported from Peru or harvested from mesquite trees in the southwestern U.S. and parts of Mexico. A staple for our Native American ancestors, mesquite has long provided humans with digestible protein, lipase, and the trace minerals calcium, magnesium, iron, and zinc. Mesquite is commonly used as a mildly sweet gluten-free flour. It can also be added to Nut/Seed Mylks (page 470) and combined well with (natural, not artificial) vanilla and other sweet-bean seasonings.

Lucuma powder (Phase 1.5) is a common ice-cream flavor in South America. High in iron, powdered lucuma root lends a caramel-like flavor and light texture to living foods.

Jerusalem artichoke syrup (Phase 1.5, for minimal use) is a raw sweetener with a lower glycemic index than other liquid sweeteners such as maple syrup. Jerusalem artichoke contains probiotics that are helpful for digestion, and can also be found in powdered form.

Coconut sugar and palm sugar (Phase 2, for minimal use) are considered to be moderate-glycemic sweeteners. These come in granular form. Palm sugar can be used in place of brown sugar or turbinado sugar.

Yacon syrup (Phase 2, for minimal use) comes from the yacon root of South America. The syrup is slightly lighter in color and thickness than molasses.

Coconut nectar syrup (Phase 2, for minimal use) is sap from coconut palm trees that has been dehydrated at low temperatures. It resembles agave syrup in appearance and taste, but is considered to have a lower glycemic index. This can be a replacement for high-fructose corn syrup (which has a strong link to the diabetes epidemic), agave syrup, maple syrup, and honey (all of which are high-glycemic).

Dried fruit paste (Phase 2, for minimal use) is a whole-food sweetener made by soaking dried fruit in water until soft, and then blending the fruit and soakwater to form a paste or thick syrup. Goji berries (Phase 1.5), raisins, dried cherries, blueberries, apples, apricots, prunes, and dried figs are lower in glycemic index than dates or dried mangos and bananas. With the exception of goji berries, dehydrated fruits are most healthful when added to low-glycemic foods and eaten very sparingly, followed by a thorough toothbrushing. It is helpful to see dried fruits as a natural candy, to be eaten in limited amounts, rather than a children's health food to be eaten freely.

It's Not Easy Being Green

What if our kids aren't used to healthy foods because they've developed other eating habits? How can we inspire them to "liven" things up? Just as our children's first baby steps required trial, error, and endurance, so does the major milestone of finding greater nutritional balance for the family. As we keep going, we too gain momentum, and naturally find ourselves running, skipping, dancing, and playing in the kitchen!

General recommendations for introducing something new to a child:

- **Keep things positive.** If the parent, grandparent, or teacher is overflowing with joy, whatever is being presented will be more readily received. If we love living foods, and stay light about the challenges, then we are more likely to appeal to the loving, trusting, and courageous nature of the child.

  At times, children and even adults may balk at the beneficial changes we are making, often because of their fear of the unknown. If this is the case, remember that by staying positive and secure within ourselves, our family and friends will also experience our shining example. If, for example, you're eating salad for breakfast alongside Junior's little bowl of cereal, he may tell you that you're *really weird*. Rather than getting defensive, try laughing and joking that it must be *backwards day!* You never know—he may want to play Backwards Day with you.

Or you could explain that you are not a TV commercial where they entice you to eat "junk" for profit and that, as a person who loves yourself, you want to eat the best foods for health and strength. A child may also respond well to a thoughtful explanation that your job as a parent is to protect your children by good guidance, and that those who do not understand this may indeed think it is weird.

- **Offer unspoken support.** Staying positive also means holding space for others. In other words, when we hold in our hearts and minds the prayer of well-being for others, we remove the obstacle of our own negativity. While this may take some practice, it is very profound, especially when it comes to more challenging relationships. We can also let the food do the talking!

  The first time Leah ever tasted fresh cucumber slices was at a friend's house as a child; her playmate's mom had set out a plateful for her and the other children to nibble on while she was busily cooking dinner. No one had said anything to the kids about eating their veggies, but their tummies were rumbling, and the fresh food did the calling. Dr. Gabriel was always exposed to fresh veggies, and as a live-food vegan for over forty years (and now the grandfather of three), both he and Leah (now a mother to two), both delight in setting out attractive displays of fresh snacks and silently watching the children and adults enjoy them.

- Help the child by starting with what is known, and moving experimentally, one step at a time, into the unknown. The one-step-at-a-time approach is the key to gentle and sustainable success in every aspect of life. As with a well-worn security blanket, this might look like gradually reducing the blanket's size, bit by bit, until there's little more than a scrap of fabric left to tote around, rather than suddenly taking the whole beloved "blankie" away all at once. With the family diet, this might look like starting with something known, like a favorite breakfast cereal, and serving it with almond "mylk" instead of dairy milk.

Once this is accepted, other breakfast options might appear on the table alongside the child's cereal bowl—which, by the way, might also gradually decrease in size, all the way down to doll-sized china! Inviting a child to help with the gardening and preparation is also helpful for bonding with new foods. When there is something in the environment that is familiar to children, they can move forward with greater confidence, feeling more secure within themselves. But if everything is new all of a sudden, with nothing familiar as a point of reference, they can easily feel overwhelmed, disoriented, and disempowered.

What we are suggesting are gentle, graceful, and lasting enhancements to family life, rather than dramatic culture shocks that may cause a family to boomerang back into old habits.

- **Tap into your creative genius:** Foods with lively colors, familiar appearances, playful names, and fun shapes help to set a positive tone for adult and child alike, thus defusing tension that may arise from lifestyle changes.

- **Provide the right dose of choice:** While our children need us to set the parameters of what foods are served in the home, such as healthy, natural, organic and plant-sourced foods versus junk food and pesticided, herbicided, irradiated, dead-animal offerings, children of all ages need to develop decision-making skills of their own.

Conscious parents are like a movie theatre showing a variety of healthy movies, and children are empowered by being able to choose their own movie. For a very young child, being asked an open-ended "What do you want for dinner?" tends to put a lot of unnecessary pressure on them, whereas having a few options set out on the table may result in a more joyful experience. Older children with experience in the kitchen, on the other hand, might absolutely love preparing the family meal all on their own. This is almost always empowering. To guide you in the options you present, consider what the child is able to understand and do at their current stage of development.

- **Don't think of a monkey:** In Prakashananda's book *Don't Think of a Monkey and Other Stories My Guru Told Me,* there is a story of a devotee who, upon receiving a mantra from his teacher, was commanded, "Don't think of a monkey." As a result, the devotee could not stop thinking about a monkey each and every time he sat down to meditate and use the sacred mantra. Retold by the nineteenth-century Hindu monk Swami Rama Tirtha, this story was used to illustrate the teaching that whatever instructions we give a child should be accompanied by a clear explanation that does not set us up for unconscious resistance.

- If we merely say, "Don't eat junk food," without explaining why that is undesirable, we may be encouraging the opposite result. Clear communication about family changes in diet helps the child to integrate the experience without going into unconscious resistance. Our kids appreciate it when we let them in on what's going on, and why. It helps them know that their feelings matter to us, as well as giving them more information for when it comes to making decisions of their own.

- **Sometimes it's all about the timing:** There may be times in a child's life when he loves berries, and then all of a sudden he doesn't want them. Or maybe she won't get close to sea veggies for months, but then out of the blue is asking for more. So take heart, and keep offering healthy options. Perhaps it may not hurt, just this once, to offer sea veggies at bedtime when you see her searching for stalling tactics.... Or perhaps some sunflower sprouts might be timed just right for a long car ride, when he's buckled into the car seat looking for signs of life.

- **The "thank-you bite."** In *Stop Reacting and Start Responding: 108 Ways to Discipline Consciously and Become the Parent You Want to Be* by parent educator Sharon Silver, we read that most children need seven to ten exposures to a new food before they're willing to begin to accept it. So rather than insisting that the child eat the food, like it or not, or deciding "this food is simply something their child doesn't like, and add it to a growing list of other foods that child hates, making it more and more difficult to cook one meal for the entire family," Silver suggests the "thank-you bite" rule. This means that, as a courtesy for the person who has lovingly prepared the food, each family member tries one to three bites of the new food.

- In order to provide choice, Silvers recommends cutting the bites into small pieces, and having the child choose which bite(s) they will take "without parental commentary." She also recommends familiar dipping sauces as a way to mediate the new food energies with familiar tastes. It is less confusing if this plan is carried out in your own home. At another person's house where the diet is different, the children/grandchildren should never be expected to eat a polite bite of something inconsistent with their ethical views or commitment to care for their bodies. In this context, it is very positive to respectfully decline, and this can be a very empowering movement of individuation for the child.

- **Ambiance:** We can also provide a peaceful atmosphere for mealtime by turning off the television or radio, and setting a central candle or vase of flowers on the table. Children often love to help with this. Mealtime and "family meeting" times are also best kept as two different occasions, to minimize the possibility of a negative experience in one affecting the other.

- **Child-chefs:** Food preparation can be a favorite activity in the home and classroom. Including the child in this daily rhythm gives them a sense of competency as well as being part of something vital to the family or community. In a classic Montessori preschool, food preparation is also used to support the young child in developing fine and gross motor skills, independence, following a logical sequence, carefulness and attention to detail, social graces, decision-making, and observation skills. It also initiates the child into relationships with foods, raises awareness of all that goes into making a meal—and yes, encourages them to eat new foods.

As one student of the "I'm Alive! Food-Prep Class for Kids" put it, "I wanted to taste it, after doing all the work of making it!" As Rabbi Dr. Gabriel says, "Food can be more easily understood as a love note from God." Before introducing a new culinary skill to the child, first assess the child's readiness for the particular task: Has the child developed the required strength or coordination? Are they calm and careful with potentially dangerous objects? Can they follow a sequence? Demonstrate how it's done first, slowing down your movements and making sure that what your hands are doing is visible to the child. If you are using a child-friendly knife or veggie peeler, you will want to mention which part of the tool we do not touch because it is sharp; but otherwise let the motions of your hands do the talking, especially for young children.

After your careful, precise, and focused demonstration, invite the child to take a turn, staying right there to observe their progress and silently support their very first attempts. They may need you to help them to get a feel for the sawing motion of a serrated knife at first, or a gentle prompting on what step comes next— but the idea is to offer the child the opportunity to think and do it on their own while the adult watches for safety. As much as possible, allow children to correct their own technique, especially if they are happy with the fruits of their labors. (See "Resources," page 485, for child-friendly knives and other appropriately sized kitchen tools.)

- **Recipes!** The following are recipes that have helped families we know to liven up their mealtimes, including the most important ingredient—love for the child.

Note: New research by one of Dr. Gabriel's "Spiritual Nutrition Masters" students has shown that anything blended for more than ten seconds loses a significant amount of energy, according to Kirlian photography. For this reason, we recommend keeping the blending as close to ten seconds or less as possible.

Living Water

I thank the water for nourishing my soul.

—**Tucson Botanical Gardens**

The Earth is approximately 75% water. A baby's body is also approximately 75% water. With age, we gradually dehydrate to 55–60%.

Our bodies are like our garden beds where, no matter how nutrient-dense the soil is, nothing will grow without water. Not only does water hydrate, it also helps our bodies to derive essential vitamins and minerals from our food. Proper hydration is of particular importance for children because the division and expansion of cells as they grow requires even more water. The child's body temperature is also less regulated than the adult's, which means children get overheated more easily. This could account for why swimming pools, sprinklers, and icy treats have such appeal for children in the summertime.

Children are drawn to water. It moves, sparkles, swirls, ripples, and gurgles with messages from the cosmos. We thirst for water not only because it brings hydrogen into our bodies but, as Masaru Emoto's book *Hidden Messages in Water* has made visible, water is also a carrier of subtler frequencies. These may be life-affirming transmissions such as love and joy, or unfortunate frequencies such as pollution and/or negative thought forms.

Even after toxins such as chlorine, pesticides, and herbicides have been removed from our drinking water, the subtler frequency of those toxins can still be present in the water, as in homeopathic remedies, and have an effect on those who consume it. Water is an interdimensional transducer of frequencies. In Judaism, we see the practice of blessing water for ceremonial handwashing, and of *mikvah,* or sacred bath, as practiced by John the Baptist. Stemming from its Hebrew roots, we see in Christianity the integral role of water in baptism for the loving dedication of infants.

In some denominations we also see the use of holy water that has been ritually blessed. In Hinduism, the newborn is bathed as part of a sacred naming ceremony.

Throughout the ages, we have been utilizing the precious gift of water not only to meet our physical requirements but to uplift one another spiritually. This insight gives us yet another perspective on living foods for the living family: Living foods are the highest in biologically active water. They are therefore able to transmit more love, if we are putting love into our water and into the well-hydrated living foods that we feed our family.

HOW DO WE BEST SUPPORT OUR
CHILDREN WITH LIVING WATER?

Children thrive on structure. As described in Dr. Gabriel's book *Spiritual Nutrition,* the best way to erase pollutants and subtle frequencies—many of which may be toxic—from water is through distilling. Once water has undergone distillation, it is free of even subtle toxic frequencies. Distilled water is a highly potent solvent, but it is also "immature." It will pull out toxins and heavy metals from the body; however, it may also leach out essential minerals. This is why distilled water needs to be matured, or "structured," before consumption.

We can restructure the water by mimicking Nature's ways: After distillation, place water in a clay or glass, egg- or cylinder-shaped jar. (The shape affects the way in which the water flows.) Add 25 drops of Crystal Energy™ (silica nanoparticles) per gallon, 12 drops of Active Ionic Minerals™ and one dropper of tachyon water. Stir the water in the egg-shaped or cylindrical container several times in one direction, and then the other, with quick reversals. This mimics water's natural flow over rocks in a stream.

Next, place your hands on the container and bless the water, saying a loving prayer aloud. Set the container outside overnight, in view of the moon and stars. Store in a cool place over a Tachyon Silica Disk™. If there is a place in nature that is especially nurturing to your family, a stone from that place can also be placed inside the water container to share that love with the family.

If structured distilled water is not available, the second-best water for drinking is reverse-osmosis (RO) filtered water, assuming that the filters have been checked regularly. Further discussion of water quality may be found in the "Living Water" chapter of Rabbi Dr. Gabriel's book *Spiritual Nutrition*. Because of the current global contamination of water by radiation, zeolite shower filters can also be purchased at the www .DrCousensOnlineStore.com.

Mass fluoridation of water is also a threat to healthy human development, which is why this practice has been banned in every nation in Europe except Ireland. The dangers of fluoride have been discussed earlier. By the time a child is eighteen years old, with regular consumption of fluoridated water the pineal gland (a.k.a. third eye) will be significantly calcified with toxic calcium fluoride buildup. This can be reversed by taking a high-quality iodine supplement such as Illumodine, which breaks up the calcium fluoride and forces it out of the system by competitive inhibition and displacement.

THE BETTER HYDRATED OUR CHILDREN ARE, THE HEALTHIER THEY WILL BE

- **Raw plant-sourced living foods are naturally more hydrating** because they are biologically active, and the zeta-potential water content of the plants has not been lost in the cooking process, though it is also lost by dehydrating raw foods. The zeta-potential can be understood as the life-force in enzymes and live foods, as well as a measure of their subtle organizing electronic fields (SOEF), part of the energy matrix that connects the organism to the cosmos and is the template for the building of the human body.

  Hot weather is the natural time to minimize dehydrated foods, increase fluids, and eat more high-water content fruits and veggies, such as watermelons, grapes, cucumbers, tomatoes, strawberries, and lettuce—the garden goodies that are in season at that time. Living foods are also high in electrons, which makes their water more hydrating and energizing. Water that has been heated to the boiling point, by contrast, has become molecularly disorganized, and therefore less helpful to bodily function, and needs to be restructured with Crystal Energy™.

- **Replace Hydration Saboteurs:** Although heavily marketed to children, beverages containing artificial colors, BVO (brominated vegetable oil, an additive used to bind artificial colors to liquid, which has been banned in ten countries), artificial flavors, corn syrup, sugar, or caffeine tax their body fluids as the body tries to flush out their harmful ingredients. Furthermore, caffeine actually bonds to the hydrogen in water, preventing hydration by making hydrogen inaccessible to our cells. Carbonated beverages also interfere with hydration, because a false acidity is created as H_2O and CO_2 combine to form HCO_3 (carbonic acid). This acidity also binds the hydrogen in water, making it unavailable to the body.
- **Add a squeeze of citrus:** The natural acids in lemons, limes, and grapefruit are a good source of natural electron-donating hydrogen.
- **Keep high-quality water available for frequent fluid breaks,** especially while children are playing sports. Avoid bottled water, as forty percent or more of these, according to the FDA, have turned out to be tap water. What's more, not only do the plastic containers tend to leach out harmful chemicals but, because the water is stagnant, in contrast to a flowing spring, and shelved under fluorescent lights, it lacks the life-force energy that makes living water so revitalizing.
- **Flavored Water:** Some children tend to consume more fluid if it's flavored with something they enjoy. Have you ever tried stevia? This sweet-leafed herb can be purchased in liquid form, plain or in yummy flavors including grape, lemon, orange, berry, vanilla, chocolate, hazelnut crème, English toffee, and even root beer.

Because stevia is a zero-glycemic-index sweetener (Phase 1), it is safe for diabetics, and also means that our children aren't put on the emotional roller coaster of sugar's well-known highs and lows. Stevia-sweetened water can also go into a baby bottle or sippy cup without promoting tooth decay, as does fruit juice. You only need a few drops to flavor your fluids, and it's nonperishable, so stevia's sweet little bottle can be easily packed inside your tote for on-the-go flavored water. If you are lucky enough to have a source of pure spring water, this will also lend a sweeter flavor.

How do you know whether or not your child is getting enough fluids? Urination should occur every hour or two. Infants urinate much more frequently. Signs of dehydration include tiredness, mood swings, difficulty concentrating, dry mouth and tongue, sunken eyes, sunken soft spot on an infant's head, constipation, and decreased urination. Severe dehydration can be life-threatening.

Hydration Station Recipes for Kids

While slightly (50 parts per million) mineralized, structured distilled water or RO (reverse-osmosis-filtered) water are the most hydrating and energetically mature beverages, providing other options can also be helpful to ensure proper hydration.

Fresh-Squeezed Lemonade (Phase 1)

1 quart structured or filtered water (see "Living Water," page384)

juice of 3–4 lemons

lemon-flavored liquid stevia to taste (from 3–4 drops up to 2–3 full droppers)

Stir together and enjoy.

Grapefruit-Rosewater Refresher (Phase 1.5)

> juice of 2 pink grapefruits
>
> 2 teaspoons rosewater
>
> 2 cups structured or filtered water (see "Living Water," page 384)
>
> stevia to taste (optional)

Stir together and enjoy.

Prickly Pink Drink (Phase 1.5)

This brightly colored superfood beverage looks and sounds like something out of a Dr. Seuss book. If your family lives in or visits the desert, you may enjoy cultivating or wild-harvesting prickly pear fruit together. Harvesting requires precautionary measures, as the fruit is protected by prickly spines—this is not an activity for toddlers. The ruby-ripe fruit can be removed with tongs and placed in a bucket. Prickly pear fruit can sometimes also be found in rural desert coops and farmer's markets.

> 8–10 prickly pear cactus fruits
>
> juice of 4 lemons
>
> 1 quart structured or filtered water (see "Living Water," page 384)
>
> lemon-flavored or unflavored liquid stevia, to taste

Using tongs, run prickly pear fruit through a Champion juicer using the juicing screen. The small seeds within the fruit are very hard, and make a big racket inside the juicer. The Champion handles them just fine, however, and the prickles end up in the pulp—so do not eat the pulp. The juice will be thick and gelatinous. Mix it with lemon juice, water, and stevia.

Mild Child Green Juice (Phase 1)

MAKES 4 SERVINGS

> 5 cucumbers
>
> 2 celery stalks
>
> 2 leaves of baby bok choy, or 1 cup sunflower seed sprouts
>
> 1 cup structured or filtered water (see "Living Water," page 384)

Juice all ingredients in a juicer, and serve with a curvy straw. This drink is good for bottles and sippy cups for the little ones, as green juices contain oral health-promoting chlorophyll, and no sugars.

Variation: If you don't have a juicer, blend ingredients in a blender, and then strain out the pulp with a nut-mylk bag (a drawstring bag made of fine-mesh fabric, available at www .DrCousensOnlineStore.com).

Lime Green Slushy (Phase 1)

INSPIRED BY A DRINK MADE IN HMONG COMMUNITIES

Cucumbers are a member of the melon family, and lend a unique freshness to this non-glycemic dessert.

> 2 medium-large cucumbers, peeled and cubed (or 1 giant homegrown cucumber)
>
> juice of 3 limes
>
> 4 cups ice cubes
>
> 1 cup parsley, stems removed
>
> liquid stevia to taste (2–3 droppers)
>
> erythritol or xylitol to taste (optional)
>
> 1 cup structured or filtered water (see "Living Water," page 384)

If the cucumber has very large, coarse seeds, you will want to seed them first; but small, soft seeds will blend up just fine. Place cucumbers into a blender on high speed, then add remaining ingredients and blend until desired consistency. Then enjoy this refreshing zero-glycemic delight.

Strawberry Slushy (Phase 1.5)

Cool as a cucumber and fruity as a berry, this refreshing icy beverage is not only loved by kids but is grownup-friendly too. It doubles as a light, alcohol-free strawberry daiquiri.

> 2 medium-large cucumbers, peeled and cubed (or 1 giant homegrown cucumber)
>
> 1½ cup frozen strawberries
>
> 3 cups ice cubes
>
> 1 cup structured or filtered water (see "Living Water," page 384)
>
> juice of 1 lime
>
> 3 full droppers berry-flavored liquid stevia
>
> erythritol or xylitol to taste (optional)

If the cucumber has very large, coarse seeds, you will want to seed them first; but small, soft seeds will blend up just fine. In a blender on high speed, blend until slushy. Serve immediately.

Kid Teas

Herbal teas offer numerous benefits—they include vitamin C-rich rose hips and hibiscus, fever-cooling and tummy-settling mint, immunity-boosting elder and echinacea, and calming and antiinflammatory chamomile—but they don't necessarily count as hydrators, because they are high in total dissolved solids (TDS), and if the TDS in a liquid are too high, this may interfere with hydrating.

Red Hibiscus Cool-Aid (Phase 1)

> 3–4 tablespoons dried hibiscus leaves (available from bulk tea suppliers)
>
> 1 gallon structured or filtered water (see "Living Water," page 384)
>
> berry-flavored liquid stevia to taste (3–5 drops to 3–4 droppers)
>
> 1–2 drops food-grade lemon essential oil (optional)

Place hibiscus leaves in a nut-mylk (mesh-fabric) bag, or tea balls. Float in a gallon jar full of structured or filtered water. Cover, and set to steep on the counter rather than in the sun (as sunlight tends to destructure the water) for 1–2 hours, or until the tea is deep-red in color. Remove tea leaves and sweeten with stevia. Chill, drink at room temperature, or pour into popsicle molds.

Peppermint-Cucumber Juice (Phase 1)

> 3 cups peppermint tea (prepared as in the previous recipe)
>
> 2 cucumbers, chopped
>
> erythritol or xylitol to taste (optional)

Blend cucumbers in a blender with the peppermint tea. Strain out pulp using a nut-mylk (mesh-fabric) bag or cheesecloth. Stir in sweetener.

Bright-Eyed Breakfasts

Many children are accustomed to something sweet and/or creamy for breakfast. We've also included some breakfast salad ideas, as we've found that this too can be a happy way to start the day for parent and child alike. Begin by serving something that is familiar to your child, and set salad on the table too. When mom or dad delights in fresh breakfast greens, or Chia Porridge with a Nut/Seed Mylk and some bee pollen, the child will take in this impression whether or not she ventures a bite. The key is to always set the stage for a positive adventure experience, free from undue pressure.

Coconut Kefir (Phase 1.5)

BY ELAINA LOVE

This probiotic beverage is best ingested first thing in the morning, on an empty stomach, to support digestive-system health. It can be combined with fresh juices, blended into smoothies, or blended with young coconut meat and cultured for a dairy-free yogurt.

See Coconut Kefir recipe on page 473.

Zoom-Bloom Blueberry Juice (Phase 1.5)

2 cups Hibiscus Red Cool-Aid (see "Kid Teas," above)

½ cup blueberries, fresh or frozen

1 tablespoon E-3 Live, gently thawed to liquid form, or 1 teaspoon of E-3 Live powder. Chlorella or spirulina may be substituted for E-3 Live.

Blend blueberries with Hibiscus Cool-Aid in a blender. Pour through a small sieve to strain out the blueberry seeds, or just leave the seeds in.

Stir in E-3 Live, and zoooooom around in spandex and a cape!

Breezy Breakfast Muesli Mix (Phase 2)

The following recipe makes a nice big batch, so you can keep some on hand for times when briefer prep is needed. This is a good one for pregnant women to stock in the pantry for after baby arrives. Rotating fresh fruit options keeps this standby breakfast exciting.

5 cups shredded coconut

3 cups Buckwheaties (recipe below)

2 cups rolled oats

2 cups goji berries, dried cherries, dried mulberries, golden
raisins, and/or dried currants

1 cup hemp seeds

Stir all ingredients together in a large mixing bowl, then transfer
into large glass storage jars. Serve with fresh fruit such as banana
slices, blueberries, strawberries, or chopped peaches or apples,
and vanilla-almond Nut/Seed Mylk (page 470) or Young Coconut
Yogurt (page 474).

Variation: During Leah's "I'm Alive! Food-Prep Class" for kids,
the muesli ingredients were set out separately in bowls, and the
children enjoyed making their own mixes.

Buckwheaties (Phase 1, gluten-free)

5 cups buckwheat groats (or any desired amount)

Soak groats in water overnight. Drain off water, and dehydrate
sprouted buckwheat at 115° or in the sun, until dry and crunchy
(about 5 hours). Store at room temperature in an airtight container.
Serve with various sauces or seasonings on top, to the child's
taste.

Cinnamon Buckwheaties (Phase 1.5 or 2)

FROM THE TREE OF LIFE CAFÉ

4 cups sprouted buckwheat

1 ½ cups shredded coconut

¼ cup "Sweet-E" (erythritol)

1 dropper hazelnut stevia

1 dropper vanilla stevia

2 pinches salt

1 tablespoons lemon juice

⅓ cup structured or filtered water (see "Living Water,"
page 384)

2 tablespoons cinnamon

Blend all ingredients together except buckwheat and shredded coconut. Once blended, combine in a bowl with the buckwheat and coconut.

Dehydrate for 6–8 hours at 115° until it resembles crispy cereal. Ingredients above are for Phase 1.5.

For Phase 2: Same as above, but add 1½ cups of raisins.

Rawnola (Phase 1)
FROM THE TREE OF LIFE CAFÉ

For a large batch, multiply all ingredient amounts by 4.

> 4 cups nuts and seeds of your choice, soaked in water overnight, or 6–8 hours.
>
> ½ cup shredded coconut
>
> ¼ cup chia seeds, soaked in 2 cups water for 2 hours
>
> 1 tablespoon cinnamon
>
> 1 tablespoon pumpkin spice
>
> 1 teaspoon ground cardamom
>
> 1 teaspoon star anise powder
>
> 1 teaspoon stevia powder (optional)
>
> Pinch of salt

In a food processor, process only the soaked nuts into large chunks, using the pulse setting. The seeds will remain whole. Be sure the chia and water are well incorporated, forming a gel.

Combine all ingredients in a mixing bowl, and stir with your hands to incorporate everything very well.

Spread on dehydrator trays and dehydrate for 2 hours at 145°, then dehydrate at 115° for 24 hours, or until all the moisture has completely disappeared.

Note: Rawnola can be saved in a glass container for 1–3 months.

Rooti-Fruiti Granola (Phase 2)

A colorful breakfast cereal that's rooted in wholesomeness! The beet root, maca root, and ginger root lend their gentle sweetness—but that's not all. Along with its cheery color, red beet offers radiation protection. An adaptogen, maca boosts the immune and endocrine systems by helping the body handle stress and maintain hormonal balance. In Ayurvedic medicine, childhood is classified as the kapha stage of life, in which astringent, bitter, and pungent herbs such as ginger and turmeric root are particularly beneficial to balance the excess mucus associated with kapha. This fun and flavorful granola is great by itself, or in a dairy-free yogurt; however, it is not a granola that hold its crunch in liquids unless you add more nuts and/or seeds (see Classic Granola Variation). Save the crumbs! They double as party sprinkles for decorating festive desserts.

Rooti-Fruiti Granola—Pink Batch

    2 cups dried coconut flakes

    1 cup rolled oats

    1 large golden apple, cored and chopped

    ¼ cup hemp seeds

    ¼ cup red beet root, peeled and chopped

    ¼ cup granulated coconut sugar

    1 tablespoon red maca root powder (red is milder in flavor
    than other varieties)

    1 teaspoon dried ginger root powder

    ¼ teaspoon freshly ground nutmeg

    ¼ teaspoon Himalayan or other high-mineral raw salt

In a food processor, process the beet with the dry ingredients (coconut flakes, oats, coconut sugar, maca, salt, and seasonings) into a dry meal. Then add the chopped apple and process again; you should now have a moist dough. Crumple dough onto a dehydrator tray lined with a nonstick sheet, and dehydrate at 115° overnight, or until crunchy. Use one dehydrator tray per batch.

Rooti-Fruiti Granola—Golden Batch

Use the same ingredients as for the Pink Batch, but substitute peeled and chopped golden beet root for the red beet root, or omit beet altogether if golden beets are not available. Also add ½ teaspoon of turmeric root powder to the dry ingredients, and ½ teaspoon orange zest, plus the juice of one orange, to the wet ingredients. Process and dehydrate, separately from the other colored batches, following the instructions for the Pink Batch.

Rooti-Fruiti Granola—Green Batch

Use the same ingredients as for the Pink Batch, but omit the beet and add 1 teaspoon of powdered spirulina or chlorella to the dry ingredients. Process and dehydrate, separately from the other colored batches, following the Pink Batch instructions.

Now that you have three colors of granola, you can mix them, or not, as you like. Store in airtight containers and keep on hand in the pantry. Eat for breakfast, or pack for munching on the go. If your child's school has a no-sugary-foods policy, this might be mistaken for a no-no, so label sugary-food lookalikes with a note, or an ingredients list. Also see the Classic Granola Variation.

Valentine's Day Variation: Make a granola dough following the Pink Batch recipe, and form into heart shapes by hand or with a heart-shaped cookie cutter before dehydrating. You will have big, pink, heart-shaped granola clusters!

Classic Granola Variation: If you want a more traditional-looking granola, simply omit the colorful ingredients such as beets, turmeric, and spirulina. Add favorite chopped nuts or seeds, after soaking them for 6–8 hours so that they start to germinate.

Banana-Split Birthday Breakfast (Phase 2)

This recipe was inspired by a breakfast banana split in The Vegan Table by Colleen Patrick-Goudreau.

For your child's special day, simply split a banana. If you can find them, the wildcrafted red Mexican bananas are a nice size, and lower-glycemic than the hybridized yellow variety. Dollop one of the Raw Vegan Yogurts (page 473) on top, and a festive sprinkle of Rooti-Fruiti Granola (just Pink Batch, or all three colors together), and top with a fresh cherry. Children also delight in assembling this for a surprise Mother's Day breakfast in bed.

Berry-Yogurt Parfaits (Phase 2)

Into small clear drinking glasses, show your child how to layer Breezy Breakfast Muesli Mix (above), Rooti-Fruiti Granola (or its Classic Granola Variation, both above), fresh berries, then one of the Raw Vegan Yogurts (page 473), with additional berries on top as garnish.

Zucchini Bread (Phase 1 or 2)

    2 cups chopped zucchini
    1 lemon, juiced
    ¼ cup xylitol
    ½ cup flax seeds
    2 cups walnuts
    ¼ teaspoon vanilla powder
    1 teaspoon cinnamon
    ¼ teaspoon allspice
    ¼ teaspoon ginger root powder

Grind flax seeds into meal using a coffee grinder or blender on high speed. Grind walnuts the same way. In a food processor, process zucchini with xylitol and lemon juice until smooth. Add ground flaxseed and walnut meal, vanilla powder and spices, and process until thoroughly mixed into dough. Form into bread pieces onto nonstick sheets or waxed paper, and dehydrate at 115° for 8 hours, until crispy on the outside and soft (but not gooey) on the inside.

Variation (Phase 2): Stir ¼ cup soaked raisins or black currants into the dough just before forming into slices to dry.

Apple-Cinnamon Bread (Phase 2)

Here's a good recipe for using the nut pulp that is strained out when making Nut/Seed Mylk (page 470). Finger food-loving toddlers especially seem to enjoy this gently warmed bread.

> 2 cups golden flax seeds
>
> 2 cups wet almond (or almond-coconut) pulp
>
> 3 apples, grated
>
> ½ cup soaked dried fruit (such as sulfur-free raisins or dried apricots)
>
> ½ teaspoon cinnamon
>
> ¼ teaspoon vanilla powder (optional)
>
> ¼ teaspoon Himalayan or other high-mineral raw salt

Grind flax seeds into meal using a coffee grinder or high-power blender. Soak the dried fruit in ½ cup filtered water until soft (at least 2 hours), then blend it with the soakwater to make a paste. Mix paste with the remaining ingredients.

Form into small bread loaves, and dehydrate at 115° for 4 hours, or until dry on the outside and slightly moist on the inside. Slice and enjoy with Dairy-Free Salted Butter (page 481).

Variation 1: Add ½ cup goji berries to the mixture before forming loaves and dehydrating.

Variation 2: Instead of the almond pulp, use coconut flakes that have been ground in a blender at high speed.

Mesquite Bread (Phase 1.5)

FROM THE TREE OF LIFE CAFÉ STAFF

> 1½ cups raw mesquite powder (see "Natural Low-Sugar
> and No-Sugar Sweeteners," page 376)
>
> 3½ cups nut pulp (what's left after making Nut Mylk)
>
> ¼ teaspoon salt
>
> ½ cup warm water
>
> 3 droppers English-toffee-flavored stevia
>
> ½ cup powdered Sweet-E (erythritol) (optional, for a
> sweeter bread)
>
> ½ cup coconut oil, plus a little extra to mix with the stevia
>
> ⅓ cup powdered chia seeds

Warm a little coconut oil and mix in the stevia. Mix all the other
ingredients in a food processor, then mix the stevia in a little
coconut oil and add while the processor is still running. Place in
large mixing bowl, and fold in powdered chia. Dehydrate at 115°
overnight.

Cinnamon Bread or Rolls (Phase 1)

FROM THE TREE OF LIFE CAFÉ STAFF

> 4 cups nut or seed pulp (what's left after making Nut/Seed
> Mylk)
>
> ½ cup coconut oil
>
> ½ cup nut butter
>
> ½ cup ground chia seeds
>
> ¼ cup Sweet-E (erythritol)
>
> 8 drops vanilla stevia
>
> 2 teaspoons cinnamon
>
> 1½ teaspoons pumpkin spice
>
> 1 teaspoon star anise

Blend the erythritol for a few seconds, then add 1–2 tablespoons hot water to make a syrup. Mix everything in a bowl until you it forms a dough. Roll out the dough on a cutting board into a loaf, and slice into inch-thick slices.

Place on a dehydrator sheet and dehydrate for 2 hours at 145°, and then 6 hours at 115°. Your bread should remain moist, not wet, in the center. Serve with coconut butter or berry jam.

Cinnamon-roll dough

Roll out the cinnamon-bread dough between two sheets of plastic wrap, into a rectangular shape about ½-inch thick. Sprinkle the stuffing (below) across the center, and roll into a log using the plastic wrap around the outside. Slice into 1-inch rounds, and dehydrate as above.

Cinnamon-roll stuffing

1 cup sun-dried tomatoes

½ cup nut/seed butter (such as almond, cashew, or pumpkin-seed)

½ cup coconut cream (see below)

1 tablespoon cinnamon

¼ cup Sweet-E (erythritol)

Pinch of salt

Blend Sweet-E into a powder. Make coconut cream by blending ½ cup coconut chips with ¼ cup melted coconut oil. Mix all ingredients together and stuff cinnamon rolls as above.

Variations: You may also add apples, pears, cardamom, walnuts, raisins, nut butter, etc., according to your diet.

Shortbread (Phase 1)

FROM THE TREE OF LIFE CAFÉ STAFF

6 cups nut pulp (left over from making Nut Mylk)

1 cup flaxseeds

1 cup + 2 tablespoons Sweet-E (erythritol) powder

1 cup coconut oil

3½ tablespoons maca (add this for Phase 1.5)

½ teaspoon salt

⅛ teaspoon liquid stevia

⅛ teaspoon hazelnut stevia

⅛ teaspoon vanilla stevia

Grind flaxseeds in a coffee grinder or high-power blender to make about ¼ cup flaxmeal. Mix all ingredients except ground flax in a bowl. Once mixed, add flax, form into shapes, and dehydrate for 1 hour at 145°, then for 6–8 additional hours at 115°.

Pecan Waffles (Phase 1)
FROM THE TREE OF LIFE CAFÉ STAFF

10 cups pecans

5 cups coconut flour or shredded coconut

2 cups Nut/Seed Mylk (page 407)

½ cup chia seeds

¼ cup coconut oil

1½ tablespoons vanilla bean powder

3 droppers vanilla stevia

45 drops liquid stevia

1 teaspoon salt

Spices to taste (cinnamon, pumpkin pie, nutmeg, cardamom, etc.)

Grind pecans in a food processor to make about 8 cups of pecan meal. Grind chia seeds to make about ¾ cups of chia meal. Then process the pecan meal, coconut oil, stevia, vanilla, and salt into a smooth consistency.

In a mixing bowl, combine the pecan mixture with the spices and coconut flour or shreds. Whisk in the Nut/Seed Mylk, then add chia meal and use hands to mix well. Line the top and bottom of the waffle iron with plastic wrap. Add a scoop of the mixture to the waffle iron and press. Transfer formed waffles to a dehydrator tray, and dehydrate at 145° for 2 hours, then at 115° for an additional 7–9 hours.

Raspberry Jam (Phase 1.5)

> 1 cup fresh or frozen raspberries
>
> ½ cup goji berries
>
> 1 teaspoon fresh lemon juice

Process ingredients in a food processor until mixed. Store in refrigerator in an airtight container. Serve over dehydrated bread.

Festive Grapefruit Halves (Phase 1.5)

MAKES 4 SERVINGS

> 2 grapefruits
>
> 4 Snow-Dusted Cranberries (page 461)
>
> 1 teaspoon xylitol (optional)

Cut grapefruits into halves. Place one half each onto 4 small serving plates, and garnish with one candied cranberry in the center of each grapefruit. If grapefruits are tart, you may also want to sprinkle a little xylitol on top.

Orange You Glad I Didn't Say Banana? Smoothie (Phase 2)

We're not knocking banana-based smoothies but—as in this oft-told kid joke—sometimes you're ready for something a bit different!

> flesh of 1 young Thai coconut, along with its coconut water
>
> 1 cup fresh-squeezed orange juice (from about 4 oranges)

1 large carrot, chopped into chunks

1 cup frozen peaches

¼ teaspoon vanilla powder (optional)

Blend all ingredients until smooth.

Strawberry Super-Shake (Phase 1.5)

Traditionally, maca root has been used by Peruvian mothers to ensure healthy birth weight for their babies, because infants living in higher altitudes are statistically smaller. Maca also helps mommies with hormonal balance as well as vital adrenal support.

2 cups Nut/Seed Mylk (page 407)

2 cups frozen strawberries

1–2 teaspoons golden maca root powder

½ cup goji berries

Blend Nut/Seed Mylk of choice with strawberries and maca powder until smooth. Goji berries can be blended in too, or stirred in at the end.

Green Smoothies (Phase 1.5 or 2)

These can double as baby food—just omit the citrus and fermented ingredients for children under twelve months.

Man-Go Green (Phase 2)

MAKES 4 SERVINGS

Man, this smoothie's good! This creamy-tangy combination tastes like a yogurt-based smoothie, but with greens instead of dairy. The healthy fats and greens also help little bodies balance the sweetness of tropical fruits such as mango.

2 cups thick pumpkin seed-coconut Nut/Seed Mylk (page 407); use 1½ cups water for creamier consistency

2 cups frozen mango

½ ripe, juicy lime (the yellower the better), peeled

1½–2 cups loosely packed parsley and/or baby Swiss chard

1 dropper vanilla stevia

pinch Himalayan salt

Blend all ingredients together in a blender on high speed until smoothie-textured.

Optional garnish: additional mango chunks and goji berries.

Variation 1: Add a 1-ounce cube of frozen E-3 Live. To have E-3 Live readily available for smoothies, let the frozen bottle of E-3 Live thaw in the refrigerator (no longer than 1 day) and then put into ice cube trays and re-freeze. Once frozen, transfer E-3 Live cubes into a glass jar or freezer bag for airtight storage. Each ice cube equals about one ounce of E-3 Live.

Variation 2: Blend in a 1-inch length of freshly filleted aloe vera leaf. To fillet: cut off serrated edges on each side, as well as the green skins on the top and bottom of the leaf. You should have a slippery and transparent piece of aloe vera gel. Rinse thoroughly before adding to blender.

Wild-Child Smoothie (Phase 2)

3 (preferably wildcrafted) bananas, peeled

1 cup wild mulberries or wild raspberries

1 cup wild edible greens such as lamb's quarters, amaranth, or purslane

½ ripe avocado*

1 cup structured or filtered water (see "Living Water," page 384) or Nut/Seed Mylk (page 470)

1 cup ice cubes

Blend all ingredients in a blender until smooth.

Coconut Spin (Phase 1.5)

MAKES 4 LARGE SERVINGS

> 1½–2 cups young Thai coconut flesh (from about two coconuts) plus their coconut water
>
> 1 generous handful fresh Italian parsley (stems included)
>
> ½ cup fresh spinach
>
> juice of 1 small lime
>
> berry or lemon stevia to taste (1-2 droppers) or ⅙ teaspoon powdered stevia.

Open the coconuts with a cleaver (demonstration videos can be found online for the technique), and pour coconut water into the blender (straining out any shell shards). Scoop out supple coconut flesh and remove any shell shards. Add coconut flesh and remaining ingredients to blender, and blend until smooth. Fresh strawberry slices make a nice garnish for each glass.

Zucchini-Genie (Phase 2)

> 3 large, ripe pears, cored and cut into chunks
>
> ½ small zucchini, cut into chunks
>
> 1 cup parsley (stems included)
>
> 1 cup spinach
>
> 2 droppers lemon stevia, or ⅙ teaspoon powdered stevia and the juice of ½ lemon
>
> 1 cup structured or filtered water (see "Living Water," page 384)

Blend all ingredients until smooth, and serve.

Probiotic Supersonic (Phase 2)

> 2 ripe d'Anjou pears
>
> 2 cups parsley
>
> 1 ripe avocado

juice of 1 lime

2 cups Coconut Kefir (page 473)

1 teaspoon powdered spirulina, chlorella, or E-3 Live

2 cups ice cubes

1 full dropper of berry stevia (or flavor of your choice), or
   $1/8$ teaspoon powdered stevia

Blend all ingredients together. Pour into glasses, and garnish with red berries and a thin slice of pear.

Key-Lime Pudding (Phase 1)

2 large avocados

juice of 4 small limes

$1/2$ cup mild green juice or structured or filtered water
   (see "Living Water," page 384)

$1/4$ teaspoon lime zest (optional)

$1/4$ cup parsley (optional)

4 heaping tablespoons xylitol

2 droppers lemon or unflavored liquid stevia, or
   $1/6$ teaspoon powdered stevia

Blend all ingredients in a blender until smooth.

Green Cream (Phase 2)

MAKES 4–5 SERVINGS

3 young Thai coconuts

$1/2$–2 teaspoons (to taste) spirulina powder, blue-green
   algae powder, E-3 Live, and/or barley-green powder

Open the coconuts with a cleaver (find a demonstration video online for the technique), and pour the water from one coconut into the blender, using a strainer to catch any shell shards. Pour water from the other two coconuts into a separate container and reserve for other uses. Scoop out the flesh of all three coconuts, removing any shell shards, and place in blender. Add green food of choice, and blend until creamy. Eat as a breakfast pudding, or pour over fresh peaches, pears, strawberries, and/or wildcrafted bananas.

Strawberry-Salba Pudding (Phase 1.5)

This hearty breakfast is rich in EFAs, and has a lovely, tangy flavor that appeals to children who like yogurt—and the color pink.

> 2 cups fresh Nut/Seed Mylk (page 470)
>
> ½ cup salba seeds or white chia seeds
>
> 1 cup whole strawberries, fresh or frozen
>
> ½ cup strawberries, chopped
>
> 1 tablespoon erythritol or xylitol

Blend 1 cup whole strawberries with strained Nut/Seed Mylk, and transfer to a large mixing bowl. Stir in chia seeds and set aside for 20 minutes, or until liquids have been absorbed by the seeds. Stir in chopped strawberries, and serve.

Variation (Phase 2): After the seeds have absorbed the liquids, stir in ¼ cup dried coconut flakes.

Just-Your-Style Chia Porridge (Phase 1)

Grownups could eat a bowl of creamy chia everyday for breakfast, as does Dr. Gabriel. The children like it too, but tend to enjoy more variety. Here's what we came up with—a family-size batch of chia pudding (not necessarily for every day) plus various condiments and toppings so each individual can choose. The possibilities are endless!

Note: This recipe is Phase 1 with no condiments and toppings. Toppings, if used, are marked below for other phases.

Chia porridge base
2 cups fresh Nut/Seed Mylk (page 470)

½ cup chia seeds

1 tablespoon erythritol or xylitol

⅛ teaspoon vanilla powder (optional)

¼ teaspoon Himalayan or other high-mineral raw salt
(optional)

Thoroughly stir all ingredients together. Serve chilled, at room
temperature, or gently heated in a double boiler on the stove.

Chia porridge condiments and topping options:
- banana slices (Phase 2)
- bee pollen (Phase 1.5)
- wild blueberries (Phase 1.5)
- carob powder—stir in about 1 teaspoon per small bowl
(Phase 1.5)
- cherries, pitted (Phase 1.5)
- goji berries (Phase 1.5)
- lucuma powder (Phase 1.5)
- maca powder—start out with a very small amount, and add
more as desired (Phase 1.5)
- mesquite powder (Phase 1.5)
- fresh nectarines, pitted and chopped (Phase 2)
- raspberries (Phase 1.5)
- strawberries, sliced (Phase 1.5)
- your choice of Raw Vegan Yogurts (page 473)

Quick and Easy Chia Porridge (Phase 1)

Keep soaked chia seeds in the refrigerator (using enough water
for your preferred consistency) for up to 4 days. Each morning,
spoon into a bowl (or a double boiler, to gently heat it) and stir in
tocotrienols (vitamin E-rich, raw, rice solubles, available at www
.DrCousensOnlineStore.com) to make it creamy, plus a pinch
of Himalayan or other high-mineral raw salt, vanilla, and Sweet-E
(erythritol) to taste. Add any of the above toppings.

Peaches and Cream (Phase 2)

Slice fresh peaches, and serve with coconut crème (blend ½ cup coconut chips with ¼ cup melted coconut oil), Macadamia-Pear Crème (page 478), or Almond Yogurt (page 474).

Grapefruit Lettuce Salad (Phase 1.5)

MAKES 4 SERVINGS

2 small heads of Bibb, buttercrunch, or green leaf lettuce

1 grapefruit

2 avocados, cubed (optional)

½ cup pecans, soaked, dehydrated and chopped (optional)

¼ leek (white end), thin-sliced, or fresh chives (optional)

Tear the lettuce onto individual plates. Cut grapefruit into halves and spoon out sections on top of the lettuce. Add desired toppings and dress with Grapefruit Salad Dressing, below.

Grapefruit Salad Dressing (Phase 1.5)

1 grapefruit, juiced

1 cup olive oil

¼ cup apple cider vinegar

½ teaspoon powdered stevia (or 2 tablespoons Jerusalem artichoke syrup or coconut syrup)

1 teaspoon *hing* (also known as asafetida, an Indian spice with a flavor similar to leeks)

1 teaspoon Himalayan or other high-mineral raw salt

freshly cracked black pepper, to taste (optional)

Blend all ingredients in a blender, or whisk in a small mixing bowl or jar. Keeps for one week if refrigerated.

Strawberry Breakfast Salad (Phase 1.5)

MAKES 2–3 SERVINGS

> 1 head of Bibb or buttercrunch lettuce, or a small bunch of romaine, torn into bite-sized pieces
>
> 1 cup strawberries, sliced
>
> ½ cup goji berries (optional)

Toss ingredients together, and drizzle on Pretty Pink Strawberry Dressing or Creamy Coconut Dressing, both below.

Pretty Pink Strawberry Dressing (Phase 1.5)

> ½ cup fresh or frozen strawberries
>
> ½ cup cold-pressed olive oil
>
> ¼ cup erythritol or xylitol
>
> juice of 1 lemon or lime
>
> pinch of Himalayan or other high-mineral raw salt

Blend strawberries, sweetener, salt, and lemon or lime juice. While blender is running, *slowly* pour in olive oil, blending until emulsified.

Creamy Coconut Dressing (Phase 2)

This sweet breakfast dressing doubles as a delicious lemony kefir-like drink. For a thick and creamy fruit dip, use only ½ of the coconut water.

> 1 young Thai coconut
>
> juice of one lemon
>
> 1 teaspoon xylitol

Open the coconut with a cleaver (find a demonstration video online for the technique), and pour out coconut water into blender through a strainer to remove any shell shards. Scoop out the coconut flesh (it should still be supple), and dip into water to remove any shell shards. Add lemon juice and xylitol, and blend until smooth. For a thicker dressing, use less coconut water.

Confetti Lettuce (Phase 2)
MAKES 2–3 SERVINGS

> 1 head of Bibb or buttercrunch lettuce, or a small bunch of romaine, torn into bite-sized pieces
>
> 1 apple, chopped
>
> ½ cup mixed black raisins and sulfur-free golden raisins
>
> ½ cup macadamia nuts, chopped
>
> 1 celery stalk, diced

Toss all ingredients high into the air (over a large salad bowl) and serve with Creamy Coconut Dressing (above).

"I'm Alive!" Breakfast Salad (Phase 2)
MAKES 2–3 SERVINGS

> 2 small heads Bibb or buttercrunch lettuce, or 1 bunch romaine lettuce
>
> 2 apples, chopped
>
> olive oil, to taste
>
> apple cider vinegar, to taste
>
> Himalayan or other high-mineral raw salt, to taste
>
> cayenne pepper, to taste

Tear lettuce onto individual plates. Divide apples onto each plate of lettuce, and drizzle on desired amounts of vinegar, oil, salt and pepper.

Love-Packed Lunchboxes, Snacks, and Sides

We've included a few recipes for lunches at home that are too messy for on-the-go meals; however, most of these lunch/snack items are very packable. Some children love to open up a scrumptious salad with a side of dressing (see "Super Suppers," page 432), while others prefer finger food.

Dehydrated foods can also help to make the snack or meal more substantial. If a child is very fond of dried foods, you may wish to pack extra drinks for proper hydration (see "Hydration Station Recipes," page 388, and "Dairy-Free Recipes," page 467). A thermos will help keep Nut/Seed Mylks fresh.

Even if we pack our children's favorite foods, lunchtime can present challenges if their own lunchbox, full of healthy food, differs from their peers.' In order to bond and make friends, our children are naturally looking for common ground with one another. Leah has observed apple-munching preschoolers at the lunch table declaring, "If you have and apple in your lunch, you can play with me!" It was as if they were saying, "Hooray! We're the same!" You know the game called "Memory"? The joy is in finding matches. Children often really appreciate "look-alike" foods that match what their classmates are eating, such as organic raisin boxes, baby carrots with nut-based ranch dressing, yogurt, pudding, or "jello" (see "Dairy-Free Recipes," page 467, and "Dare to Be Different Desserts," page 452).

Classmates may also become "envious"—in a good way!—of tasty foods that seem more special than what is in their lunches. Depending on their age, it gives our vegan kids a chance not only to share their food but to explain its vegan specialness. This is also a subtle lesson in interface integrity, for being supernormal in a "normal" world.

Sharing one's unique specialness with others is also part of childhood development. It is fortunate that some schools do not permit

blatant commercial influences on campus, even in students' clothing; yet many of our children still have more than ample exposure
to a culture of flashy labeling and cartoon characters advocating
unhealthy choices.

Especially in this context, a simple-to-make radish mouse, cherry-
tomato ladybug, or rabbit-shaped apple slice can mean a lot to our
fun and social children. (See *Play With Your Food* by Joost Elffers,
or websites on the Japanese art of *bento* boxes, for more creative
ideas.) If your child is slurping her smoothie while surrounded by
burgers and fries each day, she may also enjoy the book *The Secret
Life of Mitch Spinach* by Hillary Feerick and Jeff Hillenbrand in collaboration with Joel Fuhrman, MD. More creative ideas for healthy
fun with friends can be found in the "Supporting the Child's Social
Development" chapter (page 187).

Packing a little playfulness also helps us parents to be in a happy
mood while preparing food for our child. Eating can become an
adventure. Lunch-packing the night before can also help to prepare
the meals more consciously, taking time to center oneself as well as
to be in a conscious state of blessing of our children's food.

Cucumber Boats with Nori Sails (Phase 1 or 2)

MAKES 4 SERVINGS

*This recipe is Phase 1 if using the Sunflower Dip, or Phase 2 if using
the Cheeze Whiz.*

> 2 cucumbers
>
> 2 cups Cheeze Whiz (page 479) or Sunflower Dip (page 480)
>
> 1 sheet nori
>
> 4 skewers or thin dowels (not for sending to school, as they
>   may be perceived as a weapon)

Cut cucumbers lengthwise, and scoop out the seeds. Cut nori
sheet into 4 large triangles, and attach to skewers to look like sails.
Use a pastry bag or spoon to fill the cucumber with your spread
of choice, and insert the nori sails!

Black Olive Sunflower Hummus (Phase 1)

    1 cup soaked sunflower seeds

    ¾ cup dry sesame seeds

    juice of 2 lemons

    1 cup structured or filtered water (see "Living Water,"
        page 384)

    2 tablespoons olive oil

    1 teaspoon Himalayan or other high-mineral raw salt

    ½ cup sun-dried black olives, pitted and chopped

Soak the sunflower seeds 3–8 hours, then drain and rinse. Blend all ingredients except for the olives, adding just enough water to run the blender if needed. When smooth and creamy, stir in the olives.

Simple Sauerkraut (Phase 1)

The softened texture and pickled flavor of cultured cabbage appeals to many children, even those who don't usually care for cabbage. Raw sauerkraut can be purchased in some health food stores, if you want to try it before making your own. If it's a winner, make a double, triple, or quadruple batch and eat it daily with crackers and apple slices, soups, salads, or stuffed in avocado with a sprinkling of savory sunflower seeds (recipes to follow).

If this simple sauerkraut recipe is well-received, you can try making it with other flavors like garlic-dill, wild-harvested juniper berry (add 1 tablespoon) with caraway seed (add 3 teaspoons), or by adding another vegetable such as grated Brussels sprouts or wild-harvested sunchoke (Jerusalem artichoke) root.

Dehydrated sauerkraut is also a very tasty, packable, and kid-friendly snack—simply dehydrate sauerkraut until crunchy. While cultured vegetables are known to be highly beneficial for the mature intestinal tract, it is usually recommended to introduce them gradually, and not until after the child is one year old.

5 pounds cabbage

3 tablespoons Himalayan or other high-mineral raw salt

Grate cabbage by hand or in a food processor, or cut into fine strands with a knife. Transfer into a mixing bowl, add salt, and massage the salt in with clean hands. Transfer salted cabbage into a crock or food-grade plastic container, and pack it down firmly.

Place a plate on top of the packed cabbage so that it covers the cabbage completely, and place a weight, such as a jar of water, on top of the plate. Cover with a clean towel, and store at 70°. After 6 hours, check to make sure the cabbage is producing brine.

The sauerkraut will be ready in 1–4 weeks, depending on how strong you like it; more time fermenting gives it a stronger flavor. Transfer the sauerkraut into sterile canning jars, and store refrigerated for 3–4 months.

Savory Sunflower Seeds (Phase 1)

2 cups soaked sunflower seeds

1 tablespoon onion powder

1 teaspoon Himalayan or other high-mineral raw salt

½ teaspoon garlic powder

Soak the sunflower seeds overnight, then drain and rinse. Toss all ingredients together, and spread evenly onto dehydrator trays. Using a nonstick sheet will make cleanup easier. Store in an airtight container and keep on hand for packing in lunchboxes or sprinkling on salads, soups, and wraps.

Curried Sunflower Seeds (Phase 1)

2 cups soaked sunflower seeds

1 tablespoon curry powder (less if your curry powder is very spicy)

1 tablespoon tomato powder (buy in bulk-spice sections
of natural food stores, or from organic-herb suppliers
online—or make your own by grinding sun-dried tomatoes
in a coffee grinder or high-power blender)

1 teaspoon Himalayan or other high-mineral raw salt

Soak the sunflower seeds overnight, then drain and rinse. Toss
all ingredients together, and spread evenly onto dehydrator trays.
Using parchment paper or a nonstick sheet will make cleanup
easier. Store in an airtight container and keep on hand for packing
in lunchboxes or sprinkling on salads, soups, and wraps.

Pizza Pumpkin Seeds (Phase 1)

2 cups soaked hulled pumpkin seeds

1 teaspoon Himalayan or other high-mineral raw salt

2 teaspoons pizza seasoning blend, such as garlic powder,
basil, oregano, and fennel

1 teaspoon tomato powder (buy in bulk-spice sections of
natural food stores, or from organic-herb suppliers
online; or make your own by grinding sun-dried tomatoes
in a coffee grinder or high-power blender)

Soak the pumpkin seeds overnight, then drain and rinse. Toss all
ingredients together, and spread onto dehydrator trays; parchment paper or nonstick sheets will make cleanup easier. Pack in
lunches, or eat as a snack.

Avocado-Olive Lettuce Boats (Phase 1)
MAKES 4 SERVINGS

2 small heads of Bibb or buttercrunch, or one bunch of
romaine lettuce

4 avocados, cubed

1 jar of raw green olives, halved and pitted

½ cup seasoned sunflower seeds

dulse flakes, to taste

alfalfa or clover sprouts, for garnish

Arrange lettuce leaves onto individual plates. Mix the remaining ingredients and add them into each leaf "boat."

Avocado-Collard Mini-Wraps (Phase 1)

6 freshly picked young collard leaves (milder-tasting than mature leaves)

2 large avocados

1 cup salt-smoked almonds, chopped (recipe below)

dried onion flakes to taste (optional)

Himalayan or other high-mineral raw salt, to taste (optional)

Arrange collard leaves onto plates. Cut avocado in half. Remove pit, and slice each half into 3 sections (6 total). Remove peel. Place an avocado slice and some of the almonds in the center of each collard leaf. Salt and season to taste. Fold ends of leaves before rolling up into mini-wraps.

Smoke-Salted Almonds (Phase 1)

3 cups almonds, soaked overnight

½ teaspoon smoked sea salt

½ teaspoon Himalayan or other high-mineral raw salt

Drain water from almonds, and discard water. Add salt for structured high mineral content and smoked sea salt for smoky flavor, and dehydrate at 118° for 5–8 hours or until crunchy.

Chickpea Noodle Soup (Phase 1)

1 package kelp noodles (available in many health food stores)

5 cups structured or filtered water (see "Living Water," page 384)

5 heaping tablespoons South River brand or other chickpea (not soy-based) miso

1 cup frozen peas (optional)

1 teaspoon coconut oil

½ teaspoon kelp powder

Remove peas from freezer and thaw. Stir miso into water in the top of a double boiler to dissolve it. Add remaining ingredients, and gently heat on low; if you can't hold your finger in the soup, it's hot enough to destroy enzymes. Serve warm, or pack in a thermos.

Coconut-Sesame Butter (Phase 1.5)

2 cups grated coconut

1 cup hulled sesame seeds

Put sesame seeds into a blender on high speed, then pour in grated coconut, pushing down the mixture with a tamper as you blend for up to 10 seconds. (The energy of food has been shown to significantly decrease after 10 seconds in a blender.) The result is a mild and buttery spread. Serve with wildcrafted banana, or spread onto sprouted bread.

Bruschetta (Phase 2)

Using sprouted-oat pizza-dough recipe (see "Super Suppers," page 432), form dough into flat, bite-sized squares, rectangles, or rounds. Dehydrate as you would pizza dough, until pliable but not gooey. Serve crusts with chopped garden tomatoes, minced fresh basil, and salt and pepper to taste.

Dinosaur Kale Chips (Phase 1)

These are crunchy, oily, and salty like potato chips, but won't raise blood-sugar levels like white potatoes. The olive oil is heated to low temperatures rather than fried, and therefore is not carcinogenic. Not to mention that this is the nutrient-packed super-green—kale!

    1 large bunch dinosaur *(lacinato)* kale

    1 tablespoon olive oil

    1 teaspoon Himalayan or other high-mineral raw salt

Remove kale stalks. Add olive oil and salt, and mix thoroughly. Spread kale onto dehydrator trays and dehydrate for 3–4 hours, or until crispy.

Variation: If you do not have a food dehydrator, kale can be spread onto a stainless-steel cookie sheet and dried in a conventional oven at 170° (or at the lowest temperature), or even under a sunlamp, for 1–2 hours.

Cheezy Dino Kale Chips (Phase 1.5)

    10–12 cups loosely packed dinosaur *(lacinato)* kale

    Cheezy Sauce (below)

Remove kale stalks and place leaves into a very large mixing bowl. Pour Cheezy Sauce over kale, and toss thoroughly. Lay wet, cheezy kale leaves evenly onto dehydrator trays. Dehydrate for 4–5 hours, or until crispy.

Cheezy Sauce (Phase 1.5)

    1 cup carrot, chopped

    ¾ cup soaked sesame seeds

    1 teaspoon Himalayan or other high-mineral raw salt

    ¼ teaspoon cracked black pepper (optional)

    ¼ teaspoon onion powder

    ¼ teaspoon cumin

    ¼ teaspoon kelp powder (or desired amount to your child's taste)

    ¾ cup structured or filtered water (see "Living Water," page 384)

    juice of 1 lemon or lime

Soak sesame seeds in water overnight. Place the carrot, sesame seeds, salt, pepper, onion powder, cumin, and water into a blender; add small amounts of additional water if needed to keep it blending. This sauce doesn't taste "cheezy" until after it is dehydrated.

Dilly Dino Kale Chips (Phase 1)
FROM THE TREE OF LIFE CAFÉ STAFF

8–10 bunches of dinosaur *(lacinato)* kale
Dilly Dressing (below)

Remove stalks from 8–10 bunches of kale, and massage in the dressing. Place in a dehydrator for 2 hours at 145°, then lower to 115° and leave for 12–24 hours, or until totally dry. Store at room temperature in a metal box or glass jar. Chips will keep 2–3 weeks at room temperature.

Dilly Dressing (Phase 1)

1 cup lemon juice
½ cup filtered water
3 tablespoons dried dill
1 teaspoon black pepper
¼ teaspoon cayenne
½ teaspoon Sweet-E (erythritol)

Make a thick dressing with all the ingredients in a blender.

Noritos (Phase 1 or 1.5)

These are Phase 1 if made with bell peppers, or Phase 1.5 if made with carrots.

2 cups carrots or bell peppers (red or orange), chopped
1 tomato

¼ cup fresh lime juice

1 cup brazil nuts

1 cup soaked sesame seeds

1 clove fresh garlic

1 teaspoon onion powder

paprika to taste

nori sheets

Soak sesame seeds in water overnight. Blend all ingredients except nori in a food processor until thoroughly mixed but still chunky. Tear nori sheets into chip-size pieces. Spread a thin layer of sauce onto nori pieces, and sprinkle paprika on top. Place on dehydrator trays and dry for 3–4 hours, or until crispy.

Variation: Garnish with minced fresh chives before dehydrating.

Dulse in Olive Oil (Phase 1)

This tastes similar to olives packed in oil.

Buy whole, dried dulse rather than flakes. Break dulse into bite-sized pieces, and pack in a small glass jar with cold-pressed olive oil. Allow dulse to marinate in the oil for a few hours before serving.

Sprouts (Phase 1)

There's something about little sprouting greens that is loved by little sprouting people. First try milder sprouts like clover, broccoli, sunflower, buckwheat, and pea shoots, then try expanding the taste horizons. Children enjoy growing sprouts in a classroom windowsill, bringing tasty life to existing food-prep and science lessons. If you grow sprouts with little ones, you may enjoy singing this song that Leah wrote (sung to the tune of "Twinkle, Twinkle, Little Star"):

Sprinkle, sprinkle, little sprout.

Water helps your leaves come out.

Sun shines down from up above,

And we give to you our love.

Sprinkle, sprinkle, little sprout,

Water helps your leaves come out.

Spirulina Crunchies (Phase 1)

These treats are available at www.DrCousensOnlineStore.com. Eat them straight out of the bag, or sprinkle onto salads or an avocado. We know kids who really love these packed in their lunches—they must not mind standing out, because these crunchy supertreats turn your whole mouth blue-green naturally.

Okra Crunchies (Phase 1)

Okra is not only fun and beautiful to grow in the family garden; it also provides essential fatty acids for growing bodies. Simply pick and munch it fresh, or try these okra dehydrates.

4 cups okra, sliced

1 tablespoon ground brazil nuts

2 teaspoons fresh lime juice

2 teaspoons Frontier brand Cajun Seasoning Mix

1 teaspoon Himalayan or other high-mineral raw salt

Toss all ingredients together in a mixing bowl, and spread onto dehydrator trays using parchment paper or nonstick sheets. Dehydrate until crunchy, approximately 5 hours. Eat as is, or toss onto salads.

Happy Camper Trail Mix (Phase 1.5 or 2)

This is Phase 1.5 or 2, depending on the variety of dried berries used. (See food lists in Phase Chart, page 372.)

4 cups sunflower seeds

½ teaspoon Himalayan or other high-mineral raw salt

4-cup mixture of any of the following dried berries: goji berries, gooseberries (also called golden berries or Inca berries), mulberries, currants, raisins (black or sulfur-free golden)

Soak the sunflower seeds in water overnight, then drain and rinse. Toss sunflower seeds with salt, then spread evenly onto dehydrator trays. Dehydrate until dry and crunchy, so that it has a texture like roasted seeds. Mix with dried berries of choice, and keep on hand in glass storage jars for quick snacks and backpacking.

Savory Trail Mix (Phase 1)

1 cup dry almonds, soaked for two days

2 celery stalks, chopped

1 cup Peruvian sun-dried black olives

After almonds have soaked for two days (changing water daily), they will have doubled in size to 2 cups in volume. At this point, their brown skins can be slipped off by gently squeezing them between fingers and thumb. Discard the hulls and toss the almond whites with the remaining ingredients. Eat as a snack, or pack in lunch boxes.

Variation: Substitute Smoke-Salted Almonds (page 418) for the soaked and peeled almonds.

'Nilla Nuts (Phase 1)

3 cups pecans or walnuts

½ teaspoon vanilla powder

3 full droppers English toffee or hazelnut-flavored liquid stevia

3 full droppers vanilla-flavored liquid stevia

Himalayan or other high-mineral raw salt, to taste

Soak nuts in structured or filtered water overnight (see "Living Water," page 384), then drain and rinse. Toss nuts with vanilla, flavored stevia, and salt. Spread seasoned nuts onto dehydrator sheets using nonstick sheets to prevent liquid from dripping. Dehydrate at 110° for 3 hours, or until dry and crunchy.

Strawberry-Zucchini Sauce or Fruit Leather (Phase 1.5)

It's berry pink and yummy—tastes like applesauce!

    1 cup plus 4–5 large, fresh strawberries

    2 medium-sized zucchini or yellow summer squash, peeled

    1 teaspoon freshly minced or grated red beet, for a bright pink color

    juice of 1 small lemon or lime

    berry-flavored stevia, to taste (try 1–2 full droppers)

Blend all ingredients together until very smooth. Serve as is, or dehydrate for a low-glycemic fruit leather, following directions below.

Lemon-Drop Fruit Leather (Phase 1)

    ½ cup fresh lemon juice

    2 medium-sized zucchini, peeled and chopped to make about 4 cups

    2 tablespoons xylitol

    2–3 full droppers lemon-flavored stevia

    ⅛ teaspoon turmeric, for a bright yellow color

Blend all ingredients together until very smooth. Pour soupy fruit leather mixture onto a nonstick sheet laid on top of a dehydrator tray. Using a spatula, spread into a thin layer and dehydrate at 115° until pliable and firm, but not brittle. Use scissors (a child-sized pair is handy if you have small helpers) to cut fruit leather into bars.

Handful of Rubies (Phase 1.5)

Anti-oxidant gems for little princes and princesses.

> 1 cup pomegranate kernels

Serve in a fancy little dish.

Moon and Stars (Phase 1)

> macadamia nuts (these need to be refrigerated to stay
> fresh) and/or truly raw cashews
> bell pepper

Use a small star-shaped cookie/veggie cutter to punch out colorful bell pepper stars, using red, orange, yellow, green, and purple
bell peppers for rainbow stars! Combine with little full moons
(macadamia nuts) and/or half-moons (cashews).

Variation: In place of the bell-pepper stars, cut nori sheets into
star shapes with scissors.

Apples with Pumpkin-Seed Butter (Phase 2)

> apples
> pumpkin-seed butter, or other preferred nut butter such as
> almond or pecan

Slice apples and serve them on a plate, or pack them up to go,
with a dollop of zinc-rich raw pumpkin-seed butter. If they are
to be eaten later, pre-soak the apple slices for a few minutes in
saltwater, fresh lemon juice, or orange juice to prevent browning.

Phase 1 variation: Replace apple slices with celery sticks.

Fresh Pickles (Phase 1)

> 2 cucumbers
> 1 tablespoon apple cider vinegar
> 2 tablespoons cold-pressed olive oil
> ½ teaspoon Himalayan or other high-mineral raw salt

Peel and slice the cucumbers, and toss with the remaining ingredients. Arrange on a plate, or pack them up to go.

Fresh Pickle Deluxe (Phase 1.5)

After arranging your fresh pickle plate (above), garnish with julienned carrots, minced raw olives, and snips of fresh garden chives. Best eaten just after preparation.

Beet Pickles (Phase 1.5)

> 2 medium-sized beets, thin-sliced
>
> 2 tablespoons cold-pressed sesame oil
>
> 1 tablespoon apple cider vinegar
>
> ¼ teaspoon onion powder
>
> ¼ teaspoon garlic powder
>
> Himalayan or other high-mineral raw salt, to taste
>
> fresh cracked pepper, to taste
>
> fresh dill for garnish (optional)

Toss all ingredients together, and place in a sealed container in the refrigerator to marinate for 1–8 hours. Eat with utensils, as pickled beets will dye your fingers pink.

Quick Cucumber-Miso Snack (Phase 1)

Cut fresh cucumbers into rounds (can be peeled before cutting if desired). Spread a thin layer of mild white or chickpea miso onto each cucumber slice, and eat immediately.

Quick Cucumber-Miso Snack Deluxe (Phase 1)

Add ripe avocado and dulse flakes to your Cucumber-Miso Snack rounds (above).

Lemon Cucumbers (Phase 1)

Lemon cucumbers are round and yellow-colored on the outside. They can be found at farmer's markets, or grown in your garden. Pack them in lunches and eat like an apple.

Carrot Confetti (Phase 2)

Doubles as party food!

2 carrots, grated

1 apple, grated

½ lime, juiced

½ cup dried goji berries

¼ cup dried coconut flakes

½ cup mango, chopped

⅛ teaspoon vanilla powder (optional)

Toss all ingredients together and serve with breakfast or lunch, or as a snack.

Green Grapes with Celery (Phase 2)

green grapes

celery

Cut grapes in half, and chop celery into small bite-size pieces; toss together and serve.

Chipotle-Tomato Crisps (Phase 1)

3 cups fresh tomatoes

1½ cups golden or brown flax seeds

1 teaspoon Himalayan or other high-mineral raw salt

¼ teaspoon kelp powder

¼ teaspoon chili powder or chipotle powder (chipotle is a bit more spicy)

½ teaspoon ground cumin

Grind flax seeds into meal using a coffee grinder or blender on high speed. Blend the resulting flaxmeal with tomatoes, salt, chili or chipotle, and cumin. When thoroughly mixed, spread evenly onto dehydrator trays covered with nonstick sheets. Score the tomato-flax spread into squares or triangles with a table knife; this will help you break the crisps apart when they are dry. Dehydrate at 110° for 15–24 hours, or until crisp. Serve with fresh salsa or guacamole.

Guacamole (Phase 1)

Little hands can do it all!—mash, juice, measure, mix, and snip chives and cilantro with a child-sized pair of scissors.

> 4 small or 3 large avocados
>
> juice of one lime
>
> 1 tablespoon fresh chives, minced
>
> 1 tablespoon fresh cilantro, minced (optional)
>
> ¼ teaspoon chili powder or chipotle powder (chipotle is a bit more spicy)
>
> ¼ teaspoon powdered cumin (optional)
>
> ¼ teaspoon powdered kelp
>
> Himalayan or other high-mineral raw salt, to taste (optional)

Mash avocados with a fork, and mix in the remaining ingredients.

Garden Veggie Salsa (Phase 1)

This recipe is basically a thick gazpacho soup. It is very mild, for a child's palate. For a hotter salsa, add more jalapeño. For regular gazpacho soup, add blended tomatoes and other garden vegetables.

> 2 cups fresh garden tomatoes, chopped
>
> 1 cup red, orange, or yellow bell pepper, finely minced
>
> ½ cup cucumber, minced
>
> ½ cup zucchini or yellow summer squash, minced

½ cup fresh spring onions or chives, finely minced

¼ teaspoon fresh jalapeno pepper, finely minced, with seeds removed

½ teaspoon garlic powder

1 teaspoon Himalayan or other high-mineral raw salt

¼ teaspoon kelp powder

1 teaspoon olive oil (optional)

½ cup loosely packed minced cilantro (optional)

Stir all ingredients together in a bowl. Allow to marinate, so the flavors can blend, for at least 20 minutes before serving.

Ninja Chips (Phase 1)

This is a great recipe for introducing sea veggies into the diet. Ninja Chips are very popular with kids and adults alike!

9 sheets nori

2 cups soaked sesame seeds

2 tablespoons chickpea miso

1 teaspoon (or desired amount) kelp powder

1 teaspoon dulse flakes (or Maine Coast Sea Vegetables' triple blend of dulse, laver, and sea lettuce flakes)

2 tablespoons Prepared Mustard (recipe below)

Soak the sesame seeds overnight, then drain and discard soak-water. Soaking them ahead of time germinates the seeds and enhances the nutrition. If you're in a pinch for time, however, the chips can be made with dry sesame seeds.

Place seeds in a medium-sized mixing bowl, and stir in miso, Prepared Mustard, and additional sea veggies until well mixed. Cut nori sheets into squares. Spread a small amount of sesame mixture onto each square, and place onto dehydrator trays. Dehydrate at 115° for 2 hours, or until crispy.

Prepared Mustard (Phase 1)

4 tablespoons dry mustard

¼ teaspoon wasabi powder (optional)

pinch turmeric (optional)

¼ cup water

2 tablespoons apple cider vinegar

juice of 1 lemon

½ cup olive oil

Whisk or blend all ingredients together. Store in an airtight container in the refrigerator, as you would other mustards.

Sea Veggie-Walnut Crackers (Phase 1)

The EFA-rich walnuts lend a buttery flavor to these crackers, while the flaxseed binds everything together. The sea veggies add a salty flavor, trace minerals, and radiation-protective support.

3 cups soaked walnuts

¼ cup golden flax seeds

3 stalks celery

2 teaspoons kelp powder

¼ cup dulse flakes

1½ teaspoon Himalayan or other high-mineral raw salt

Soak walnuts overnight, then drain and rinse. Grind flaxseed into meal using a coffee grinder or blender on high speed; use freshly ground flaxmeal for this recipe. Grind walnuts in a food processor until they resemble wheat bulgur or couscous. Transfer into a large mixing bowl.

Process the celery until finely minced, then stir in salt, sea vegetables and ground walnuts. Spread onto dehydrator trays using nonstick sheets, and dry at 115° for about 12 hours, or until crisp. Store in airtight containers. Eat with avocado for a snack, pack in lunchboxes, or serve with salad.

Tomato-Flax Crackers (Phase 1)

FROM THE TREE OF LIFE CAFÉ STAFF

2½ cups flaxseed

8 cups tomato chunks

¾ teaspoon salt

½ teaspoon pepper

herbs of your choice—fresh basil, rosemary, tarragon, dill, cumin, smoked paprika, etc.

Blend tomato chunks into a purée. Soak flaxseed in tomato purée for 4 hours. Mix the seasonings together, then add into the seed mixture. Layer on a nonstick sheet using a wet spatula, and score with a knife into square pieces. Dehydrate at 115° for 24 hours, turning over halfway through drying time.

Bumps on a Log, Savory-Style (Phase 1)

Perhaps you've tried the nut-butter and raisin (or dried-currant) version. Here's a zero-glycemic option.

6 long sticks of celery (leaves removed)

1 or 2 avocados

1 heaping tablespoon mild, light chickpea miso

squeeze of lemon juice (to keep the avocado from oxidizing)

1 teaspoon black sesame seeds

Invite little hands to mash the avocado, squeeze the lemon, and mix in the miso with a fork in a bowl. Fill celery wands with the mixture, and sprinkle with black sesame seeds.

Super Suppers

A hearty, build-your-own salad is a good standby meal. It is wise to vary the salad bar offerings a bit each day. Setting the table as a salad bar helps individual family members choose what their own body may be asking for, without having to make more than one meal.

To help with serving salads at suppertime, we've started with child-friendly dressing recipes. Mild, baby-green mixes and/or lettuces such as romaine or buttercrunch make a good base. Strong, peppery greens like mature arugula or mustard can be set aside for grownups whose taste buds are less sensitive.

For additional recipes, see Dr. Gabriel's books *Rainbow-Green Live Food Cuisine, Conscious Eating,* and *There is a Cure for Diabetes,* Leah's book *Baby Greens,* and the recipe books listed in our "Resources" section (page 485).

Salad Bar Suggestions

- greens (see note above)
- chopped tomatoes
- cherry or pear tomatoes
- fresh or frozen (and thawed) peas*
- pea sprouts
- sunflower sprouts
- clover sprouts
- micro greens (such as broccoli or kale sprouts)
- sliced okra or Okra Crunchies (page 423)
- bell pepper, sliced, chopped, or cut into shapes with a cookie cutter
- carrot curls (use a veggie peeler)
- radish rounds
- kohlrabi, peeled and sliced
- chopped celery
- cucumber circles or half-circles
- green or black olives (sun-dried, or brined and unheated, pitted)
- chives, chopped
- fresh or dehydrated sauerkraut
- sunflower seeds (raw or soaked overnight), salted and dehydrated until crunchy

- pine nuts
- black or golden raisins
- minced cabbage
- broccoli
- cauliflower
- grated beets
- Young Coconut Yogurt (page 474)
- Sunflower Dip (page 480)
- steamed quinoa, black rice, wild rice, brown rice, and/or sprouted and steamed lentils, if cooked food is desired

* **Note:** Frozen foods are suggested for occasional use only. According to Kirlian photography, food loses about 2/3 of its energy when frozen.

Macadamia Ranch Dressing (Phase 1)

1 cup macadamia nuts

1½ cups filtered water

¼ cup apple cider vinegar

Himalayan or other high-mineral raw salt, to taste

1–2 tablespoons freshly minced garden chives

small bunch fresh basil

cracked black pepper (optional)

¼ teaspoon kelp powder (or desired amount)

Blend all ingredients except the fresh herbs in a blender for 10 seconds, until creamy and smooth. Pulse or stir in fresh herbs, just enough to mix and not completely blended. Chill until served.

Variation: Peeled almonds or truly raw cashews can be substituted for macadamia nuts.

French Tomato Dressing (Phase 1)

4 fresh garden tomatoes

1 cup olive oil

¼ cup apple cider vinegar

Italian seasoning, to taste

Himalayan or other high-mineral raw salt, to taste

¼ teaspoon kelp powder

⅛ teaspoon powdered stevia leaf (optional)

Blend all ingredients together in a blender until smooth. Chill until served.

Creamy Miso Dressing (Phase 1)

¼ cup olive oil

¼ cup lemon juice

2 tablespoons chickpea miso

½ teaspoon Himalayan or other high-mineral raw salt

¼ teaspoon kelp powder

Whisk all ingredients together in a jar, or blend in a blender until smooth.

Creamy Sesame Dressing (Phase 1)

This is a delicious and more economical version of tahini dressing.

½ cup hulled and soaked sesame seeds

1 cup structured or filtered water (see "Living Water" section, page 384)

2 tablespoons apple cider vinegar

1 teaspoon Himalayan or other high-mineral raw salt

¼ teaspoon kelp powder

½ teaspoon dried basil

cracked pepper, to taste

Soak hulled sesame seeds overnight, and drain. Place seeds in a blender with water, vinegar, salt, and seasonings. Blend until creamy. Keeps for a few days in the refrigerator.

Papaya-Chipotle Dressing (Phase 2)

This delicious dressing has a little kick. The unique contribution of papaya seeds adds a peppercorn-like flavor, and is also said to help rid the body of parasites. Drizzle over salads or lettuce tacos.

2 cups fresh papaya, peeled, seeded, and cubed (reserve seeds)

½ cup cold-pressed olive oil

juice of one medium-size lime

2 tablespoons apple cider vinegar

¼ teaspoon chipotle powder

½ teaspoon Himalayan or other high-mineral raw salt

Add back 1 teaspoon of the papaya seeds. Blend all ingredients together in a blender until smooth and creamy (no more than 10 seconds).

Hummus (Phase 1)

FROM THE TREE OF LIFE CAFÉ STAFF

4 cups hulled raw sesame seeds

1 cup olive or sesame oil

2 medium to large zucchinis

½ cup lemon juice

another ¼ cup olive oil

⅛ teaspoon *hing* (also known as asafetida, an Indian spice with a flavor similar to leeks)

1 teaspoon salt

1 tablespoon cumin

⅛ teaspoon cayenne

½ teaspoon white pepper

1 cup chopped parsley or cilantro

Peel the zucchini, and chop it into small chunks. To make tahini: Blend 4 cups sesame seeds with 1 cup olive or sesame oil. Then purée all other ingredients in a blender. This may need to be done in batches, depending on the blender. Blend in the tahini last. Fold in the parsley.

Variations: Add ½ cup chopped olives. For Red Pepper Hummus, substitute 3 red bell peppers for the zucchini. For Spicy Hummus, substitute chipotle for cayenne, and then add 1½ teaspoon smoked paprika.

Black Olive Paté (Phase 1)

2 cups hulled sesame seeds

½ cup olive oil

1 cup sunflower seeds

6 cups peeled and chopped zucchini

another ½ cup olive oil

¼ cup filtered water

½ cup lemon juice

1 cup chopped parsley

1 cup pitted black kalamata olives

1 cup fresh chopped basil

½ teaspoon black pepper

⅛ teaspoon cayenne

⅛ teaspoon *hing* (also known as asafetida, an Indian spice with a flavor similar to leeks)

1 teaspoon salt

Peel, chop, and measure the zucchini. Blend sesame seeds with ½ cup olive oil in a blender to make about 1½ cups tahini. Place all remaining ingredients with the tahini in a food processor, and incorporate very well together to form a paté.

Variation: Rather than salt and olives, use 1¼ cup olives and ¼ cup olive brine.

Dino Kale Salad (Phase 1)

    1 large bunch dinosaur kale

    2 tablespoons olive oil

    Himalayan or other high-mineral raw salt, to taste

    ½ cup hemp seeds

    1 teaspoon onion powder (optional)

Remove kale stalks, and place leaves into a medium to large salad bowl. Add olive oil and salt, and massage into the leaves by hand to soften the kale. Stir in hemp seeds and onion powder.

Israeli Salad (Fatoush) (Phase 1)

FROM THE TREE OF LIFE CAFÉ STAFF

    2–3 cucumbers, peeled and chopped

    5 cups chopped tomatoes

    2 cups mixed fresh cilantro, parsley and mint, chopped

    1 cup diced radishes

    ¼ cup olive oil

    1 teaspoon sea salt

After peeling and chopping the cucumber, rub it with sea salt and let sit 1 hour, then drain. Prepare and combine remaining ingredients. After 1 hour, add cucumber and serve.

Bundle-It-Up Winter Salad (Phase 1)

    1 head green cabbage

    1 cup dark leafy greens such as kale or collard greens, broken into bite-sized pieces

    1 cup almonds, chopped

    1 cup sunflower sprouts (these and other micro-greens can be grown year-round indoors by a sunny window)

    1 cup raw, sun-dried or brine-cured, chopped olives

½ cup hemp seeds

olive oil or sesame oil

apple cider vinegar

Himalayan or other high-mineral raw salt

kelp powder and dulse flakes, to taste

nori sheets

Toss all ingredients together in a salad bowl. Swaddle inside nori sheets for a hearty veggie wrap. Can also be simply served as a salad.

Raw Pizza (Phase 2)
MAKES 6 PERSONAL-SIZED PIZZAS

Pizza Crust (Sprouted Oat-Coconut, Phase 2)
With the addition of coconut, these personal-size crusts resemble white-flour bread crusts in appearance; however, this whole-grain recipe is rich in flavor. Light toppings such as those suggested below are a good complement to these crusts, rather than adding an equally rich seed-cheeze topping.

2 cups soaked oat groats

2 cups shredded coconut

3 tablespoons coconut oil, liquid form

1 teaspoon Himalayan or other high-mineral raw salt

2 teaspoons pizza-seasoning dried-herb mix (you can make your own with dried herbs such as garlic, onion, basil, oregano, thyme, caraway, sage, etc.)

¼ cup parsley leaves

Soak oat groats for 2–3 days, changing water each day, so they begin to sprout. Grind the coconut into a creamy but grainy paste in a food processor. Grind sprouted oat groats in a food processor, and pour in coconut oil while processor is running. When thoroughly mixed, scrape into a medium-sized mixing bowl, and stir in shredded coconut paste, salt, and pizza seasonings. Knead the dough by hand to mix thoroughly, and form into 6 balls the size of a small fist. Flatten dough balls by hand, and dehydrate at 118° for 5–8 hours, or until dry yet still soft in consistency. Do not let them get crispy.

Sun-Dried Tomato Sauce (Phase 1)

½ cup sun-dried tomatoes

1 cup fresh tomatoes

Himalayan or other high-mineral raw salt, to taste

pizza seasoning dried-herb mix, to taste

⅛ teaspoon kelp powder (or desired amount)

¼ cup olive oil

Blend all ingredients together in a blender, and use as pizza sauce.

Fresh pizza-topping suggestions:

- green or black pitted olives, stored in brine or sun-dried (these are now available raw)
- baby arugula, broken up into small pieces
- hemp seeds or ground brazil nuts (similar to Parmesan cheese)
- thin-sliced bell pepper
- broccoli florets, chopped small
- Caramelized Onions (recipe below)
- thin-sliced zucchini

Caramelized Onions (Phase 2)

1 onion

1 tablespoon coconut sugar

1 teaspoon coconut oil

Himalayan or other high-mineral raw salt, to taste.

Thin-slice the onion. Toss in the coconut sugar, oil, and salt, and mix well. Dehydrate on a nonstick sheet until soft but slightly crunchy.

Tree of Life Pizza (Phase 1 or 1.5)

FROM THE TREE OF LIFE CAFÉ STAFF

MAKES 3 PIZZAS

Pizza Crust (Nut-Seed, Phase 1)

> 4 cups sunflower seeds
>
> 2 cups walnuts
>
> 3 cups peeled zucchini, puréed
>
> 2–3 tablespoons olive oil
>
> 2–3 tablespoons lemon juice
>
> ¼ cup mixed fresh herbs such as rosemary, oregano, and thyme, to taste, or 2 tablespoons dried Italian seasoning
>
> 1½ teaspoon salt
>
> ½ teaspoon black pepper
>
> 1 cup ground flaxseed
>
> 1 cup filtered water

Purée zucchini in food processor or blender. Process all remaining ingredients except ground flax in food processor with puréed zucchini. Transfer to a mixing bowl, then add flax. Let sit 10–15 minutes, then spread on nonstick dehydrator sheets. Dehydrate for 8–12 hours at 115°, flipping the crusts over halfway through. They should be dry, but not crispy.

Pizza Crust (Buckwheat-Nut-Seed, Phase 1.5)

> 4 cups sprouted buckwheat
>
> 2 cups carrot juice, or 3 cups puréed zucchini
>
> 2 cups any type of nuts or seeds

¼ cup fresh mixed herbs of your choice, or 2 tablespoons Italian seasoning

1 teaspoon salt

½ teaspoon pepper

¼ cup olive oil

3 tablespoons lemon juice

1 cup ground flaxseed

Process sprouted buckwheat, carrot juice, nuts, and herbs in a food processor until fully creamed. Place in a mixing bowl with the rest of the ingredients, and proceed as for Phase 1 Pizza Crust recipe above.

Cheeze (Phase 1)

5 cups Brazil nuts, or 3 cups Brazil nuts plus 3 cups cashews or soaked and peeled almonds

¼ cup lemon juice

2 tablespoons dried oregano, or 1 small bunch fresh oregano

1 teaspoon sea salt

1 teaspoon *hing* (also known as asafetida, an Indian spice with a flavor similar to leeks)

½ teaspoon white pepper

1 cup filtered water (more as needed)

Blend all ingredients into a cream in half-batches, or use a food processor. If using a Vitamix, add more water as needed. This is a basic recipe—add fresh or dried herbs to your liking!

Pizza Sauce (Phase 1)

6 cups fresh tomatoes, chopped, or use grape tomatoes

2 cups sun-dried tomatoes

1 red bell pepper

1–2 tablespoons fresh rosemary

1 bunch fresh basil

¼ cup olive oil

1½ tablespoon lemon juice

1½ teaspoon salt

⅛ teaspoon chili pepper flakes

Blend together no more than 10 seconds.

Mac 'n' Cheeze (Phase 1.5)

FROM ELAINA LOVE

See recipe on page 480.

Lasagna (Phase 1)

FROM THE TREE OF LIFE CAFÉ STAFF

Lasagna Noodles (Phase 1)

10–12 small zucchini

Himalayan or other high-mineral raw salt

Slice zucchini lengthwise into thin strips with a mandoline. Salt, let sit for a couple hours, pat dry, and set aside.

Cheeze (Phase 1)

See Cheeze recipe above.

Marinara Sauce #1 (Phase 1)

3 cups fresh tomatoes

3 cups sun-dried tomatoes

¼ cup olive oil

¼ cup lemon juice

1 red bell pepper

2 cups fresh basil leaves, loosely packed

2 tablespoons fresh rosemary

2 teaspoons sea salt

1 teaspoon pepper flakes

Blend ingredients into a thick sauce. Add more sun-dried tomatoes if it's too thin, or water if it's too thick.

Parmesan Cheeze (Phase 1)

½ cup Brazil nuts or hemp seeds

¼ teaspoon salt

¼ teaspoon Italian seasoning

⅛ teaspoon *hing* (also known as asafetida, an Indian spice with a flavor similar to leeks)

1 tablespoon lemon zest (optional)

Pulse in food processor to get a Parmesan-cheese-like texture.

To assemble the Lasagna:

Place a layer of zucchini in a baking dish, and top with a layer of Cheeze, followed with Marinara. Continue until dish is full, finishing with a layer of Marinara. Place some crumbled Parmesan Cheeze on top, and dehydrate at 105° for 3–4 hours, or until warm all the way through. Lasagna should not be watery.

Optional: Massage 8 cups of spinach or kale with salt, let sit for 1 hour, drain off as much water as possible, then layer spinach or kale in between Cheeze and Marinara.

Spaghetti and Neat Balls (Phase 1)

FROM THE TREE OF LIFE CAFÉ STAFF

Spaghetti Noodles (Phase 1)

12 medium zucchini

Himalayan or other high-mineral raw salt

Spiralize zucchini using a small blade of a vegetable spiralizer. (The Saladacco vegetable spiralizer is a tool created by the Joyce Chen company. This and other brands can be purchased online at www.Amazon.com.) Sprinkle and toss gently with salt. Let sit for at least 2 hours. Drain.

Neat Balls (Phase 1)

MAKES 30–40 BALLS

4 cups mixed nuts, such as walnuts and sunflower seeds

2 stalks celery

1 tablespoon apple cider vinegar

½ cup fresh fennel

¼ cup parsley

2 tablespoons olive oil

¼ cup ground flaxseed

1 tablespoon Italian seasoning

1 tablespoon dried oregano

1 tablespoon dried sage

1 tablespoon dry marjoram

1 tablespoon dry thyme

¾ teaspoon salt

⅛ teaspoon *hing* (also known as asafetida, an Indian spice with a flavor similar to leeks)

¼ cup water, or just enough to help it mix well

Pulse all ingredients in a food processor to form a paste. Roll into small balls the size of a walnut. Dehydrate for 4–6 hours at 115°.

Marinara Sauce #2 (Phase 1)

2 cups fresh tomatoes, with seed pulp removed if juicy

2 cups sun-dried tomatoes plus ½ cup of the soakwater

½ cup olive oil

1 cup packed fresh basil

2 red bell peppers

1 teaspoon Himalayan or other high-mineral raw salt

1 tablespoon lemon juice

½ teaspoon red pepper flakes

½ cup fresh herbs such as rosemary or oregano

½ teaspoon stevia powder (optional)

Prepare in a blender on medium-low speed for no more than 10 seconds.

Parmesan Cheeze

See recipe under Lasagna, above.

ELT/ZLT (Eggplant or Zucchini, Lettuce, and Tomato) Sandwich (Phase 1)

Sandwich Bread (Phase 1)

3 cups pumpkin seeds

3 cups sunflower seeds

1 medium to large zucchini, chopped

1 cup sun-dried tomato

2 tablespoons dried basil

1 teaspoon salt

3 tablespoon olive oil

3 cups water

¼ cup apple cider vinegar

1 cup ground chia seeds

Note that this batch is too large for blenders, so process by half-batches. Blend all ingredients except chia until creamy. Place in a mixing bowl, and add enough chia to form a soft, spreadable mix. Spread evenly, 1-inch thick, on nonstick sheets on a dehydrator tray. Dehydrate 6–8 hours at 115°, flipping bread over halfway through. They should be dry all the way through, but not as hard as a cracker.

Avo Mayo (Phase 1)

> 3 ripe avocados
>
> ¼ cup olive oil
>
> 2 tablespoons lemon juice
>
> 2 tablespoons apple cider vinegar
>
> 1 teaspoon mustard
>
> ½ teaspoon salt
>
> ½ teaspoon white pepper

Blend all ingredients until smooth (no longer than 10 seconds).

Barbecued Eggplant or Zucchini (Phase 1)

> 3 large eggplants or medium-large zucchinis
>
> ½ cup sun-dried tomatoes
>
> 1 cup sun-dried tomato soakwater
>
> ½ cup olive oil
>
> 2 tablespoons apple cider vinegar
>
> ¼ teaspoon *hing* (also known as asafetida, an Indian spice with a flavor similar to leeks)
>
> 2 tablespoons lemon juice
>
> 2 tablespoons sage
>
> 2 teaspoons smoked paprika
>
> ¼ teaspoon chipotle powder
>
> 1 tablespoon Italian seasoning
>
> 1 teaspoon cumin
>
> 1 ½ teaspoons Himalayan or other high-mineral raw salt
>
> additional salt for preparing eggplant/zucchini

Slice eggplants or zucchinis with a mandoline. Salt and let sit 2–3 hours. Rinse and pat dry. Blend remaining ingredients into a sauce. Cover eggplant or zucchini with the sauce, and place on a dehydrator tray. Dehydrate at 115° until desired crispiness is achieved (at least 6–8 hours). Serve on Sandwich Bread (above) with Avo Mayo, lettuce, and sliced tomatoes.

Chipotle Lentils (Phase 1 or 1.5)

This recipe is hearty and warming for the winter months. Serve for dinner, potlucks, and fiestas. This dish is Phase 1 if bell peppers are used, and Phase 1.5 if carrots are used.

    2 cups dried lentils

    1 cup black olives (salt-cured, or raw olives in brine)

    2 ripe avocados (optional; preferably not, if out of season)

    ½ cup fresh cilantro, minced

    ¼ cup cold-pressed olive oil

    2 cups cherry tomatoes, halved (optional, if out of season)

    ripe bell pepper or carrot, minced (optional)

    ⅛ teaspoon kelp powder

    ½ teaspoon cumin powder (best if ground fresh)

    ¼–½ teaspoon chipotle powder; depending on degree of
      heat desired

    ½ teaspoon Himalayan or other high-mineral raw salt, to
      taste

Soak dried lentils for 1–2 days. (Two full days of soaking helps to ensure that even the late bloomers sprout.) Drain the lentils and lightly steam them; or simply rinse and place them into a large mixing bowl. Mix in all of the remaining ingredients.

Kelp-Noodle Pad Thai (Phase 1)

MAKES 4 SERVINGS

This raw version is MSG-free; chickpea miso, smoked seasonings, and dried herbs are used for depth of flavor rather than soy sauce, shoyu, or soy-based liquid aminos.

Veggie Medley with Kelp Noodles (Phase 1)

> 1 carrot, julienned
>
> 1 cup sugar snap peas, whole or chopped
>
> 1 cup baby bok choy, chopped (optional)
>
> ½ cup freshly sprouted pea shoots (optional)
>
> ¼ cup fresh cilantro, minced (can be served on the side)
>
> ¼ cup fresh garlic chives or spring onions minced
>
> 12-ounce package of kelp noodles

Toss all ingredients together in a medium to large mixing bowl, and set aside.

For julienning the carrots, The Pampered Chef carries a small, handy tool called the julienne peeler, which can be used by children under adult supervision. Though this tool is much safer than a mandoline slicer or a chef's knife, it is still somewhat sharp. It works like a veggie peeler, but juliennes as it peels. Because of its size, it is easy to store and clean.

Pad Thai Sauce (Phase 1)

> ½ cup raw almond butter or wild jungle peanut butter (see note below)
>
> juice of 1 small lime
>
> 1 teaspoon onion powder
>
> ¼ teaspoon garlic powder
>
> ⅛ teaspoon chipotle
>
> ½ teaspoon smoked paprika, to taste (optional)

2 teaspoons chickpea miso

2 tablespoons cold-pressed sesame oil

¼ cup structured or filtered water (see "Living Water," page 384) or mild lemongrass tea, if needed, to thin the sauce

hot pepper flakes (for garnish only)

In a small mixing bowl, combine all of the Pad Thai sauce ingredients except hot pepper flakes, and mix with a fork or a whisk. Pour this sauce onto the Veggie Medley, and toss to mix. Garnish the grownups' plates with hot pepper flakes, and serve immediately.

Variation: Kelp noodles are available online and in many health food stores, but can be replaced with thin-sliced green cabbage, or zucchini noodles sliced angel-hair pasta-thin. (These can be prepared with a tool called the Saladacco spiral slicer, made by Joyce Chen. Other online companies make similar tools, if you prefer a larger noodle.)

Note: Wild jungle peanut butter is not only raw but, because it comes from a wild strain of peanut, it is also aflatoxin-free. This item is carried by an online company called Viva Pura.

Avocado-Tomato Soup (Phase 1)

FROM THE TREE OF LIFE CAFÉ STAFF

2 pints cherry tomatoes

3 small or 2 large avocados

2 cups sun-dried tomatoes

1½ cups sun-dried tomato soakwater

¼ teaspoon green stevia powder

1 teaspoon white pepper

1 teaspoon Himalayan or other high-mineral raw salt

¼ teaspoon *hing* (also known as asafetida, an Indian spice that tastes similar to leeks)

¼ cup lemon juice

3 tablespoons dulse flakes

2 tablespoons olive oil

2 tablespoons fresh rosemary

3 tablespoons fresh basil

1 tablespoon fresh marjoram or thyme

If no fresh herbs are available, you may use dried herbs, reducing the amounts by half. Blend all ingredients except herbs in blender. Mix in herbs, and serve cold; or warm the soup in a dehydrator for a couple of hours; or heat slowly and gently in the top of a double boiler. If it's too hot to finger-touch, then enzymes and nutrients are probably being lost.

Red Pepper Soup (Phase 1)

FROM THE TREE OF LIFE CAFÉ STAFF

4 tomatoes

3 red bell peppers

1 bunch oregano

1 teaspoon Himalayan or other high-mineral raw salt

¾ cup chickpea miso

½ cup olive oil

1 tablespoon lemon juice

1 teaspoon smoked paprika

dash cayenne (optional)

Blend everything except the fresh herbs together until smooth. Fold in the herbs after blending.

Dare to Be Different Desserts

The first three cookie recipes are vegan variations on the classic icebox cookie.

Vanilla Snowflake (Low-) Sugar Cookies (Phase 2)

2½ cups dried coconut flakes

½ cup sesame seeds

½ cup lucuma powder (see "Natural Low-Sugar and No-Sugar Sweeteners," page 376)

2 tablespoons coconut oil

4 tablespoons coconut nectar syrup

1 teaspoon vanilla powder

pinch Himalayan or other high-mineral raw salt

powdered xylitol for dusting*

If coconut oil is solidified, gently melt the oil in a double boiler over low-heat, or in a small stainless-steel bowl in a dehydrator. Grind sesame seeds and coconut flakes together in a high-power blender, pushing the mixture downward with the tamper until it forms a thick and creamy paste. Be careful not to overblend or overheat the mixture. Scrape the sesame-coconut paste into a medium-sized mixing bowl, and add the remaining ingredients; stir together until thoroughly combined. This is your cookie dough.

Roll out cookie dough by placing it between two nonstick sheets (for lining dehydrator trays) or waxed paper, and rolling over it with a rolling pin or round jar. Use snowflake cookie cutters, hearts, or other desired shapes, to cut the cookies. Remove excess dough, keeping the cookie shapes on the nonstick sheets or waxed paper. Dust cookies with powdered xylitol.

Once cookies are decorated, slide a tray underneath the sheet so you can transfer the cookies into the refrigerator without breaking them. Chill until hardened. Once hardened, the cookies can be transferred onto a serving plate or tray without breaking. Chill until just before serving.

*Powdered xylitol can be purchased online or in many health food stores. You can also make this alternative to confectioner's sugar by grinding small amounts of xylitol in an electric coffee grinder or high-power blender; or use goji berry powder. Fresh mint leaves and whole goji berries make a lovely holly-berry garnish.

Grandma's Oatmeal Raisin Cookies (Phase 2)

MAKES ABOUT 20 SMALL COOKIES

This recipe is inspired by Leah's mom, who made nut butter-coconut-oat refrigerator cookies for her as a child. Her grandkids love 'em too.

1 cup almond butter

1½ cup rolled oats

1 cup coconut flakes

⅓ cup lucuma powder (see "Natural Low-Sugar and No-Sugar Sweeteners," page 376)

⅓ cup date paste or coconut nectar syrup

2 tablespoons structured or filtered water (see "Living Water," page 384)

2 tablespoons coconut oil, in liquid form

½ teaspoon vanilla powder

1 teaspoon cinnamon

pinch Himalayan or other high-mineral raw salt

½ cup raisins

In a medium mixing bowl, stir dry ingredients together. Mix in wet ingredients. Roll by the tablespoonful into balls, and flatten. Moistening your hands before rolling can be helpful. Chill until firm, and serve with Nut/Seed Mylk, or a cup of warm tea.

Kumquat Eggs in Carob Cookie Nests (Phase 2)

MAKES ABOUT 10 SMALL COOKIES

- 1 cup raw almond or pumpkin seed butter
- 1 cup rolled oats
- 1 cup coconut flakes
- ½ teaspoon vanilla powder (optional)
- 5 tablespoons carob powder
- 4 tablespoons coconut oil, softened
- pinch Himalayan crystal salt (omit if using salted nut butter)
- 4 tablespoons date paste or coconut nectar syrup
- 1–2 tablespoons structured or filtered water (see "Living Water," page 384)–use just enough to help to hold the dough together
- 10 kumquats or 20 blueberries

Stir dry ingredients together in a medium mixing bowl. Mix in wet ingredients. Roll into balls, and press with thumb to shape into nests. Chill until firm. Place 1 kumquat or 2 blueberry "eggs" in the center of each nest, and serve.

Soft, Chewy, Warm, Apple Raisin Cookies (Phase 2)

MAKES 24 MEDIUM-SIZED COOKIES.

Nut-free, gluten-free, raw, vegan, and yummy.

- 2 cups dried coconut flakes
- 1 cup golden flaxseed
- 2 cups chopped apples
- 1 cup raisins
- ¼ cup xylitol or palm sugar
- 2 droppers unflavored stevia; or use vanilla and/or cinnamon-flavored stevia to substitute for the next two ingredients

¼ teaspoon cinnamon powder (optional)

¼ teaspoon vanilla powder (optional)

1 tablespoon coconut oil

Grind the coconut and flaxseed into flour, about one cup at a time, in a coffee grinder or high-power blender. Process the chopped apples and raisins in a food processor until apples are in small chunks. Stir xylitol or palm sugar into the apple-raisin mixture until dissolved, and add the stevia, cinnamon, and vanilla powders. Stir in the coconut-flax flour. Mix the coconut oil into the dough; this will be easier if it is slightly softened first in a dehydrator or double boiler.

Once all ingredients are thoroughly mixed, form into flat cookies and place directly onto the mesh screens of a food dehydrator; there is no need to use nonstick sheets. Dehydrate at least 4 hours until cookies are gently warmed, still soft and chewy rather than crisp and crunchy.

Caramel-Apple Slices (Phase 2)

Serve apple slices with Jerusalem artichoke syrup or coconut nectar syrup, and enjoy.

Choc-o-Lanterns (Phase 2)

oranges

Carob Hazelnut Pudding (page 455)

one cinnamon stick for each orange

Cut, hollow out, and carve oranges as you would pumpkins for jack-o-lanterns. Kid-friendly pumpkin-carving tools work great for this. Fill with the pudding, put the tops back on the oranges, and insert a cinnamon stick for a "pumpkin stem."

True-Blue Jello (Phase 1.5)

Thanks to Michela Casey, a former Tree of Life Café manager, for demonstrating this quick and easy recipe in her inspiring dessert class. Children love it!

All you need is fresh, organic blueberries. Simply blend the desired amount of blueberries into a smooth sauce, pour into serving dishes, and chill before serving. The pectin from the blueberries firms up the sauce into jello!

Very Cherry Jello (Phase 1.5)

1 cup Hibiscus Red Cool-Aid (page 392)

2 cups frozen dark, sweet cherries, thawed

3 tablespoons ground psyllium seed

Put half of the cherries (1 cup) into a shallow mold, or divide them into individual serving dishes. Place the remaining cup of cherries, along with the Hibiscus Cool-Aid and psyllium seed meal, into a blender, and blend until smooth. Pour this onto the cherries in the mold or serving dishes. Chill until gelatinous, and serve.

Yellow Jello (Phase 1)

MAKES 6 SERVINGS

This jiggly, lemony dessert is diabetic-friendly—and kid-approved. You'll never look at tomatoes the same way again!

3 small-to-medium yellow tomatoes

juice of 2 lemons, including pulp

4 tablespoons ground psyllium seed

6 tablespoons xylitol

3 full droppers lemon-flavored stevia

Blend all ingredients together thoroughly in a blender, and pour into dessert bowls. Chill until firm, and serve. Serve with favorite whipped topping (see "Dairy-Free Recipes," page 467). Please be aware that both xylitol and psyllium seed may have a natural laxative effect!

Lemon Ice (Phase 1)

MAKES 6 SERVINGS

> $3/4$ cup fresh lemon juice (juice of 3–4 lemons)
>
> 2 cups structured or filtered water (see "Living Water," page 384)
>
> 3 full droppers liquid stevia or lemon-flavored stevia, or $1/4$ teaspoon powdered stevia
>
> 3 heaping tablespoons erythritol or xylitol

When juicing the lemons, save the peel halves. Stir all ingredients together until xylitol is dissolved. Pour into a shallow pan such as a glass cake dish or pie plate, and place in freezer. After 1 hour, ice crystals will just be starting to form. With a fork, break up the ice crystals and return to the freezer. Check every hour, breaking up the ice each time. When it has become crushed lemon ice, remove from freezer and serve in emptied lemon peel halves, snow-cone cups, or serving dishes.

Variation 1: Replace lemons with limes for a fresh Lime Ice, or use ½ cup lemon juice and ½ cup lime juice to make Lemon-Lime Ice.

Strawberry Popsicles (Phase 1.5)

Blend fresh or frozen strawberries, using just enough water to run the blender. Sweeten to taste with berry-flavored stevia, and pour into popsicle molds. Freeze and serve.

Strawberry Cream Popsicles (Phase 1.5)

> 2 cups fresh or frozen strawberries
>
> 1 large ripe avocado

½–1 cup structured or filtered water (see "Living Water,"
page 384), or just enough to run the blender

2 full droppers berry-flavored liquid stevia

Blend until smooth and pour into popsicle molds. Freeze and
serve.

Basic Cheezecake (Phase 1)

FROM THE TREE OF LIFE CAFÉ STAFF

Cheezecake Crust

2¼ cups granola or soaked and dehydrated nuts

1–3 tablespoons coconut oil (just enough for crust to stick
together)

¼ teaspoon salt

2 teaspoons cinnamon (optional)

Pulse all ingredients in a food processor until crumbly. Press into
bottom of a springform pan, and set aside in fridge while you make
the cake filling.

Cheezecake Filling

2½ cups cashews, or soaked and peeled almonds
(3½ cups if not using agar-agar)

1 cup agar-agar paste (below) if you want a lower-fat filling

1 cup structured or filtered water (see "Living Water,"
page 384)

1 cup coconut oil

½ cup Sweet-E (erythritol) powder

16 drops vanilla-flavored stevia

pinch of salt

Mix all ingredients in a food processor, along with your choice of
flavor options below. Put into the crust, and refrigerate for 6–8
hours or until it has set.

Cheezecake Flavor Options:

¼ cup lime juice

- 1 cup carob powder
- 1 tablespoon pumpkin spice
- 1½ teaspoons cinnamon
- 1 teaspoon cardamom
- ¼ cup ginger juice

Agar-Agar Paste (Phase 1)

8 cups cold water

½ cup agar-agar flakes

Place flakes in water and whisk. Heat on the stovetop on high heat. Bring to a boil, stirring for 4–6 minutes, or until flakes are all dissolved. Allow to cool off, then refrigerate. It should be hard, like a thick gelatin.

Coconut Cream Pie (Phase 1)

FROM THE TREE OF LIFE CAFÉ STAFF

Coconut Cream Pie Crust

Prepare a crust of your choice (see Cheeze Cake Crust above as an example) in a pie dish or springform pan.

Coconut Cream Pie Filling

3 cups young coconut meat*

1–1½ teaspoons vanilla-flavored stevia

½ cup Sweet-E (erythritol) (optional)

¾ cup coconut oil

1½ teaspoons vanilla powder

1 tablespoon ground chia seed

½ cup structured or filtered water (see "Living Water," page 384)

3 tablespoons agar-agar (prepared as above and stored in fridge)

Blend all ingredients until smooth and creamy, using tamper to help blend them. Pour filling into pie dish, and allow to set for a few hours in the refrigerator.

*Frozen young coconut meat can be purchased at some health food stores and thawed for this recipe. Fresh young coconuts are available at many Asian and health food stores. These can be opened with a cleaver (find a demonstration video online for the technique).

Alive and Low-Sweet Candies

Quinn's Candy—Berries! (Phase 1.5 or 2)

When Leah's daughter was three, she and her mother were standing in the checkout line together when a huge bag of colorful round candies caught her eye. "Look, Mommy!" she exclaimed. "Berries!"

Why do so many candies look, smell, and taste like berries? Because children love berries! They have not lost their primordial instinct for the gems of nature. Be a kid in a candy store—harvest berries together in a local garden or orchard, or forage a trustworthy wild-berry source and witness the sheer joy—the love of the berries, and the experience of communing with Divine creation. It could be blueberries, raspberries, blackberries, strawberries, goji berries, gooseberries, Incan berries, boysenberries, mulberries, red currants, black currants, grapes, or acai berries—just to name a few. Berries are Phase 1.5; grapes are Phase 2.

Eat the berries—scrumptious as-is—or dip them into Macadamia Nut Whip (page 478).

Bowl Full of Cherries (Phase 1.5)

Simply wash and dry desired amount of fresh organic cherries, serve in a bowl, and enjoy!

Snow-Dusted Cranberries (Phase 1.5)

Serve these simple sweets for a holiday gathering. They look very festive held in a little candy dish, or as garnish on a plate of Vanilla Snowflake (Low-) Sugar Cookies (page 452).

    2 cups fresh cranberries
    ½ cup xylitol
    small dish of water

In a coffee grinder or blender on high speed, grind the xylitol into "powdered sugar." You can make a bigger batch if you like; powdered xylitol keeps unrefrigerated in a sealed container. Dip cranberries into water to moisten them, and then into the powdered xylitol.

Fruit Lollies (Phase 1.5 or 2)

This recipe was inspired by fun and fruity photos posted at Littlefood-junction.com by Smita Srivastava.

    bananas
    grapes
    strawberries
    apples, or any fruit that can be cut into slices
    melon balls
    narrow ribbon to decorate the sticks (optional)

Cut bananas into thick rounds. Cut strawberries in half lengthwise to form heart shapes. Cut apples or other fruit into star-shaped or other artfully carved slices. Stack fruit on thin wooden craft sticks (similar to very thin dowels). Decorate with ribbon if desired.

Candied Edible Flowers (Phase 1)

> handful of pansies
>
> 1 cup powdered xylitol
>
> small bowl of water

The xylitol can be purchased powdered, or ground in a coffee grinder or high-power blender. Dip pansies into water, and then gently press into powdered xylitol.

Dried Fruit (Phase 2)

There's something that feels special about opening up a little package. This recipe is just for fun. Use these sparingly, and remember to brush those pearly whites!

Fill an empty candy tin with goji berries, golden raisins, or dried gooseberries. You can also wrap up dried apricots, figs, or pitted dates in a crinkly wrapper, put them into the tin as is, or tuck a nut nugget inside.

Rumor has it that there's an edible candy wrapper made of kelp out there. If you find it, let us know!

Party Sprinkles (Phase 1.5)

> bee pollen!

Bee pollen can be purchased from health food stores or local beekeepers selling honey at farmer's markets. The color and flavor of different pollens vary. Jarrah Bee Pollen (from Australia) tastes like a kids' breakfast cereal, and the yummy Cascadian Mix (from Washington State) comes in a confetti mix of colors. The nuggets can be eaten by the handful, or sprinkled into smoothies, live ice creams, and other desserts.

Bee pollen contains the primordial life-force of the plant world. It is high in B vitamins (except B12). It contains fifty-six minerals and thousands of enzymes, and is an exceptional source of non-soy lecithin, which is needed to support brain development. For strict vegans, pollen is available that is harvested from the flowers by suction, without the intermediation of the bee world.

Carob Candies (Phase 1.5 or 2)

MAKES ABOUT 1 DOZEN SMALL CANDIES, DEPENDING ON THE SHAPE AND SIZE OF THE MOLDS

Raw carob powder comes in differing textures. For this recipe, we want a finely ground carob powder (such as that available at www.Purejoy-planet.com, or in bulk at www.Azurestandard.com). The orange peel powder is what gives these candies a bit of a bitter taste, like chocolate. These are Phase 1.5 with goji berries, or Phase 2 with raisins and dried cherries.

> 1 cup black raisins, dried cherries, or goji berries
>
> ½ cup raw carob powder
>
> ½ cup coconut oil in liquid form
>
> 2 teaspoons orange peel powder

To make your own orange peel powder, simply save your organic peels (scrub before peeling), dehydrate until brittle, then grind into a powder using a coffee grinder or high-power blender. Store in an airtight container.

If coconut oil is solid, place it in the dehydrator or double boiler to gently liquefy it. Combine all ingredients in a food processor until chunky, with bits of raisin or dried cherry remaining. Spoon mixture into candy molds, and chill until firm. Eat just after removing from the fridge, as it melts in your mouth and hands.

Xylitol Gum and Hard Candies (Phase 1)

These are Phase 1, but not a raw food. Look for brands that use xylitol made from birch trees, with no artificial colors or flavors. You might like to keep a pack in your purse or glovebox for surprise candyland encounters with a clown or bank teller, or for a piñata or parade. Chewing on xylitol gum can be helpful for oral hygiene when a toothbrush is not at hand. The Rescue Remedy homeopathic company now makes a xylitol-sweetened chewing gum for use after a trauma.

Pixie Dust Straws (Phase 1.5 or 2)

For a special occasion. Whether these are Phase 1.5 or 2 depends on the choice of fruit powder (see food lists in "Phase Chart," page 372).

For pixie dust, use pomegranate, cherry, goji berry, and/or other dried berry powders, now available through many live-food companies. Buy biodegradable paper straws, available online in many colors and patterns. Cut them to the desired length, fill them with "pixie dust," and seal the ends with beeswax. Some companies even sell nametags that match the paper straws, to use as special party favors.

Food Guidelines for Babies

For sterility and safety, all vegetables, fruits, and seeds, as well as nut-mylk strainer bags, must be soaked in 3% food-grade hydrogen peroxide (H_2O_2) for twenty minutes minimum, using one teaspoon of H_2O_2 for each quart of pure distilled water or spring water. Rinse thoroughly with water after sanitizing.

Introduce recipes to babies in small amounts—about 1/2 ounce for the first four to eight times. Work up to a normal serving size gradually, to allow the baby's body and tastes ample time to acclimate. (Mommy or Daddy can drink the balance of the baby food.)

A thorough monitoring of the baby's assimilation of nourishment includes using growth, developmental, and health measurements to assess their appetite, weight, age, and signs of healthy eating.

BABY'S APPETITE

Appetite is the most important indicator of when and how much to feed the baby. Babies will have variable feeding needs depending on growth spurts—typically ten to fourteen days after birth, and about every three weeks after that. Babies will want less food between growth spurts.

Signs of hunger include rooting, smacking of the lips, or crying when dry, warm, and rested. If baby seems hungry after completing the serving amount, wait twenty minutes and then offer an additional ounce or two. Note that breast milk normally fluctuates in fat and nutrient content. By paying attention to hunger signs, you can also adjust the live Nut/Seed Mylk recipe for baby. If the baby is hungry, you can increase the fat, protein, or sweetening. You could also make a small decrease in the proportion of water in the recipe.

CALCULATING SERVING SIZES FOR BABIES

Multiply baby's weight in pounds by 2.5 ounces to get the total daily serving: A 7-pound baby would get 17.5 ounces in a 24-hour period, and a 10-pound baby would get 25 ounces. We recommend making one 16-ounce recipe each 24 hours for a 6-pound baby, or each 12 hours for larger babies up to 12.5 pounds. The recipe can be doubled for older babies. Make fresh batches whenever the baby requires more than 24 ounces in a 24-hour period.

FEEDING TIMES

Newborns take about 1–2 ounces every 2–3 hours in the first week. The number and spacing between feedings gradually increase according to each baby's growth patterns. At four months of age, this will be about 6–7 ounces every 6–8 hours. Let the baby determine the amount. Be attentive to the baby's signals, rather than trying to follow a protocol or empty a bottle. Note that babies who are experiencing growth spurts will want more, in a sudden burst, to coincide with their growing needs.

SIGNS OF HEALTHY NOURISHMENT

A baby who is relaxed and satisfied after feeding has been well nourished. The baby will urinate at least six to eight times a day. The baby gains weight starting at about two weeks, and continues to do so. The baby shows signs of good digestion—the stomach feels soft, not bloated or cramped; the skin is clear, without diaper rash or eczema; and the baby is free of constipation and diarrhea.

Research at Mount Sinai Hospital in New York City found advanced glycation end products (AGEs) in high concentrations in some infants. AGEs occur when glucose is excessive and combines unnaturally with lipids or protein in various forms, including enzymes in the system. This unnatural situation damages the protein complexes, making them unable to perform their functions properly.

A high amount of AGEs is found in type 2 diabetics. These toxic components were also high in some infants whose mother's blood was high in AGEs. They found that the AGEs were high in the breast milk, especially of diabetics, and in baby formulas as well. These increased AGEs are potentially associated with increased rates of type 2 diabetes.

Studies in *Diabetes Care* (December 2010) showed that babies can have elevated AGEs at birth. These AGEs are inflammatory, and are also associated with increased insulin resistance. They have been shown to pass on to babies from mothers who are diabetic or have high blood sugar. In a study of sixty infants, it was found that AGEs in the pregnant mother were transferred to the baby; AGE levels in infant blood were the same as those of the mothers.

When the babies switched from breast milk to infant formula, which is highly processed, highly cooked, and highly sweetened, the AGEs in the infants' blood doubled, similar to the levels of diabetics. These children were also found to have higher insulin levels. The researchers also found that baby formulas had at least 100 times more AGEs than breast milk. So using our raw mylk formulas is a safer way to proceed, from this perspective.

The following recipe for Live Vegan Baby Mylk has been helpful to mothers who are unable to breastfeed, or who need supplemental formula and do not have a breast milk supply from a trusted source. Please note that this formula has not been tested with double-blind studies.

Dairy-Free Recipes

Live Vegan Baby Mylk (Phase 1 or 1.5)

FROM SUSAN MILLER MADELEY, MASTER'S GRADUATE OF THE TREE OF LIFE CENTER U.S., UNDER THE GUIDANCE OF DR. GABRIEL

MAKES 24 OUNCES (3 CUPS)

Important note: Please also see "Food Guidelines for Babies," above. Compared to mother's milk, this is equal in calories, B vitamins, calcium, and Vitamins A, C, and E. It is higher in assorted omega-3 fatty acids, protein (including relaxing tryptophan), Vitamin K, iron, magnesium, and zinc. It is lower in carbohydrates and selenium. This recipe is Phase 1 unless sweeter Phase 1.5 flavorings are added (see Phase Chart, page 372).

  raw organic pumpkin seeds

  ¾ cup pure spring water, or structured or filtered water
    (see "Living Water," page 384)

  1¾ cups fresh young coconut water

  2 tablespoons soaked goji berries (with soakwater)

  ¼–½ teaspoon Udo's Choice™ Infant's Blend probiotic
    powder

Soak pumpkin seeds in spring, structured, or filtered water for 6–8 hours, and drain. Blend coconut water with pumpkin seeds and goji berries. Strain through a sterilized nut-mylk (mesh-fabric) bag. Stir in probiotic powder. Adjust to 3 cups liquid if needed, with additional spring, structured, or filtered water, or coconut water.

Once baby acclimates to the simple recipe, you can substitute a "nursery tea" for the coconut water, using any of the following baby-friendly herbs:

- **Elderberries:** Antiviral, for immune support, respiratory support, and flu prevention.
- **Bilberries:** For the cardiovascular system, and for lowering blood sugar.
- **Chamomile:** Antiinflammatory, antibacterial, antiviral, antiparasitic; relaxes the stomach and intestines.
- **Stevia leaf:** For a sweet flavor; stevia has no known side effects.

You can also gradually introduce sunflower seeds (blend in with other ingredients) for additional selenium and carbohydrates, and eventually (also gradually) algae and phytoplankton.

Optional: The following nutritional supplements can also be added to the Baby Mylk:

- **Blue-green algae** (1/8 teaspoon per 16–32 ounces**):** Provides antimicrobial, antiviral, and antifungal support, DHA, ALA, Vitamins B and C, protein, the antioxidant phycocyanin, PEA, iron, DNA,RNA, enzymes, and beta-carotene. It is uniquely good for supporting brain development and IQ.
- **Spirulina** (1/8 teaspoon per 16–32 ounces): Provides chlorophyll, protein, iron and trace minerals, Vitamins A, B1, B2, B6, E, and K, GLA, EFA, RNA, DNA, antioxidants, and immune-system support.
- **Golden algae** (1/8 teaspoon per 16–32 ounces): Provides long-chain omega-3 fatty acids.
- **Phytoplankton** (1 drop per 16–32 ounces of milk): Provides antiviral, antifungal, antibacterial, and antiinflammatory support, DHA, nucleotides, DNA, EPA, RNA, protein, vitamins A, B, and K, minerals, and polysaccharides.
- **Vitamin D3** (1,000 IU, or 1 drop every 2 days if using Premier Research brand liquid): Spending 5 minutes per day naked in sunlight or under a sunlamp, or 20 minutes per day clothed, is also recommended for vitamin D production by the body.
- **DHA/ALA** (300 milligrams a day): Provides brain and nervous system developmental and functional support.

- **Vitamin K** (1.5–12 micrograms): Essential for formation of at least three proteins involved in blood clotting, and other proteins found in plasma, bone, and kidney.
- **Vitamin B12** (3 micrograms per feeding, or ¼ teaspoon Max-ND by Premier Research Labs).

Instant Rice Mylk (Phase 1)

This recipe is Phase 1 as long as it is sweetened with xylitol or stevia. It not only tastes just like the Mexican drink horchata, but also offers a super option for traveling with children, and for children with nut allergies.

1½ cups structured or filtered water (see "Living Water," page 384)

¼ cup tocotrienols*

3 tablespoons erythritol or xylitol (omit for babies)

⅛ teaspoon vanilla powder

¼ teaspoon cinnamon (omit for babies)

1 pinch Himalayan or other high-mineral raw salt

Blend in a blender until creamy (no more than 10 seconds) or shake in a travel blender bottle (see "Resources," page 485).

If you are making this for a baby, omit the cinnamon and erythritol/xylitol, as these can irritate the developing digestive system. The rice (in the tocotrienols*) has a mild sweetness of its own, so sweetener is not essential for flavor. Please note that this raw beverage is not a breast-milk replacement, but it can be used in solid baby-food recipes.

*Tocotrienols are stabilized rice-bran and rice-germ solubles. They are a vitamin E source that does not raise blood sugar levels, as do other grains, and are available through Dr. Cousens' Online Store (www.DrCousensOnlineStore.com). Tocotrienols can also be added to any of the following Nut/Seed Mylks for nutritional benefits.

Nut/Seed Mylk (Phase 1 or 2)

This is Phase 1 if made with unsweetened nuts or seeds, or Phase 2 if coconut is used. **Note:** *In order to avoid allergic reactions, we do not recommend nuts for children under two years of age.*

> 1 cup raw nuts and/or seeds of your choice
>
> 3 cups structured or filtered water (see "Living Water," page 384)
>
> 1 pinch Himalayan or other high-mineral raw salt
>
> 1–2 pitted dates, or 1 tablespoon xylitol or stevia, to taste (omit if made for babies)
>
> ¼–½ cup fresh fruit, or 1 teaspoon vanilla powder or extract, or other desired flavoring, to taste

Soak nuts and/or seeds overnight, and strain. Place in a blender with water, and blend thoroughly. Strain out pulp using a nut-mylk bag (a drawstring bag made out of fine-mesh fabric): Pour the liquid into the bag while holding it over a bowl, and squeeze the bag over the bowl to remove as much liquid as possible. Use pulp for other recipes, or compost it. High-quality nut-mylk bags may be purchased at www.DrCousensOnlineStore.com.

Pour strained mylk into the blender again, and add salt, any desired sweeteners, fruit, or flavors such as vanilla, and blend again. Hemp seeds, if used, can be blended with the already-strained Nut Mylk; there is no need to strain out hemp-seed pulp.

Here are just a few Nut/Seed Mylk possibilities:

- almond
- almond-hemp seed
- brazil nut-sesame
- coconut (use shredded, dried coconut as you would nuts or seeds)
- coconut-almond
- coconut-hazelnut
- coconut-pumpkin seed
- coconut-sesame

- coconut-walnut
- hazelnut
- hazelnut-pumpkin seed
- pecan-pumpkin seed
- pine nut-almond
- pumpkin seed-sesame
- sesame-almond

Pink Mylk (Phase 1.5)

2 cups coconut-pumpkin seed mylk, or almond mylk

1 cup strawberries, leaves/stems removed

1 tablespoon erythritol or xylitol, or 4–8 drops liquid stevia (berry-flavored or unflavored), or ⅙ teaspoon powdered stevia

Blend until smooth, and serve.

Variation: For an even brighter color—and added radiation protection—add ¼ inch of peeled fresh red beet root.

Carob Mylk (Phase 1.5)

2 cups Nut/Seed Mylk of choice (above)

2 tablespoons carob powder

1 tablespoon mesquite powder

Blend until smooth, and serve.

Super-Bee Sesame Mylk (Phase 2)

Have you ever observed bees as they carry pollen? Look closely at their little pollen-laden legs when they buzz by or land on your picnic table. Thank you, bees, for pollinating the fruit trees! Note that bee pollen is from plants, not bees, so many people consider it vegan. Bees help gather it, however—unless it is machine-harvested from plants using a suction machine.

3 cups sesame mylk, strained

3 tablespoons carob powder

2 tablespoons local bee pollen

4 tablespoons hemp seeds

1 teaspoon cinnamon (optional)

1–2 tablespoons coconut syrup or xylitol

pinch Himalayan or other high-mineral raw salt

Blend all ingredients together, and serve.

Sweet Cardamom Mylk (Phase 1)

INSPIRED BY THE TREE OF LIFE CAFÉ

3 cups almond Nut/Seed Mylk (recipe above)

½ teaspoon cardamom powder

½ teaspoon vanilla powder

½ dropper hazelnut-flavored liquid stevia, or to taste

Stir or blend seasonings and sweetener into almond mylk. Chill and serve, perhaps with Grandma's Oatmeal Raisin Cookies.

Rich and Creamy Steamers (Phase 1 or 2)

This recipe is Phase 1 if made with almonds, or Phase 2 if almond-coconut.

almond or almond-coconut Nut/Seed Mylk (recipe above)

flavored liquid stevia

Using two parts water and one part nuts, make a thick batch of almond mylk or almond-coconut mylk. After straining out the nut pulp, stir in flavored stevia to taste. Good steamer flavors are hazelnut, English toffee, vanilla, chocolate raspberry, or a combination of flavors. Warm the mylk *gently* in the top of a double boiler. (If it's too hot to keep your finger in it, it's destroying the enzymes.) Serve warm on a wintry eve.

Variation (Phase 2): Replace flavored stevia with vanilla powder or almond extract (⅛ teaspoon per cup), and sweeten to taste with palm sugar.

Coconut Kefir (Phase 2)

MAKES 4 CUPS

Kefir cleans and strengthens the immune system, improves digestion, cultivates friendly flora in the intestines, reduces food and sugar cravings, moisturizes the skin, and helps reverse the aging process by breaking down undigested proteins. Kefir is a complete protein, and an excellent source of amino acids and enzymes. Coconut water is considered a sweetener because it has 29 grams of glucose per coconut.

> 4 cups unsweetened coconut water, or 2 cups coconut water plus 2 cups Nut/Seed Mylk (recipe above)
>
> 1 tablespoon kefir starter or proteolytic probiotic, or ¼ cup cultured kefir

Place all ingredients in a blender, and process for no more than 10 seconds. Transfer it to a jar, put the lid on, and leave in a warm (60–80°) location for 8–12 hours. For faster results, warm the mixture to 80° before placing it in the jar. The beverage is ready when it is slightly effervescent and/or tastes sour.

Note: Kefir starter and proteolytic probiotics (Master Culture Blend) are available at www.DrCousensOnlineStore.com.

Variation: For solid, yogurt-like kefir, blend the culture for 10 seconds with 2–4 cups of coconut meat, or nuts/seeds blended with enough water to form a cream. The yogurt is ready when it tastes sour or looks spongy. Enjoy in a salad dressing, over fruit, in a smoothie, or alone, flavored with stevia and vanilla powder.

Raw Vegan Yogurts (Phase 1, 1.5, or 2)

These are great for breakfast, lunch boxes, or snacks.

Young Coconut Yogurt (Phase 2)

   1 young Thai coconut

   1 teaspoon vanilla powder or extract (optional)

   1 cup fresh fruit, such as strawberries, cherries, or peaches

   2 teaspoons probiotic powder, such as Ultra Blend (this
      is not a starter such as the Master Culture Blend used for
      kefir), available at www.DrCousensOnlineStore.com.

Open young coconut using a cleaver (find a demonstration video online for the technique). Pour coconut water into blender, straining out any shards of coconut shell. Scoop out supple coconut flesh, and dip in water to remove any shell shards. Add coconut flesh, vanilla, and probiotic powder into blender, and blend until smooth. Pulse in fresh fruit until the mixture reaches the desired consistency (can be chunky or creamy), and serve.

Almond Yogurt (Phase 1 or 2)

This recipe is Phase 1 if using lemon, or Phase 2 if using coconut kefir. It is very rich, like a whole-milk yogurt, but made only with healthy, plant-sourced fats.

   1 cup almonds (2 cups after soaking)

   2 cups (use more if needed to run the blender) structured
      or filtered water (see "Living Water," page 384), or
      Coconut Kefir (recipe above)

   juice of 2 medium-sized lemons or limes (reduce to one
      lemon or lime if using kefir)

   4 tablespoons coconut oil

   2–3 droppers vanilla-flavored liquid stevia

   5 tablespoons erythritol or xylitol

   2 teaspoons probiotic powder, such as Ultra Blend (this is
      not a starter such as the Master Culture Blend), available
      at www.DrCousensOnlineStore.com

Soak almonds for two days, then squeeze them to slip the brown skins off; or place almonds in boiling water for 30 seconds and skin them immediately. Place almond whites in blender, add remaining ingredients, and blend until smooth and creamy. Chill to thicken, or eat as-is.

Variation (Phase 1.5): Pulse in 1 cup of fresh or frozen blueberries.

Apricot-Hempseed Yogurt (Phase 2)

> 6 fresh apricots
>
> 10 ounces frozen strawberries
>
> ½ cup hemp seeds
>
> 1 cup structured or filtered water (see "Living Water," page 384) or Coconut Kefir (recipe above)
>
> 1 teaspoon vanilla powder (optional)
>
> 1 dropper apricot-flavored liquid stevia
>
> 2 teaspoons probiotic powder, such as Ultra Blend (this is not a starter such as the Master Culture Blend), available at www.DrCousensOnlineStore.com

Blend until thick and creamy, and serve.

Avocado-Hempseed Yogurt (Phase 1.5)

> 1 large ripe avocado
>
> 10 ounces frozen dark, sweet cherries
>
> 1 cup Coconut Kefir (recipe above)
>
> ⅓ cup hemp seeds
>
> juice of ½ lemon
>
> 1 dropper lemon-flavored or unflavored stevia
>
> 2 teaspoons probiotic powder, such as Ultra Blend (this is not a starter such as the Master Culture Blend), available at www.DrCousensOnlineStore.com

Blend until thick and creamy, and serve.

Strawberry Sunflower Yogurt (Phase 2)

MAKES 4 SERVINGS

1½ cups sunflower seeds, soaked overnight

juice of ½ lemon

juice of 1 orange

3 tablespoons erythritol or xylitol

1–2 full droppers berry-flavored liquid stevia

1 cup strawberries, fresh or frozen

½ cup structured or filtered water (see "Living Water," page 384) or Coconut Kefir (page 473)

Soak sunflower seeds overnight. Drain, and blend with fresh water, xylitol, lemon juice, orange juice and ½ cup of the strawberries. Pulse or stir in the remaining ½ cup of strawberries, and serve.

Carob Hazelnut Pudding (Phase 1.5)

MAKES 5 SERVINGS

3 avocados

½ cup carob powder

1 cup hazelnut mylk (see Nut/Seed Mylk recipe, page 470)

2 droppers hazelnut or chocolate-flavored stevia

1 teaspoon orange-peel powder (optional)

¼ cup xylitol

Blend all ingredients together in a blender until creamy and smooth. You may need to add more mylk to get the blender to run. Or you can try stopping the blender, stirring the contents, and starting it again. If you have a Vitamix, the tamper feature works well for thick consistencies such as this pudding. Chill until ready to serve.

To make your own orange-peel powder, simply save your organic orange peels (scrub oranges before peeling), then dehydrate them until hard and dry, and grind into a powder using a coffee grinder or blender on high speed. Store in an airtight container.

Chia Pudding (Phase 2)

MAKES 4 SERVINGS

This pudding resembles tapioca.

> 2 cups of your favorite Nut/Seed Mylk (page 470), or young coconut mylk
>
> ½ cup chia or salba (white chia) seeds
>
> ½ cup black raisins
>
> ¼ teaspoon cinnamon
>
> ⅛ teaspoon vanilla powder
>
> 1 teaspoon erythritol or xylitol (omit if young coconut mylk is used)

To make young coconut mylk, if used instead of Nut/Seed Mylk, just blend young coconut meat with its coconut water. Because coconut milk is already sweet, it is not necessary to add sweetener.

Stir all ingredients together in a medium-sized mixing bowl, and let sit for 15 minutes or until the chia seeds and raisins have soaked up most of the mylk. Serve at room temperature, chilled, or warmed in the dehydrator.

Variation: Replace ½ cup black raisins with ¼ unsulfured golden raisins plus ¼ cup fresh pineapple cut into small chunks.

Better Than a Cheese Stick (Phase 1)

Young coconut meat tends to go over big with kids. It's a little sweeter than cheese, and is both creamy and firm like mozzarella. It feels fresh and clean in the body.

Vegan Vanilla Ice Cream (Phase 1.5 or 2)

Depending on the flavorings added, this recipe may be either Phase 1.5 or Phase 2 (see Phase Chart, page 372).

- 2 young Thai coconuts
- 2 tablespoons coconut syrup (optional, depending on desired sweetness)
- 1 teaspoon vanilla powder

Open coconuts and pour coconut water into a blender. Scoop out the meat, removing any shell pieces. Add coconut syrup and vanilla powder. Blend until smooth, and follow directions for your ice-cream maker. If you don't have an ice-cream maker, pour mixture into ice cube trays, freeze, and then run through a juicer (using the blank screen for a Champion juicer), or blend again in a high-powered blender.

Macadamia Nut Whip (Phase 1)

- 1 cup macadamia nuts
- 2 cups structured or filtered water (see "Living Water," page 384)
- 2 tablespoons erythritol or xylitol
- 1 teaspoon vanilla powder

Blend all ingredients in a blender. Chill and serve.

Macadamia-Pear Crème (Phase 2)

MAKES 4 SERVINGS

INSPIRED BY THE TREE OF LIFE CAFÉ STAFF

Serve with breakfast or dessert.
- 3 fresh pears
- 1 cup macadamia nuts
- 1 cup structured or filtered water (see "Living Water," page 384)

½ teaspoon vanilla powder (optional)

juice of ½ lemon

Blend until smooth and creamy. Chill, or serve at room temperature.

Strawberry Shake (Phase 2)
MAKES 2 SERVINGS

5 ounces frozen strawberries

⅓ cup hemp seeds

1 cup structured or filtered water (see "Living Water,"
page 384)

1 dropper berry-flavored or unflavored stevia, or to taste

Blend all ingredients in a blender until smooth, and serve.

Cheeze Whiz (Phase 1 or 1.5)
FROM ELAINA LOVE

MAKES 4 SERVINGS

This recipe is Phase 1 if using bell pepper, Phase 1.5 if using carrot.

2 cups raw macadamia nuts

1 clove fresh garlic

1–2 tablespoons lemon juice

1½ tablespoons mellow white miso

¼ cup water, or more if needed for blending

⅓ teaspoon onion powder

2 tablespoons Premier Research nutritional yeast flakes
(We do not recommend other nutritional-yeast strains.)

1 carrot or 1 red bell pepper, chopped

Blend until smooth and creamy, adding more water if needed to
keep blender running. For best distribution, place in a quart-sized
plastic zip bag and cut a small hole in one corner. Remove all air,

and seal the top. Squeeze Cheeze Whiz out of the corner of the bag, onto crackers or veggies.

Variation: Add ¼ teaspoon chipotle powder to make Nacho Cheese Dip.

Mac 'n' Cheeze (Phase 1)

For a raw Mac 'n' Cheeze, mix Cheeze Whiz (above) with julienned-zucchini "noodles," and gently warm the mixture in a dehydrator. Cooked brown-rice macaroni can substitute for zucchini noodles—simply toss with Cheeze Whiz while macaroni is still warm.

Sunflower Dip (Phase 1)

FROM ELAINA LOVE

MAKES 8 SERVINGS

2 cups sunflower seeds (4 cups after soaking)

½ cup water (or more, for a lighter, mousse texture)

⅓–½ cup lemon juice

½ cup tahini or white sesame seeds

¼ cup light miso

1 teaspoon Himalayan or other high-mineral raw salt

1 tablespoon onion powder

1 clove fresh garlic

⅛ teaspoon cayenne

½ bunch parsley (about 1 ounce), minced

8 scallions, thinly sliced, or 2 tablespoons red onion, chopped

1–3 teaspoons kelp powder (optional, for more of a tuna-like flavor)

2 stalks celery, chopped or minced (optional)

Soak sunflower seeds. Purée or blend everything except parsley and scallions until creamy and smooth, adding extra water if necessary. Add parsley and scallions, and pulse until well incorporated.

Sour Cream and Onion Dip (Phase 1)

Yep, it's very green, and much better for a teenage complexion. Think creamy guacamole, without the picante. Eat with Dinosaur Kale Chips (page 418) or Ninja Chips (page 430).

> 2 ripe avocados
>
> juice of ½ lemon
>
> ¼ teaspoon garlic powder
>
> 1 teaspoon onion flakes
>
> Himalayan or other high-mineral raw salt, to taste

Put all ingredients in a food processor, and process until smooth.

Brazil Nut Parmesan (Phase 1)

Pulse desired amount of fresh Brazil nuts in a food processor until you have a mixture of finely chopped nuts and nut meal. Sprinkle onto raw pizza or salads for a buttery flavor.

Dairy-Free Salted Butter (Phase 1)

> ½ cup coconut oil, soft but not liquid (if liquid, chill to thicken slightly)
>
> ½ cup olive oil
>
> 1 tablespoon light miso

Stir all ingredients together until thoroughly combined.

CHAPTER 13

Conclusion

This book is about supporting the holistic physical, emotional, mental, and spiritual development of our children. By providing ourselves as parents, grandparents, teachers, or caregivers with these foundations for a healthy life, we are supporting the total aliveness of our children and grandchildren on all levels.

By supporting the child's body, mind and spirit through living nutrition, movement, touch, adequate sleep, and relationship with nature, we are supporting the developmental preconditions for aliveness by going beyond ego-identification with the body-mind complex; we are supporting the child's experience of Peace with the Body and Peace with the Mind.

By minimizing the undermining influences of the culture of death— whether GMO foods, flesh foods, fluoridated water, radiation, vaccines, or dark and violent media—we are protecting the unique aliveness and expression of the child. We are proactively honoring the child's right to develop holistically and naturally rather than to be exploited and transformed into a mere consumer, a dispensable life, a number in training for industrial-worker enslavement, or a video-game drone killer to later be hired by the military for real drone killings. Although we are all born originals, most die as copies. This book is about supporting our children to grow up and live in the world as unique expressions of the original, unique, healthy soul pattern they were meant to be.

By supporting the emotional intelligence (EQ) and development of the child through veganic, living nutrition rather than suppressing the feeling body, we are allowing emotion to move freely through the body rather than getting stuck and creating disharmony and disease. By honoring the child's feeling body, we are supporting emotional awareness that leads to the liberated experience of mastery over one's emotions, rather than being ruled by them, and that enhances their intimacy and love capacity for their own future relationships and parenthood.

By supporting the child's social development through Peace with the Ecology and Peace with Community, supporting Peace with the Body and Mind through holistic veganic dietary choices, and creating Peace with the Family by providing a loving home life, we are supporting the child's self-esteem, awareness of interconnection, intimacy, and love capacity, and the aliveness of all beings. By supporting a spiritually alive environment for both the parent and the children—one that nurtures imagination, meaningful work, wisdom teachings, silence, and sacred sound—we help our children quiet their minds and ignite their hidden Divine spark into a living flame, so that their whole life will be at Peace with the Divine.

May all children be blessed with holistic loving support for their unique and sacred journey of unfolding aliveness. And may all parents, grandparents, and teachers be blessed with the humble awareness that to serve young life during these invaluable years is a precious Divine gift.

Resources for Holistic Parenting

CONSCIOUS-PARENTING SUPPORT

- La Leche League International: www.llli.org
- Yoga DVDs for families, including videos with prenatal yoga, yoga for children, and mother-with-baby yoga: www.Gaiam.com
- Living Food Retreats (Conscious Eating, Spiritual Fasting, and our 30-Day Reversing Diabetes Program) are offered at the Tree of Life Center U.S., Patagonia, AZ, www.TreeOfLifeCenterUS.com
- "Parenting with a Fresh Perspective" coaching with Leah Lynn: www.ImAliveFoodForKids.com
- Susan Miller Madeley: www.SusanMillerCoaching.com and www.NourishingBabies.com
- Online "Raw Parenting" program by Nina Dench: www.therawfoodcoach.com/rawparentingvirtual-program/

LIVING-FOOD PRODUCTS

- Viva Pura, Patagonia, AZ: www.VivaPura.com
- Elaina Love: www.ElainaLove.com, www.PureJoyPlanet.com
- Dr. Cousens' Online Store: www.DrCousensOnlineStore.com

WHOLE-FOOD SUPPLEMENTS

- Tree of Life Rejuvenation Center online store: www.DrCousensOnlineStore.com

RAW-FOOD POTLUCK INFORMATION

- www.meetup.com
- www.rawfoodnetwork.com/potlucks.html

LIVING-/PLANT-SOURCED-FOOD RESTAURANTS

- Listings of restaurants by state available on
www.restaurantsraw.com

LIVING-FOOD KITCHEN EQUIPMENT

- Vitamix blender: www.vitamix.com
- Blender bottle (for drinks on the go): Elaina Love's Pure Joy
Planet, www.PureJoyPlanet.com
- Excalibur dehydrators: www.excaliburdehydrator.com
- Montessori Services (child-sized kitchen and garden tools):
www.MontessoriServices.com
- For Small Hands (child-sized kitchen and garden tools):
www.ForSmallHands.com

DISCOUNT ORGANIC FOOD AND
HEALTH-PRODUCT SUPPLIERS

- Azure Standard: www.azurestandard.com. Azure Standard ships
certified organic, pesticide-free, and non-GMO foods throughout the U.S. Usually, there is a pickup location where others in
your community also pick up orders on a scheduled day.
- Vita-Cost offers discounted organic and non-GMO food and
health products: www.vitacost.com

POLITICAL ADVOCACY FOR CITIZEN RIGHTS
TO ORGANIC FOODS AND SUPPLEMENTS

- The Health Freedom Alliance website includes health-related
news articles: www.healthfreedoms.org

BOOKS FOR CHILDREN

- *The Secret Life of Mitch Spinach* by Hillary Feerick and Jeff Hillenbrand, in collaboration with Joel Fuhrman, MD, is a story for
school-aged children about a boy who by all appearances lives a
"normal" life, yet behind the scenes his diet of greens gives him a
secret life of heightened abilities.

- *Mitch Spinach and the Smell of Victory* by Hillary Feerick and Jeff Hillenbrand
- *Mitch Spinach and the Tree House Intruder* by Hillary Feerick and Jeff Hillenbrand
- *Monkey Mike's Raw Food Kitchen: an Un-Cookbook for Kids* (ebook) by Joanne Newell: www.uncooking101.com/site/review/joanne-newells-monkey-mikes-raw-food-kitchen/
- *The Raw Princess Recipe and Playbook and The Raw Superhero Recipe and Playbook* by Nina Dench
- *A Boy, A Chicken and the Lion of Judah,* by Roberta Kalechofsky, is about a Jewish boy named Ari and his heartfelt decision to become vegetarian.
- Free coloring book for children from Christian Vegetarian Association (CVA) available at www.all-creatures.org/cva/img/pdf/coloringbook.pdf
- *Hope: A Pig's Tale by Randy Houk* (Humane Society of the United States).
- *Do Animals Have Feelings Too?* by Trudy L. Calvert (National Geographic Society)
- Our Farm: By the Animals of Farm Sanctuary, by Maya Gottfried, watercolor illustrations by Robert Rahway Zakanitch
- *That's Why We Don't Eat Animals: A Book About Vegans, Vegetarians, and All Living Things* by Ruby Roth
- *Vegan is Love: Having Heart and Taking Action* by Ruby Roth
- *Steven the Vegan* by Dan Bodenstein, illustrated by Ron Robrahn
- *Fruits I Love* by Victoria Boutenko, illustrated by Katya Korobkina. A poetic expression of delight in fresh fruit by a world-renowned living-food author, mother, and grandmother.
- *A Gift from Little Bear* by Victoria Boutenko, illustrated by Natalia Bazhenova
- *Green Smoothie Magic* by Victoria Boutenko, illustrated by Katya Korobkina
- *I Love Greens* by Victoria Boutenko, illustrated by Eugene Podkolzin

- *The Well Child Coloring Book* by Michael Samuels, MD. A basic anatomy coloring book. Note that the terminology is for more advanced readers, and the nutritional information may be out of date.
- *The Curious Garden* by Peter Brown. An inspiring story about a boy named Liam, who brings new green life to a gray environment.
- *My Daddy is a Pretzel* by Baron Baptiste. Introduces the yoga asanas to children.
- *God Inside of Me* by Della Reese. A story of a girl named Kenisha who learns how to let go and let God.
- *Grandfather Four Winds and Rising Moon* by Michael Chanin and Sally J. Smith. A beautifully illustrated book sharing native wisdom teachings.
- *Old Turtle* by Douglas Wood, illustrated by Cheng-Khee Chee. A story of peace with diverse religious cultures, and remembrance of Divine origin.
- *A Story of Becoming* by Ayn Cates Sullivan, PhD, illustrated by Belle Crow DuCray, is a story about transformation, discovery, and an apple tree.
- *Mama Miti: Wangari Maathai and the Trees of Kenya* by Donna Jo Napoli and Kadir Nelson. A beautiful picture book about peace with the ecology, inspired by the life of Wangari Muta Maathai, the first African woman to win the Nobel Peace Prize.
- *The Lorax* by Dr. Seuss. A Seussical tale prompting the reader to take responsibility for caring for the Earth.
- *The Dragon and the Unicorn,* written and illustrated by Lynne Cherry. A mythical story about the value of the forest ecology.
- *Anh's Anger* by Gail Silver, illustrated by Christiane Krömer. A beautifully illustrated story raising awareness about childhood emotion.
- *My Shining Light* by Nidhi Misra, illustrated by Joe Servello. A spiral-bound booklet printed by Parent Child Press that brings awareness about the inner light of the child.

- *I Want to Hear the Quiet* by Aline D. Wolf, illustrated by Joe Servello. A booklet printed by Parent Child Press that brings awareness to the numerous sounds in modern society that compete with the child's desire for silence.
- *I Know How Seeds Grow* is a spiral-bound booklet by child author Sophie Wolf, and the title is self-explanatory.
- *When I Make Silence* by Jennifer Howard, illustrated by Alicia Jewell. This booklet by Parent Child Press tells the story of a child's moments in silence, and shows children experiencing silence together in a classroom setting.
- For more vegan-friendly children's books, see www.goodreads.com (offering 90 different listings).
- Additional literature for children on gardening, ecology, peacefulness, and silence can be found at Montessori Services: www.MontessoriServices.com.

INSPIRING BOARD GAMES FOR CHILDREN

The games that we play with children can send a message about human purpose. In some games, the aim is to dominate through war or financial gain. In others (both cooperative and competitive) the goal hints at something higher.

- "The Yoga Garden Game" is a cooperative board game for children that introduces the yoga *asanas:* www.yogakids.com.
- "Wildcraft: An Herbal Adventure Game" is a cooperative board game for children that teaches about medicinal herbs, available at www.learningherbs.com.
- "Fur and Feathers" is a board game that teaches children about animals and how to take care of them.
- Search for more at www.VeganEssentials.com or www.Amazon.com.

BOOKS WITH LIVING-FOOD RECIPES
ESPECIALLY FOR CHILDREN

- *Real Life Raw: Kids in the Kitchen* by Tina Jo Stephens
- *Creating Healthy Children* by Karen Ranzi
- *Disease-Proof Your Child: Feeding Kids Right* by Joel Fuhrman, MD
- *Raw Family Signature Dishes: A Step-by-Step Guide to Essential Live-Food Recipes* by Victoria Boutenko
- *Baby Greens: A Live-Food Approach for Children of All Ages* by Michaela Lynn (Leah) with Michael Chrisemer
- *Hallelujah Kids* by Julie Wandling (http://ecommerce.hacres .com/)
- *Recipes for Life from God's Garden* by Rhonda J. Malkmus (http://ecommerce.hacres.com/)
- *Evie's Kitchen: Raising an Ecstatic Child* by Shazzie
- E-books by Tiffany Washko: *Raw Foods Recipes for Kids, Raw Baby Food Recipes*, and *Green Smoothie Recipes for Kids* (available on www.greensmoothiekid.com)
- *The Healthy Lunchbox* (e-book) by Shannon "Shakaya" Leoni
- www.TheGardenDiet.com has a series of e-books on raising children with living foods.
- *70 Best Raw Food Recipes of the Rawfoodfamily* and *Raising Raw Children* by Ka Sundance

RESOURCES FOR SUPPORTING THE EMOTIONAL BODY

- "Zero Point Workshop" at the Tree of Life US Center, Patagonia, AZ: www.DrCousens.com
- "The Journey" is a therapeutic, metaphoric forgiveness process developed by Brandon Bays (author of *The Journey* and *The Journey for Kids: Liberating Your Child's Shining Potential*) at www.thejourney.com
- Emotional Literacy Series (twenty-one books) by Enchanté productions

- www.KidsEQ.com
- "Stop Reacting—Start Responding" series on www.MomTV .com, hosted by Sharon Silver, author of *Stop Reacting and Start Responding: 108 Ways to Discipline Consciously and Become the Parent You Want to Be*
- Therapeutic puppetry arts for children: Juniper Tree Puppets, www.junipertreepuppets.com

FAMILY-IN-NATURE SUPPORT

- Children and Nature Network: www.childrenandnature.org /movement/naturalfamilies/clubs
- Richard Louv: www.richardlouv.com

INSPIRING FILMS

Note: Please refer to parent movie-review websites to determine age-appropriateness of any film before watching it with a child.

- *Impact of Fresh, Healthy Food on Learning and Behavior* (search on www.YouTube.com)
- *Simply Raw.* Filmed at the Tree of Life Center U.S. in Patagonia, Arizona, we see true stories of diabetes reversal through a zero-glycemic living-foods approach.
- *Just Choices.* A film for older children and teens about a group of students working on a social justice project. This short film follows their collective experience learning about ethical treatment of animals.
- *Ryan's Well.* The remarkable true story of a young boy's expression of service and charity.
- *The Little Red Wagon.* This docudrama is based on the true story of Zach Bonner, a boy who walked across the United States raising awareness about homeless children.
- *Dolphin Tale (and Dolphin Tale 2).* Based on a true story of healing and transformation through an extraordinary act of compassion for animals.

- *The Raw Natural,* by Rachel Hellman. Recommended for older children and teens (contains some graphic material), especially athletes and those living with a disability.
- *High School Musical.* The two main characters in this popular musical demonstrate the courage to pursue their sacred design rather than succumb to the countering pressure of family, friends, and the status quo.

Recipe Index

Notes

CHAPTER 1

1. From St. Teresa's poem "The Servant of Unity," in Daniel Ladinsky, *Love Poems from God: Twelve Sacred Voices from the East and West* (New York: The Penguin Group, 2002), 286.

CHAPTER 2

1. *1995 Search Institute Survey of Youth: 6th to 12th Graders* (Search Institute, 1997).

2. Peggy Jenkins, *The Joyful Child* (Harbinger House, Inc., 1989), 35.

3. E.M. Standing, *Maria Montessori: Her Life And Work* (London: Hollis and Carter Limited, 1957), 108.

4. K. Dorfman, *What's Eating Your Child?: The Hidden Connection Between Food and Childhood Ailments* (New York: Workman Publishing Company, Inc., 2011), 45.

CHAPTER 3

1. C.A. Boyle et al., "Trends in the Prevalence of Developmental Disabilities in U.S. Children, 1997–2008," *Pediatrics* (e-published May 23, 2011): doi:10.1542/peds.2010-2989.

2. J. Baio, "Prevalence of Autism Spectrum Disorder Among Children Aged 8 Years—Autism and Developmental Disabilities Monitoring Network, 11 Sites, United States, 2010," *Morbidity and Mortality Weekly Report (MMWR)* 63, no. SS02 (Atlanta, GA: Centers for Disease Control, March 28, 2014): 1–21.

3. Ibid.

4. S.L. Murphy, J. Xu, and K.D. Kochanek, "Deaths: Final Data for 2010," *National Vital Statistics Reports* 61, no. 4 (Hyattsville, MD: National Center for Health Statistics, 2013).

5. C.L. Ogden et al., "Prevalence of Childhood and Adult Obesity in the United States, 2011-2012," *Journal of the American Medical Association* 311, no. 8 (2014): 806–14, doi:10.1001/jama.2014.732.

6. Ibid.

7. *National Diabetes Statistics Report: Estimates of Diabetes and Its Burden in the United States, 2014* (Atlanta, GA: U.S. Department of Health and Human Services, Centers for Disease Control and Prevention, 2014).

8. W.J. Craig et al., "Position of the American Dietetic Association: Vegetarian Diets," *Journal of the American Dietetic Association* 109 (2009): 1,266–82.

9. Irma Sevilla and Nereyda Aguirre, *Study on the Effects of Wild Bluegreen™ Algae on the Nutritional Status and School Performance of First-, Second- and Third-Grade Children Attending the Monseñor Velez School in Nandaime, Nicaragua* (Nicaragua: Universidad Centroamericana, 1995).

10. Ibid.

11. Ibid.

12. Ibid.

13. Ibid.

14. Gabriel Cousens, *Spiritual Nutrition: Six Foundations for Spiritual Life and the Awakening of Kundalini* (Berkeley, CA: North Atlantic Books, 2005).

15. C.G. Perrine, *Pediatrics* 125 (March 22, 2010): 627–32.

16. Abram Hoffer, MD, *Orthomolecular Medicine For Everyone: Megavitamin Therapeutics for Families and Physicians* (Basic Health Publications, 2008).

17. H.E. Volk et al., "Residential Proximity to Freeways and Autism in the CHARGE Study," *Environmental Health Perspectives* 119 (2010): 873–7, e-published December 16, 2010: http://dx.doi.org/10.1289/ehp.1002835.

18. R.L. Hotz, "The Hidden Toll of Traffic Jams: Scientists Increasingly Link Vehicle Exhaust With Brain-Cell Damage, Higher Rates of Autism," *The Wall Street Journal* (November 8, 2011).

19. Ibid.

20. Ibid.

21. A.G. Marsh et al., "Bone mineral mass in adult lacto-ovo-vegetarian and omnivorous males," *American Journal of Clinical Nutrition* 37 (March 1983): 453–6.

22. J.T. Dwyer, "Health aspects of vegetarian diets," *American Journal of Clinical Nutrition* 48 (September 1988): 712–38.

23. Gabriel Cousens, *Conscious Eating* (Berkeley, CA: North Atlantic Books, 2000).

24. A. Pan et al., "Red Meat Consumption and Mortality: Results From 2 Prospective Cohort Studies," *Archives of Internal Medicine* 172, no. 7 (April 9, 2012): 555–63, doi:10.1001/archinternmed.2011.2287.

25. I.B. Wilkinson, I.L. Megson, H. MacCallum et al., "Oral vitamin C reduces arterial stiffness and platelet aggregation in humans," *Journal of Cardiovascular Pharmacology* 34, no. 5 (November 1999): 690–3.

26. V. Messina and A.R. Mangels, "Considerations in planning vegan diets: children," *Journal of the American Dietetic Association* 101, no. 6 (June 2001): 661–9.

27. C. Yarrington and E.N. Pearce, "Iodine and Pregnancy," *Journal of Thyroid Research* 2011, article 934104 (2011): doi: 10.4061/2011/934104.

28. Y. Lanti et al., "Iodine supplementation into drinking water improved intelligence of preschool-children aged 25–59 months in Ngargoyoso sub-district, Central Java, Indonesia: A randomized control trial," *Journal of Biology, Agriculture and Healthcare* 2, no. 5 (2012): www.iiste.org, (paper) ISSN 2224-3208, (online) ISSN 2225-093X.

29. Francesca L. Crowe, Paul N. Appleby, Ruth C. Travis, and Timothy J. Key, "Risk of hospitalization or death from ischemic heart disease among British vegetarians and nonvegetarians: results from the EPIC-Oxford cohort study," *American Journal of Clinical Nutrition* (March 2013): doi:10.3945/ajcn.112.044073.

30. R.C. Travis, N.E. Allen, P.N Appleby, E.A. Spencer, A.W. Roddam, and T.J. Key, "A prospective study of vegetarianism and isoflavone intake in relation to breast cancer risk in British women," *International Journal of Cancer* 122, no. 3 (February 1, 2008): 705–10.

31. Gabriel Cousens, *There Is a Cure for Diabetes*, revised edition (Berkeley, CA: North Atlantic Books, 2012).

32. T.J. Key, P.N. Appleby, E.A. Spencer, R.C. Travis, N.E. Allen, M. Thorogood, and J.I. Mann, "Cancer incidence in British vegetarians," *British Journal of Cancer* 101, no. 1 (July 7, 2009): 192–7, e-published June 16, 2009.

33. T.J. Key, P.N. Appleby, E.A. Spencer, R.C. Travis, A.W. Roddam, and N.E. Allen, "Cancer incidence in vegetarians: results from the European Prospective Investigation into Cancer and Nutrition (EPIC-Oxford)," *American Journal of Clinical Nutrition* 89, suppl. (2009): 1,553-7S.

34. Phillip J. Tuso, MD, Mohamed H. Ismail, MD, Benjamin P. Ha, MD, and Carole Bartolotto, MA, RD, "Nutritional Update for Physicians: Plant-Based Diets," *The Permanente Journal* 17, no. 2 (Spring 2013): 61–6, http://dx.doi.org/10.7812/TPP/12-085.

35. G.E. Fraser, "Associations between diet and cancer, ischemic heart disease, and all-cause mortality in non-Hispanic white California Seventh-day Adventists," *American Journal of Clinical Nutrition* 70, suppl. 3 (September 1999): 532–8S.

36. Teresa Norat, Annekatrin Lukanova, Pietro Ferrari, and Elio Riboli, "Meat consumption and colorectal cancer risk: Dose-response meta-analysis of epidemiological studies," *International Journal of Cancer* 98, no. 2 (March 10, 2002): 241–56, doi:10.1002/ijc.10126.

37. Francesca L. Crowe, Paul N. Appleby, Ruth C. Travis, and Timothy J. Key, "Risk of hospitalization or death from ischemic heart disease among British vegetarians and nonvegetarians: results from the EPIC-Oxford cohort study," *American Journal of Clinical Nutrition* (March 2013): doi:10.3945/ajcn.112.044073.

38. Paul N. Appleby, Gwyneth K. Davey, and Timothy J. Key. "Hypertension and blood pressure among meat eaters, fish eaters, vegetarians and vegans in EPIC—Oxford," *Public Health Nutrition* 5, no. 5 (October 2002): 645–54, doi:10.1079/PHN2002332.

39. S. Harris, *Organochlorine Contamination of Breast Milk* (Washington, DC: Environmental Defense Fund, November 7, 1979).

40. J. Furhman, MD, *Disease-Proof Your Child: Feeding Kids Right* (New York: St. Martin's Press, 2005), 95.

41. Elias E. Manuelidis and Laura Manuelidis, "Suggested Links between Different Types of Dementias: Creutzfeldt-Jakob Disease, Alzheimer Disease, and Retroviral CNS Infections," *Alzheimer Disease and Associated Disorders* 3 (1989): 100–9.

42. P. Giem et al., "The incidence of dementia and the intake of animal products: preliminary findings of the Adventist Health Study," *Neurobiology* 12 (1992): 28–36.

43. Gidon Eshel, Alon Shepon, Tamar Makov, and Ron Milo, "Land, irrigation water, greenhouse gas, and reactive nitrogen burdens of meat, eggs, and dairy production in the United States," *Proceedings of the National Academy of Sciences* 111, no. 33 (2014): 11,996–12,001, e-published July 21, 2014, doi:10.1073/pnas.1402183111.

44. Paul A. Eubig, Andréa Aguiar, Susan L. Schantz, "Lead and PCBs as risk factors for attention deficit/hyperactivity disorder," Environmental Health Perspectives 118 (2010): 1,654–67, doi.org/10.1289/ehp.0901852.

45. John Robbins, *Diet for a New America* (Walpole, NH: Stillpoint Publishing, 1987), 331.

46. Ibid.

47. Robbins, op. cit., 334.

48. Ibid.

49. A. Roslin, "Canada: Fish Eaters Threatened by Fukushima Radiation," Vancouver Sun (January 16, 2012): http://readersupportednews.org/news-section2/343-203/9463-canada-fish-eaters-threatened-by-fukushima-radiation.

50. Ibid.

51. Ibid.

52. Ibid.

53. R.L. Hotz, "U.S. Tuna Has Fukushima Taint," *The Wall Street Journal* (May 29, 2012).

54. Centers for Disease Control and Prevention staff, CDC Estimates of 2009 H1N1 Influenza Cases, Hospitalizations and Deaths in the United States, April 2009–March 13, 2010 (Atlanta, GA: Centers for Disease Control and Prevention, April 19, 2010): www.cdc.gov/h1n1flu/estimates/April_March_13.htm.

55. H.H. Reckeweg, "The Adverse Influence of Pork Consumption on Health," *Biological Therapy* 1, no. 2 (1983).

56. Leviticus 11:7.

57. L.S. Godsborough, "Pork," *Reader's Digest* (March, 1950).

58. Genesis 1:29.

59. J.N. Sofos, "Microbial growth and its control in meat, poultry and fish," *Quality Attributes and their Measurement in Meat, Poultry and Fish Products,* Advances in Meat Research series, vol. 9, A.M. Pearson and T.R. Dutson, eds. (London: Blackie Academic and Professional, an imprint of Chapman and Hall, 1994), 359–91.

60. S.F. Altekruse, M.E. Berrang, H. Marks et al., "Enumeration of *Escherichia coli* cells on chicken carcasses as a potential measure of microbial process control in a random selection of slaughter establishments in the United States," *Applied Environmental Microbiology* 75, no. 11 (2009): 3,522–7.

61. Gorman, Jim, "The 10 Dirtiest Foods You're Eating," MensHealth. com (2010), www.menshealth.com/mhlists/foodborne_illness/.

62. L. Fontana, R.M. Adelaiye, A.L. Rastelli, M.M. Miles, E. Ciamporcero, V.D. Longo, H. Nguyen, R. Vessella, and R. Pili, "Dietary protein restriction inhibits tumor growth in human xenograft models of prostate and breast cancer," *Oncotarget* 4, no. 12 (December 2013): 2,451–61, e-published November 23, 2013.

63. A.S. Hamilton and T.M. Mack, "Puberty and genetic susceptibility to breast cancer in a case-control study in twins," *New England Journal of Medicine* 348, no. 23 (June 5, 2003): 2,313–22.

64. H. Yu and T. Rohan, "Role of the Insulin-Like Growth Factor Family in Cancer Development and Progression," Journal of the National Cancer Institute 92 (200): 1,472-89.

65. J.W. Anderson et al., "Breast-feeding and cognitive development: a meta-analysis," *American Journal of Clinical Nutrition* 70, no. 4 (October 1999), 525-35.

66. A.W. Speedy, "Global Production and Consumption of Animal Source Foods," *Journal of Nutrition* 133, no. 11, suppl. 2 (November 2003), 4,048-53S.

67. A.J. Lanou et al., "Calcium, Dairy Products, and Bone Health in

Children and Young Adults: A Re-Evaluation of the Evidence," *Pediatrics* 115, no. 3 (March 2005), 736-43.

68. O. Vaarala, M. Knip , J. Paronen, A.-M. Hämäläinen, P. Muona, M. Väätäinen, J. Ilonen, O. Simell, and H.K. Åkerblom, "Cow milk formula feeding induces primary immunization to insulin in infants at genetic risk for type 1 diabetes," *Diabetes* 48 (1999): 1,389–94.

69. S. Lucarelli, T. Frediani, A.M. Zingoni, F. Ferruzzi, O. Giardini, F. Quintieri et al., "Food allergy and infantile autism," *Panminerva Medica* 37, no. 3 (1995): 137–41.

70. P. Whiteley, P. Shattock, A.-M. Knivsberg et al., "Gluten- and casein-free dietary intervention for autism spectrum conditions," Frontiers in Human Neuroscience 6 (2012): 344, doi:10.3389 /fnhum.2012.00344.

71. Lucarelli et al., op. cit.

72. *British Journal of Cancer* 61, no. 3 (March 1990): 345–9.

73. *International Journal of Cancer* (April 15, 1989).

74. *Cancer* 64, no. 3 (1989): 605–12.

75. Laura Power, "Biotype diets system: blood types and food allergies," *Journal of Nutritional and Environmental Medicine* 16, no. 2 (May 2007): 125–35.

76. R. Shears, "Girl, 14, left brain-damaged after eating KFC chicken twister forced into new court battle as food giant appeals $8M payout," Mail Online (e-published September 19, 2012): www .dailymail.co.uk/news/article-2205394/Girl-14-left-brain-damaged -eating-KFC-chicken-twister-forced-new-court-battle-food-giant -appeals-8m-payout.html.

77. A. Kijistra, W.A. Traag, L.A.P. Hoogenboom, "Effects of flock size dioxin levels in eggs from chickens kept outside," *Poultry Science* 86 (2007): 9, www.ps.oxfordjournals.org.

78. E. Olsen, "U.S. urged to educate women about foods linked to dioxin," *New York Times* (July 2, 2003): http://www.nytimes. com/2003/07/02/us/us-urged-to-educate-women-about-foods -linked-to-dioxin.html.

79. Ashley Montagu, *Touching: The Human Significance of the Skin* (New York: Harper and Row, 1978).

80. Sheehan, Nancy, "A year after miracle babies, family rejoices," *Worcester Telegram and Gazette* (October 13, 1996).

CHAPTER 4

1. C. Benbrook, X. Zhao, J. Yáñez, N. Davies, and P. Andrews, "New evidence confirms the nutritional superiority of plant-based organic foods," *The Organic Center* (March 2008).

2. H. Willer and L. Kilcher, *The World of Organic Agriculture: Statistics and Emerging Trends 2011* (Bonn, Germany: IFOAM [International Foundation of Organic Agriculture Movements] and Frick, Switzerland: FiBL [Research Institute of Organic Agriculture], 2015).

3. University of Nebraska, "Research shows Roundup Ready soybeans yield less," *IANR News Service* (2000), www.biotech-info.net /Roundup_soybeans_yield_less.html.

4. Gabriel Cousens, *Rainbow Green Live-Food Cuisine* (Berkeley, CA: North Atlantic Books, 2003).

5. E.A. Guillette, M.M. Meza, M.G. Aquilar, A.D. Soto, and I.E. Garcia, "An anthropological approach to the evaluation of preschool children exposed to pesticides in Mexico," *Environmental Health Perspectives* 106, no. 6 (June 1998): 347–53.

6. D. Steinman, *Diet for a Poisoned Planet: How to Choose Safe Foods for You and Your Family—The Twenty-first Century Edition* (Philadelphia: Running Press, 2006).

7. C. Ward and L. Reynolds, "Organic agriculture contributes to sustainable food security," *Vital Signs* (Jan. 15, 2013).

8. Guyton, K.Z. et al., International Agency for Research on Cancer (World Health Organization), "Carcinogenicity of tetrachlorvinphos, parathion, malathion, diazinon, and glyphosate," *Lancet Oncology* (2015), http://dx.doi.org/10.1016/S1470-2045(15)70134-8.

9. www.ewg.org/foodnews.

10. Gabriel Cousens, *Rainbow Green Live Food Cuisine*, (Berkeley, CA: North Atlantic Books, 2003), 87.

11. www.istpp.org/print_friendly/genetic_engineering.html.

12. R. Laws, "History of Vegetarianism: Native Americans and Vegetarianism," *Vegetarian Journal* (September 1994): www.ivu.org/history /native_americans.html.

13. Environmental Working Group, "Environmental Working Group analysis of tests of 10 umbilical cord blood samples conducted by AXYS Analytical Services (Sydney, BC) and Flett Research, Ltd. (Winnipeg, MB)," *Body Burden: The Pollution in Newborns* (July 14, 2005).

14. Bridget M. Kuehn, "Increased Risk of ADHD Associated With Early Exposure to Pesticides, PCBs," *Journal of the American Medical Association* 304, no. 1 (July 2010): 27–8, doi:10.1001/jama.2010.860.

15. J.V. Bruckner, "Differences in sensitivity of children and adults to chemical toxicity: the NAS panel report," *Regulatory Toxicology and Pharmacology* 31, no. 3 (June 2000): 280–5.

16. L.Y. Lefferts, "Pesticide residues variability and acute dietary risk assessment: a consumer perspective," *Food Additives and Contaminants* 17, no. 7 (July 2000): 511–7.

17. F.M. Pottenger, *Pottenger's Cats: A Study in Nutrition,* 2nd ed. (Lemon Grove, CA: Price Pottenger Nutrition, 1995).

18. Joel Fuhrman, MD, *Disease-Proof Your Child: Feeding Kids Right* (New York: St. Martin's Press, 2005).

19. C. Nungesser and G. Nungesser, *How We All Went Raw* (In the Beginning Health Ministry, 2004), back cover.

20. P. Nison, *Raw Knowledge: Enhance the Powers of the Mind, Body and Soul,* 3rd ed. (Three Forty Three Publishing Co., 2002).

21. M. Donaldson, "Is Johnny Getting Old Before He Grows Up?: How to Ensure Lifelong Good Habits," *Hallelujah Acres Health News* (September–October 2009).

22. Ibid.

23. Gabriel Cousens, *Spiritual Nutrition: Six Foundations for Spiritual Life and the Awakening of Kundalini* (Berkeley, CA: North Atlantic Books, 2005), 424.

24. Center for Food Safety, www.centerforfoodsafety.org/issues/311/ge-foods/about-ge-foods#.

25. Trudy Netherwood et al., "Assessing the survival of transgenic plant DNA in the human gastrointestinal tract," *Nature Biotechnology* 22 (2004): 2.

26. National Cancer Institute, www.cancer.gov/cancertopics/types/Hodgkin.

27. "Position of the American Dietetic Association: Vegetarian Diets," *Journal of the American Dietetic Association* 109 (2009): 1,266.

28. Y. Bao et al., "Association of Nut Consumption with Total and Cause-Specific Mortality," *New England Journal of Medicine* 369 (November 21, 2013): 2,001–11, doi: 10.1056/NEJMoa1307352.

29. J.C. Lovejoy et al., "Effects of diets enriched in almonds on insulin action and serum lipids in adults with normal glucose tolerance in type 2 diabetes," *American Journal of Clinical Nutrition* 76 (2002): 1,000–6.

30. *Stroke* 26 (1993): 778–82. These results were first published in *The Lancet* 343 (1994): 1,454–9 and subsequently in other reputable journals such as *Preventative Medicine* 28 (333–9), *American Journal of Clinical Nutrition* 74 (72–9), and *Annals of Internal Medicine* 132, no. 7 (538–46).

31. Federal Trade Commission, *Marketing Food to Children and Adolescents: A Review of Industry Expenditures, Activities, and Self-Regulation: A Federal Trade Commission Report to Congress* (July, 2008).

32. "Preliminary report from Harvard School of Public Health Reveals Students Prefer Healthy School Meals," *News Medical* (November 19, 2009): www.news-medical.net/news/2009119/Preliminary-report -from-Harvard-Schools-of-Public-Health-Reveals-Students-Prefer -Healthy-School-Meals.aspx.

33. K. Dorfman, *What's Eating Your Child?: The Hidden Connection Between Food and Childhood Ailments* (New York: Workman Publishing Company, April 28, 2011), 38, 53.

34. Ibid.

35. "Soy Infant Formula Could Be Harmful to Infants; Groups Want it Pulled," *Nutrition Week* 29, no. 46 (December 10, 1999): 1–2.

36. S.E. Hankinson et al., "Circulating concentrations of insulin-like growth factor I and risk of breast cancer," *The Lancet* 351, no. 9113 (May 9, 1998): 1,393–6.

37. L.R. White, H. Petrovich, G.W. Ross, and K.H. Masaki, "Association of mid-life consumption of tofu with late life cognitive impairment and dementia: the Honolulu-Asia Aging Study," *Fifth International Conference on Alzheimer's Disease* 487 (Osaka, Japan, July 27, 1996).

38. L.R. White, H. Petrovitch, G.W. Ross, K.H. Masaki, J. Hardman, J.

Nelson, D. Davis, and W. Markesbery, "Brain aging and midlife tofu consumption," *Journal of the American College of Nutrition* 29, no. 2 (April 2000): 242–55.

39. Ibid.

40. J.J. Mangano and J.D. Sherman, "Elevated airborne beta levels in Pacific/West Coast US states and trends in hypothyroidism among newborns after the Fukushima nuclear meltdown," *Open Journal of Pediatrics* 3 (March 2013): 1–9.

41. J.E. Chavarro et al., "Soy food and isoflavone intake in relation to semen quality parameters among men from an infertility clinic," *Human Reproduction* 23, no. 11 (2008): 2,584–90, doi:10.1093 /humrep/den243.

42. Joel Fuhrman, MD, *Disease-Proof Your Child: Feeding Kids Right* (New York: St. Martin's Press, 2005).

CHAPTER 5

1. Joel Fuhrman, MD, *Disease-Proof Your Child: Feeding Kids Right* (New York: St. Martin's Press, 2005).

2. J. Savage et al., "Parental Influence on Eating Behavior: Conception to Adolescence," *Journal of Law, Medicine, and Ethics* 35, no. 1 (2007): 22–34, doi:10.1111/j.1748-720X.2007.00111.x.

3. Rabbi Gabriel Cousens, *Torah as a Guide to Enlightenment* (Berkeley, CA: North Atlantic Books, 2011), 276.

4. Op. cit., 278.

CHAPTER 6

1. Gabriel Cousens, *Depression-Free for Life: An All-Natural, Five-Step Plan to Reclaim Your Zest for Living* (New York: William Morrow and Company, 2000).

2. B.L. Beezhold and C.S. Johnston, "Restriction of meat, fish, and poultry in omnivores improves mood: A pilot randomized controlled trial," *Nutrition Journal* 11, no. 9 (2012).

3. J. Fulbright, *Exploring Creation with Zoology 3: Land Animals of the Sixth Day* (Anderson, IN: Apologia Educational Ministries, Inc., 2008), 4–6.

4. Dr. Gabriel Cousens, *Conscious Eating* (Berkeley, CA: North Atlantic Books, 2000), 34–35.

CHAPTER 8

1. S. Glazer, *The Heart of Learning: Spirituality in Education* (New York: Penguin Books, 1999).

2. Maria Montessori, *The Secret of Childhood* (New York: Ballantine Books, 1966), 97–8.

3. E. Caspari and E. Wolberd, *Caspari Montessori Institute Teacher Training Manual* (Livingston, MT: Caspari Montessori Institute, 2010).

4. T. Delate et al., "Trends in the Use of Antidepressants in a National Sample of Commercially Insured Pediatric Patients, 1998 to 2002," *Psychiatric Services* 55, no. 4 (April 2004): 387–91.

5. D. Baldwin, "Psychotropic Drugs and Sexual Dysfunction," *Informa Healthcare* 7, no. 2 (1999): 261–73.

6. Gabriel Cousens, *Depression-Free for Life: An All-Natural, Five-Step Plan to Reclaim Your Zest for Living* (New York: William Morrow and Company, 2000).

7. A.F. Taylor and F.E. Kuo, "Could Exposure to Everyday Green Spaces Help Treat ADHD? Evidence from Children's Play Settings," *Applied Psychology: Health and Well-Being* 3, no. 3 (November 2011): 281–303, doi:10.1111/j.1758-0854.2011.01052.x.

8. Rabbi Nehunia ben haKana, *The Bahir,* trans. Aryeh Kaplan (York Beach, ME: Weiser Books, 1989).

9. Avraham ben HaRambam, *Hamaspik L'Ovdei Hashem* (Nanuet, NY: Feldheim Publishers, 2014).

10. S. Hart and V.K. Hodson, *The Compassionate Classroom* (Encinitas, CA: Puddle Dancer Press, 2004), 15.

11. Gabriel Cousens, *Conscious Eating* (Berkeley, CA: North Atlantic Books, 2000).

12. K. Dorfman, *What's Eating Your Child?: The Hidden Connection Between Food and Childhood Ailments* (New York: Workman Publishing Company, 2011), 38.

13. N. Sinn and J. Bryan, "Effect of supplementation with polyunsaturated fatty acids and micronutrients on ADHD-related problems

with attention and behavior," *Journal of Developmental and Behavioral Pediatrics* 28, no. 2 (2007): 82–91.

14. Jostein Holmen et al., "The Nord-Trøndelag Health Study 1995-97 (HUNT 2): Objectives, contents, methods and participation," *Norsk Epidemiologi* 13, no. 1 (2003): 19–32.

15. L.A. Bazzano, J. He, L.G. Odgen et al., "Dietary intake of folate and risk of stroke in US men and women: NHANES I Epidemiologic Follow-up Study," *Stroke* 33, no. 5 (May 2002): 1,183–9.

16. P.W. Siri-Tarino, Q. Sun, F.B. Hu, and R.M. Krauss, "Meta-analysis of prospective cohort studies evaluating the association of saturated fat with cardiovascular disease," *American Journal of Clinical Nutrition* ajcn.27725 (January 2010).

17. H.M. Krumholz et al., "Lack of association between cholesterol and coronary heart disease mortality and morbidity and all-cause mortality in persons older than 70 years," *Journal of the American Medical Association* 272 (1994): 1,335–40.

18. A. Evans, H. Tolonen, H.-W. Hense, M. Ferrario, S. Sans, K. Kuulasmaa (for the World Health Organization's MONICA Project), "Trends in coronary risk factors in the WHO MONICA Project," *International Journal of Epidemiology* 30 suppl. (2001): S35–40.

19. B. Howard, J. Manson, M. Stefanick et al., "Low-fat dietary pattern and weight change over 7 years: the Women's Health Initiative Dietary Modification Trial," *Journal of the American Medical Association* 295 (2006): 39–49.

20. Ibid.

21. H. Petursson, J.A. Sigurdsson, C. Bengtsson, T.I. Nilsen, and L. Getz, "Is the use of cholesterol in mortality risk algorithms in clinical guidelines valid? Ten years prospective data from the Norwegian HUNT 2 study," *Journal of Evaluation in Clinical Practice* (September 25, 2011): doi:10.1111/j.1365-2753.2011.01767.x.

22. L. Hooper, C.D. Summerbell, R. Thompson, D. Sills, F.G. Roberts, H. Moore, and G. Smith, "Reduced or modified dietary fat for preventing cardiovascular disease," *The Cochrane Collaboration* (July 6, 2011): doi:10.1002/14651858.CD002137.pub2.

23. G.E. Fraser and D.J. Shavlik, "Ten years of life: Is it a matter of choice?" *Archives of Internal Medicine* 161, no. 13 (July 9, 2001): 1,645–52.

24. A. Colin, J. Reggers, V. Castronovo, and M. Ansseau, "Lipids, depression and suicide," *Encephale* 29, no. 1 (January–February 2003): 49–58.

25. N. Ruljanc ic, A. Malic, and M. Mihanovic, "Serum cholesterol concentration in psychiatric patients," *Biochemia Medica* 17, no. 2 (2007): 197–202.

26. L.F. Ellison and H.I. Morrison, "Low serum cholesterol concentration and risk of suicide," *Epidemiology* 12, no. 2 (March 2001): 168–72.

27. J.A. Golier, P.M. Marzuk, A.C. Leon, C. Weiner, and K. Tardiff, "Low serum cholesterol level and attempted suicide," *American Journal of Psychiatry* 152, no. 3 (March 1995): 419–23.

28. E. Deans, "Low cholesterol and suicide: Your brain needs cholesterol—don't go too low," *Evolutionary Psychiatry* (March 21, 2011): www.psychologytoday.com/blog/evolutionary-psychiatry/201103/low-cholesterol-and-suicide.

29. S. Shrivastava, T.J. Pucadyil, Y.D. Paila, S. Ganguly, and A. Chattopadhyay, "Chronic cholesterol depletion using statin impairs the function and dynamics of human serotonin receptors," *Biochemistry* 49, no. 26 (2010): 5,426–35.

30. M. Merialdi and J.C. Murray, "The Changing Face of Preterm Labor," *Pediatrics* (October 1, 2007).

31. A. Macchia, S. Monte, F. Pellegrini et al., "Omega-3 fatty acid supplementation reduces one-year risk of atrial fibrillation in patients hospitalized with myocardial infarction," *European Journal of Clinical Pharmacology* 64, no. 6 (June 2008): 627–34.

32. J. Golding, C. Steer, P. Emmett et al., "High levels of depressive symptoms in pregnancy with low omega-3 fatty acid intake from fish," *Epidemiology* 20, no. 4 (July 2009): 598–603.

33. M.D. Lewis, J.R. Hibbeln, J.E. Johnson, Y.H. Lin, D.Y. Hyun, and J.D. Loewke, "Suicide deaths of active-duty U.S. military and omega-3 fatty-acid status: A case-control comparison," *Journal of Clinical Psychiatry* 75, no. 12 (2011): 1,585–90.

34. M.R. Garland and B. Hallahan, "Essential fatty acids and their role in conditions characterized by impulsivity," *International Review of Psychiatry* 18, no. 2 (April 2006): 99–105.

35. Ibid.

36. M. Bousquet, M. Saint-Pierre, C. Julien, N. Salem, F. Cicchetti, and F. Calon, "Beneficial effects of dietary omega-3 polyunsaturated fatty acid on toxin-induced neuronal degeneration in an animal model of Parkinson's disease," *FASEB Journal* 22, no. 4 (2007): 1,213–25.

37. J.V. Pottala, A. Garg, B.E. Cohen, M.A. Whooley, and W.S. Harris, "Blood eicosapentaenoic and docosahexaenoic acids predict all-cause mortality in patients with stable coronary heart disease: The Heart and Soul Study," *Circulation: Cardiovascular Quality Outcomes* 3, no. 4 (July 2010): 406–12.

38. G.S. Masterton, J.N. Plevris, and P.C. Hayes, "Review article: Omega-3 fatty acids—a promising novel therapy for non-alcoholic fatty liver disease," *Alimentary Pharmacology and Therapeutics* 31, no. 7 (April 2010): 679–92.

39. B. Gopinath, D.C. Harris, V.M. Flood, G. Burlutsky, and P. Mitchell, "Consumption of long-chain n-3 PUFA, alpha-linolenic acid and fish is associated with the prevalence of chronic kidney disease," *British Journal of Nutrition* 105, no. 9 (May 2011): 1,361–8.

40. R.K. McNamara, R. Jandacek, T. Rider et al., "Deficits in docosahexaenoic acid and associated elevations in the metabolism of arachidonic acid and saturated fatty acids in the postmortem orbitofrontal cortex of patients with bipolar disorder," *Psychiatry Research* 160, no. 3 (September 30, 2008): 285–99.

41. M.E. Sublette, J.R. Hibbeln, H. Galfalvy et al., "Omega-3 polyunsaturated essential fatty acid status as a predictor of future suicide risk," *American Journal of Psychiatry* 163, no. 6 (2006): 1,100–2.

42. R. DeCaterina, R. Madonna, R. Zucchi, and M.T. LaRovere, "Antiarrhythmic effects of omega-3 fatty acids: From epidemiology to bedside," *American Heart Journal* 146, no. 3 (September 2003): 420–30.

43. B. Gopinath et al., "A better diet quality is associated with a reduced likelihood of CKD in older adults," *Natural Medicines Comprehensive Database* 23, no. 10 (October 2013): 937–43, doi: http://dx.doi.org/10.1016/j.numecd.2012.07.003.

44. Joel Furhman, MD, *Disease-Proof Your Child: Feeding Kids Right* (New York: St. Martin's Press, 2005).

45. D. Hurley, "Your Gut Can Influence How You Feel: It All Starts with GABA and Serotonin," www.bodyecology.com/articles/your-gut-can -influence-how-you-feel-it-all-starts-with-serotonin (December 13, 2011).

46. Department of Medical Microbiology and Parasitology, University College Hospital, Ibadan, Nigeria, "In Vitro Antimicrobial Properties of Coconut Oil on Candida Species in Ibadan, Nigeria, *Journal of Medicinal Food* 10, no. 2 (June 2007): 384–7, www.ncbi.nlm.nih .gov/pubmed/17651080.

47. Feingold Association of the United States, "A Different Kind of School Lunch: Students of Midwestern Community are Enjoying Fresh, Delicious Food Plus a Big Change in Their Learning Environment," www.feingold.org/pf/wisconsin1/html (October 2002).

48. Parents Television Council, "It's Just Harmless Entertainment—Oh Really?" www.parentstv.org/PTC/flyers/factsheet.htm.

49. *Journal of the American Medical Association,* "Early Home Environment and Television Watching Influence Bully Behavior," *Science Daily* (April 21, 2005): www.sciencedaily.com /releases/2005/04/050420091955.htm.

50. University of Michigan study, "Kids and TV: Tuned into Unhealthy Food," www.futurity.org/kids-and-tv-tuned-in-to-unhealthy-food/.

51. Morgan Video Productions, dir. A. Barbaro and J. Earp, *Consuming Kids: The Commercialization of Childhood* (Northampton, MA: Media Education Foundation 2008).

52. University of Michigan Health System, "Television and Children," www.med.umich.edu/yourchild/topics/tv.htm.

53. Leslie Manookian, prod., Kendall Nelson and Chris Pilaro, dir., *The Greater Good* (BVP Pictures, 2011).

54. University of Michigan Health System, "Television and Children," www.med.umich,edu/yourchild/topics/tv.htm.

55. Ibid.

56. Ibid.

57. Science Daily, "Teen Pregnancy Linked to Viewing of Sexual Content on TV," www.sciencedaily.com/releases/2008/11/08110384043 .htm (2008).

58. University of Michigan Health System, "Television and Children," www.med.umich.edu/yourchild/topics/tv.htm.

59. Gabriel Cousens, *Creating Peace by Being Peace* (Berkeley, CA: North Atlantic Books, 2008).

60. P. McDonough, "TV Viewing Among Kids at Eight-Year-High," *The Nielson Company* (October 26 2009), www.nielson.com/us/en /insight/news/2009/tv-viewing-among-kids-at-an-eight-year-high .html/.

61. Stephanie LaLand, *Random Acts of Kindness by Animals* (San Francisco: Conari Press, 2008), 161.

62. http://cyber.law.harvard.edu/VAW02/mod2-6.htm.

63. American Psychological Association, www.apa.org/monitor/2009/12 /child-abuse.aspx.

64. www.irishexaminer.com/ireland/young-sex-offenders-start-off-with -child-porn-289375.html.

CHAPTER 9

1. N.Z. Miller, *Vaccine Safety Manual for Concerned Families and Health Practitioners* (Santa Fe, NM: New Atlantean Press, 2008).

2. Sayer Ji, "200 Evidence-Based Reasons Not To Vaccinate," www.greenmedinfo.com/sites/default/files/gpub_58635_anti _therapeutic_action_vaccination_all.pdf (February 22, 2015).

3. "Vaccines: Get the Full Story—Doctors, Nurses, and Scientists on Protecting Your Child and Yourself," www.vaccinationcouncil.org.

4. Peter Doshi, MD, "Are U.S. flu death figures more PR than science?" *BMJ (formerly British Medical Journal)* 331 (December 8, 2005): 1,412, doi:10.1136/bmj.331.7529.1412.

5. Ibid.

6. W.D. King et al., "Brief report: Influenza Vaccination and Health Care Workers in the United States," *Journal of General Internal Medicine* 21, no. 2 (February 2006): 181–4, doi:10.1111/j.1525-1497.2006.00325.x.

7. www.cbsnews.com/news/gardasil-researcher-speaks-out/.

8. www.medscape.com/viewarticle/833798.

9. S.H. Oh, E.H. Choi, S.H. Shin et al., "Varicella and Varicella Vaccination in South Korea," ed. S.A. Plotkin, *Clinical and Vaccine Immunology* 21, no. 5 (2014): 762–8, doi:10.1128/CVI.00645-13.

10. Ibid.

11. Miller NZ, The polio vaccine: a critical assessment of its arcane history, efficacy, and long-term health-related consequences, N.Z. Miller/Medical Veritas 1 (2004) 239–251.

12. A. Stein, "Vaccinated Kids Account for 90 Percent of Child Whooping Cough Cases in Vermont," VTDigger.org, www.vtdigger.org/2012/10/08/90-percent-of-whooping-cough-cases-in-vermont-among-vaccinated-children/ (October 8, 2012).

13. Z Wang, R. Yan, H. He et al., "Difficulties in Eliminating Measles and Controlling Rubella and Mumps: A Cross-Sectional Study of a First Measles and Rubella Vaccination and a Second Measles, Mumps, and Rubella Vaccination," ed. M. Kirk, *PLOS ONE* 9, no. 2 (2014): e89361, doi:10.1371/journal.pone.0089361.

14. C. Ma, L. Hao, Y. Zhang et al., "Monitoring progress towards the elimination of measles in China: an analysis of measles surveillance data," *Bulletin of the World Health Organization* 92, no. 5 (2014): 340–7, doi:10.2471/BLT.13.130195.

15. J.M. Warfel, L.I. Zimmerman, and T.J. Merkel, "Acellular pertussis vaccines protect against disease but fail to prevent infection and transmission in a nonhuman primate model," *Proceedings of the National Academy of Sciences* 111, no. 2 (January 14, 2014): 787–92, e-published November 25, 2013, doi:10.1073/pnas.1314688110.

16. Ibid.

17. M.A. Witt, P.H. Katz, and D.J. Witt, "Unexpectedly Limited Durability of Immunity Following Acellular Pertussis Vaccination in Pre-Adolescents in a North American Outbreak," *Clinical and Infectious Diseases* (2012), e-published March 15, 2012, doi:10.1093/cid/cis287.

18. J. Howenstine, "Why You Should Avoid Taking Vaccines," NewsWithViews.com (December 7, 2003).

19. Ibid.

20. Ibid.

21. CDC, *Morbidity and Mortality Weekly Report 33*, no. 24 (June 22, 1984): 349–51, www.cdc.gov/mmwr/preview /mmwrhtml/00000359.htm.

22. CDC, "Measles in an Immunized School-Aged Population—New Mexico," *Morbidity and Mortality Weekly Report 34*, no. 4 (February 1, 1985): 52–4, 59, www.cdc.gov/mmwr/preview /mmwrhtml/00000476.htm.

23. CDC, "Measles Outbreak among Vaccinated High School Students—Illinois," *Morbidity and Mortality Weekly Report 33*, no. 24 (June 22, 1984): 349–51, www.cdc.gov/mmwr/preview /mmwrhtml/00000359.htm.

24. Jeffry John Aufderheide, "17 Examples of Admitted Vaccine Failure," *Vactruth* (February 23, 2013), http://vactruth .com/2013/02/23/17-examples-of-vaccine-failure/.

25. *Vital Statistics of the United States 1937, 1938, 1943, 1944, 1949, 1960, 1967, 1976, 1987, 1992* (National Vital Statistics Reports); *Historical Statistics of the United States—Colonial Times to 1970, Part 1: Health* (U.S. Department of Health and Human Services, Vital Records and Health Data Development Section, Michigan Department of Community Health); *Statistical Abstract of the United States: 2003* (U.S. Census Bureau); *Reported Cases and Deaths from Vaccine Preventable Diseases, United States, 1950–2008* (CDC). See more at www.vaccinationcouncil.org/2014/06/24 /measles-and-measles-vaccines-fourteen-things-to-consider -by-roman-bystrianyk-co-author-dissolving-illusions-disease -vaccines-and-the-forgotten-history/#sthash.FL1sFqm7.dpuf.

26. Z. Wang, R. Yan, H. He et al., "Difficulties in Eliminating Measles and Controlling Rubella and Mumps: A Cross-Sectional Study of a First Measles and Rubella Vaccination and a Second Measles, Mumps, and Rubella Vaccination," ed. M. Kirk, *PLOS ONE* 9, no. 2 (2014): e89361, doi:10.1371/journal.pone.0089361.

27. J. Howenstine, "Why You Should Avoid Taking Vaccines," NewsWithViews.com (December 7, 2003).

28. William Atkinson, MD, FDA workshop (September 18, 1992).

29. P.G. Auwaerter et al., "Changes within T Cell Receptor V Subsets in Infants Following Measles Vaccination," *Clinical Immunology and Immunopathology* 79, no. 2 (May 1996): 163–70.

30. P.A. Rota, A.S. Khan, E. Durigon, T. Yuran, Y.S. Villamarzo, and W.J. Bellini, "Detection of measles virus RNA in urine specimens from vaccine recipients," *Journal of Clinical Microbiology* 33, no. 9 (September 1995): 2,485–8.

31. CDC Health Advisory "U.S. Multi-state Measles Outbreak, December 2014–January 2015," distributed by the CDC Health Alert Network (January 23, 2015).

32. P. Rota, K. Brown, A. Mankertz et al., "Global Distribution of Measles Genotypes and Measles Molecular Epidemiology," *Journal of Infectious Diseases* 204, suppl. 1 (2011): S514–23, doi:10.1093 /infdis/jir118.

33. National Vaccine Information Center, www.medalerts.org/vaersdb /index.php.

34. www.thinktwice.com/Dutch.pdf.

35. Institute of Medicine's Vaccine Safety Committee report, eds. K.R. Stratton, C.J. Howe, and R.B. Johnston, Jr., *Adverse Events Associated with Childhood Vaccines: Evidence Bearing on Causality* (Washington, DC: National Academy Press, 1994): 6, www.ncbi.nlm.nih.gov /books/NBK236288/.

36. A. Lavy, E. Broide et al., "Measles is more prevalent in Crohn's disease patients: A multicentre Israeli study," *Digestive and Liver Disease* 33, no. 6 (August–September 2001): 472–6.

37. N.P. Thompson et al., "Is measles vaccination a risk factor for inflammatory bowel disease?" *The Lancet* 345, no. 8957 (April 29, 1995), 1,071–4.

38. Brian Hooker, Janet Kern, David Geier et al., "Methodological Issues and Evidence of Malfeasance in Research Purporting to Show Thimerosal in Vaccines Is Safe," *BioMed Research International,* article ID 247218 (2014): doi:10.1155/2014/247218.

39. https://autismoevaccini.files.wordpress.com/2012/12/vaccin -dc3a9cc3a8s.pdf.

40. D.R. Francis, "Why do death rates decline?" *National Bureau of Economic Research Digest* (March 2002).

41. P. Brown, "Scientist killed Amazon Indians to test race theory," *The Guardian* (September 23, 2000), www.theguardian.com/world/2000/sep/23/paulbrown.

42. www.bewellbuzz.com/general/10-reasons-flu-shots-dangerous-flu/.

43. Ibid.

44. *Vital Statistics of the United States 1937, 1938, 1943, 1944, 1949, 1960, 1967, 1976, 1987, 1992* (National Vital Statistics Reports); *Historical Statistics of the United States—Colonial Times to 1970, Part 1: Health* (U.S. Department of Health and Human Services, Vital Records and Health Data Development Section, Michigan Department of Community Health); *Statistical Abstract of the United States: 2003* (U.S. Census Bureau); *Reported Cases and Deaths from Vaccine Preventable Diseases, United States, 1950–2008* (CDC). See more at: www.vaccinationcouncil.org/2014/06/24/measles-and-measles-vaccines-fourteen-things-to-consider-by-roman-bystrianyk-co-author-dissolving-illusions-disease-vaccines-and-the-forgotten-history/#sthash.FL1sFqm7.dpuf.

45. F. Friedrich et al., "Temporal association between the isolation of Sabin-related poliovirus vaccine strains and the Guillain-Barré syndrome," *Revista do Instituto de Medicina Tropical de São Paulo* 38, no. 1 (January-February 1996): 55–8.

46. C. Black, "MMR vaccine and idiopathic thrombocytopaenic purpura," *British Journal of Clinical Pharmacology* 55, no. 1 (January 2003): 107–11.

47. V. Suprynowicz, "$2 billion paid out for vaccine injuries to kids," *Las Vegas Review-Journal* (August 26, 2012): www.reviewjournal.com/vin-suprynowicz/2-billion-paid-out-vaccine-injuries-kids.

48. D. Malkin, "Simian virus 40 and non-Hodgkin lymphoma," *The Lancet* 359, no. 9309 (March 9, 2002): 812–3.

49. R.A. Vilchez et al., "Association between simian virus 40 and non-Hodgkin lymphoma," *Lancet* 359, issue 9309 (March 9, 2002): 817–23.

50. X.A. Bu, "Study of simian virus 40 infection and its origin in human brain tumors," *Zhonghu Liu Xing Bing Xue Zhi* 21, no. 1 (February 2000): 19–21.

51. Archie Kalokerinos, *Every Second Child* (New Canaan, CT: Keats Pub, 1981).

52. *Washington Post* (September 24, 1976).

53. N.Z. Miller, "The polio vaccine: a critical assessment of its arcane history, efficacy, and long-term health-related consequences," *Medical Veritas* (2004): 239–51, ThinkTwice Global Vaccine Institute, www .thinktwice.com/Polio.pdf.

54. P.M. Strebel et al., "Epidemiology of poliomyelitis in U.S. one decade after the last reported case of indigenous wild virus associated disease," *Clinical and Infectious Diseases* (February 1992): 568–79.

55. Ibid.

56. F.W. Rosa et al., "Absence of antibody response to simian virus 40 after inoculation with killed-poliovirus vaccine of mother's offspring with neurological tumors," *New England Journal of Medicine* 318 (1988): 1,469.

57. F.W. Rosa FW et al., "Response to: Neurological tumors in offspring after inoculation of mothers with killed poliovirus vaccine," *New England Journal of Medicine* 319 (1988): 1,226.

58. W. Carlsen, "Rogue virus in the vaccine: Early polio vaccine harbored virus now feared to cause cancer in humans," *San Francisco Chronicle* (July 15, 2001): 10. Research by Susan Fisher, epidemiologist, Loyola University Medical Center.

59. David Oshinsky, *Polio: An American Story* (New York: Oxford University Press, 2005).

60. B.E. Eddy, G.S. Borman, G.E. Grubbs, R.D. Young, "Identification of the oncogenic substance in rhesus monkey kidney cell culture as simian virus 40," *Virology* 17 (May 1962): 65–75, doi:10.1016/0042-6822(62)90082-x.

61. R. Moskowitz, "Hidden in Plain Sight: The Role of Vaccines in Chronic Disease," www.whale.to/vaccine/moskowitz.html.

62. T. Verstraeten, R. Davis, and F. DeStefano, "Thimerosal VSD study, Phase I, Update 2/29/00," CDC Confidential Report (February 29, 2000).

63. R. Schmitz et al., "Vaccination Status and Health in Children and Adolescents: Findings of the German Health Interview and Examination Survey for Children and Adolescents (KiGGS)," *Deutsche Ärzteblatt International* 108, no. 7 (2011): 99–104, www.vaxchoicevt .com/wp-content/uploads/2013/01/schmitz-KIGGS.pdf.

64. C.D. Bethell et al., "A National and State Profile of Leading Health Problems and Health Care Quality for U.S. Children: Key Insurance Disparities and Across-State Variations," *Academic Pediatrics* 11, no. 3, suppl. (May 2011): S22–33.

65. A. Bachmair, "Vaccine Free: 111 Stories of Unvaccinated Children," CreateSpace Independent Publishing Platform (November 22, 2012): www.vaccineinjury.info.

66. S. Claridge, "Investigate Before You Vaccinate: Making an informed decision about vaccinating your children," The Immunisation Awareness Society, www.ias.org.nz.

67. Hays J, *The Culling of Man: Rise of the New World Order* (Google eBook), Jan 20, 2013, p 232.

68. Shabnum Nabi, *Toxic Effects of Mercury* (New Delhi: Springer, 2014), 228.

69. Ibid., 234.

70. P. Doshi, "Influenza: marketing vaccine by marketing disease," *BMJ (British Medical Journal)* 346 (2013): f3037, doi:10.1136/bmj.f3037.

71. S.B. Hubbard, "Johns Hopkins Scientist Slams Flu Vaccine," *Vaccine Information Network* (May 16, 2013).

72. "Glaxo's Swine Flu Shot Linked to Narcolepsy in UK Kids," *Bloomberg* (February 26, 2013).

73. D. O'Flanagan, A.S. Barret, M. Foley, S. Cotter, C. Bonner, C. Crowe, B. Lynch, B. Sweeney H. Johnson, B. McCoy, and E. Purcell, "Investigation of an association between onset of narcolepsy and vaccination with pandemic influenza vaccine, Ireland, April 2009–December 2010," *Euro Surveillance* 19, no. 17, article ID 20789 (2014): www.eurosurveillance.org/ViewArticle.aspx?ArticleId=20789.

74. R.E. Thomas, T. Jefferson, T.J. Lasserson, "Influenza vaccination for healthcare workers who work with the elderly," *Cochrane Database of Systematic Reviews* 2, article no. CD005187 (2010), doi:10.1002/14651858.CD005187.pub3.

75. CDC publication, *Fluview: 2012–2013 influenza season, week 3, ending January 19, 2013* (Atlanta, GA: U.S. Department of Health and Human Services, CDC, 2013), www.cdc.gov/flu/weekly/weeklyarchives2012-2013/weekly03.htm.

76. S. B. Hubbard, "Dr. Russell Blaylock Warns: Don't Get the Flu Shot—It Promotes Alzheimer's," Newsmax, December 18, 2011.

77. Ibid.

78. D.L. Levy, "The Future of Measles in Highly Immunized Populations: A Modeling Approach," *American Journal of Epidemiology* 120, no. 1 (July 1984): 39.

79. J.M. Heffernan and M.J. Keeling, "Implications of Vaccination and Waning Immunity," *Proceedings of the Royal Society B (Biological)* 276 (2009).

80. G.A. Poland and R.M. Jacobson, "The re-emergence of measles in developed countries: time to develop the next-generation measles vaccines?" *Vaccine* 30, no. 2 (January 5, 2012): 103–4, doi:10.1016/j.vaccine.2011.11.085.

81. N.Z. Miller, "Why People Choose Not to Vaccinate," *Age of Autism* (February 24, 2015), www.ageofautism.com/2015/02/neil-miller-why-people-choose-not-to-vaccinate.html.

82. H.U. Albonico et al., "Febrile infectious childhood diseases in the history of cancer patients and matched controls," *Medical Hypotheses* 51, no. 4 (October 1998): 315–20.

83. M. Montella et al., "Do childhood diseases affect NHL and HL risk? A case-control study from northern and southern Italy," *Leukemia Research* 30, no. 8 (August 2006): 917–22, e-published January 6, 2006.

84. F.E. Alexander, "Risk factors for Hodgkin's disease by Epstein-Barr virus (EBV) status: prior infection by EBV and other agents," *British Journal of Cancer* 82, no. 5 (March 2000): 1,117–21.

85. S.L. Glaser, "Exposure to childhood infections and risk of Epstein-Barr virus-defined Hodgkin's lymphoma in women," *International Journal of Cancer* 115, no. 4 (July 1, 2005): 599–605.

86. C. Gilham, "Day care in infancy and risk of childhood acute lymphoblastic leukaemia: findings from UK case-control study," *British Medical Journal* 330, no. 7503 (June 4, 2005): 1,294, e-published April 22, 2005.

87. K.Y. Urayama, "Early life exposure to infections and risk of childhood acute lymphoblastic leukemia," *International Journal of Cancer* 128, no. 7 (April 1, 2011): 1,632–43, doi:10.1002/ijc.25752, e-published December 17, 2010.

88. Environmental Working Group, "A Benchmark Investigation of Industrial Chemicals, Pollutants, and Pesticides in Umbilical Cord Blood" (July 14, 2005), www.ewg.org/research /body-burden-pollution-newborns.

89. NIH report *Mental Health: A Report of the Surgeon General* (Rockville, MD: U.S. Department of Health and Human Services, Substance Abuse and Mental Health Services Administration, Center for Mental Health Services, National Institute of Mental Health, National Institutes of Health, 1999).

90. Survey USA, "Cal-Oregon Unvaccinated Survey," *Generation Rescue* (June 26, 2007), www.generationrescue.org/resources/vaccination /cal-oregon-unvaccinated-survey/.

91. S. Visser, M. Danielson, R. Bitsko et al., "Trends in the Parent-Report of Health Care Provider-Diagnosis and Medication Treatment for ADHD Disorder: United States, 2003–2011," *Journal of the American Academy of Child and Adolescent Psychiatry* 53, no. 1 (2014): 34–46, e2.

92. T.J. Moore et al., "Prescription Drugs Associated with Reports of Violence Towards Others," *PLOS ONE* (December 15, 2010), doi:10.1371/journal.pone.0015337.

93. Ian Sinclair, *Vaccination: The Hidden Facts* (Ryde, Australia: Ian Sinclair, 1992).

94. G.S. Goldman and N.Z. Miller, "Relative trends in hospitalizations and mortality among infants by the number of vaccine doses and age, based on the Vaccine Adverse Event Reporting System (VAERS), 1990–2010," *Human and Experimental Toxicology* 31, no. 10 (October 2012): 1,012–21.

95. M.A. Hernán et al., "Recombinant hepatitis B vaccine and the risk of multiple sclerosis: A prospective study," *Neurology* 63, no. 5 (September 14, 2004): 838–42, doi:10.1212/01. WNL.0000138433.61870.82.

96. F. Martini et al., "Simian virus 40 in humans," *Infectious Agents and Cancer* 2, no. 13 (2007): doi:10.1186/1750-9378-2-13.

97. L. Hewitson et al., "Influence of pediatric vaccines on amygdala growth and opioid ligand binding in rhesus macaque infants: A pilot study," *Acta Neurobiologiae Experimentalis* 70 (2010): 147–64.

98. Andrew J. Wakefield et al., "Ileal-lymphoid-nodular hyperplasia, non-specific colitis, and pervasive developmental disorder in children," *Lancet* 351 (1998): 637–41.

99. F. Edward Yazbak, "Autism: Is there a vaccine connection? Part I: Vaccination after delivery" (1999), "… Part II: Vaccination around pregnancy" (1999), and "… Part III: Vaccination around pregnancy, the sequel" (2000), www.whale.to/vaccine/yazbak.html or https://yazbakarticles.wordpress.com.

100. W. Schilling, "VOSI research report RR8-V50.2," Voices of Safety International (October 27, 2000).

101. Neil Miller, Vaccine Safety Manual for Concerned Families and Health Practitioners (New Atlantean Press, 2008).

102. T. Verstraeten, R.L. Davis, D. Gu, and F. DeStefano, "Increased risk of developmental neurologic impairment after high exposure to thimerosal-containing vaccine in first month of life," *Proceedings of the Epidemic Intelligence Service Annual Conference* 49 (Atlanta, GA: Centers for Disease Control and Prevention, 2000).

103. B. Hooker, J. Kern, D. Geier, B. Haley, L. Sykes, P. King, and M. Geier, "Methodological Issues and Evidence of Malfeasance in Research Purporting to Show Thimerosal in Vaccines Is Safe," *BioMed Research International,* article ID 247218 (Hindawi Publishing Corporation, 2014).

104. T. Verstraeten et al., op. cit.

105. B. Hooker et al., op. cit.

106. H.A. Young et al., "Thimerosal exposure in infants and neurodevelopmental disorders: an assessment of computerized medical records in the vaccine safety datalink," *Journal of the Neurological Sciences* 271, no. 1–2 (2008): 110–8.

107. J.P. Barile et al., "Thimerosal exposure in early life and neuropsychological outcomes 7–10 years later," *Journal of Pediatric Psychology* 37, no. 1 (2012): 106–18.

108. Ibid.

109. N. Andrews et al., "Thimerosal exposure in infants and developmental disorders: a retrospective cohort study in the United Kingdom does not support a causal association," Pediatrics 114, no. 3 (2004): 584–91.

110. T. Verstraeten et al., "Safety of thimerosal-containing vaccines: a two-phased study of computerized health maintenance organization databases," *Pediatrics* 112, no. 5 (2003): 1,039–48.

111. W.W. Thompson et al., "Early thimerosal exposure and neuropsychological outcomes at 7 to 10 years," *The New England Journal of Medicine* 357, no. 13 (2007): 1,281–92.

112. B. Hooker et al., op. cit.

113. G.S. Goldman and N.Z. Miller, "Relative trends in hospitalizations and mortality among infants by the number of vaccine doses and age, based on the Vaccine Adverse Event Reporting System (VAERS), 1990–2010," *Human and Experimental Toxicology* 31, no. 10 (October 2012): 1,012–21.

114. "Judicial Watch Uncovers FDA Gardasil Records Detailing 26 New Reported Deaths," *Judicial Watch* (October 19, 2011), www .judicialwatch.org/press-room/press-releases/judicial-watch -uncovers-fda-gardasil-records-detailing-26-new-reported-deaths/.

115. Ibid.

116. A. Ram, "128 kids died after vaccine in 2010, government can't say why," *Times of India* (May 29, 2011), http://timesofindia.indiatimes. com/india/128-kids-died-after-vaccine-in-2010-govt-cant-say-why /articleshow/8641123.cms.

117. C. Englund, "India has suspended the use of HPV Gardasil vaccines due to deaths," *American Chronicle* (April 11, 2010), www.american-chronicle.com/.

118. W.C. Torch, "Diphtheria-pertussis-tetanus (DPT) immunization: A potential cause of the sudden infant death syndrome (SIDS), American Academy of Neurology, 34th Annual Meeting, April 25–May 1, 1982," *Neurology* 32 (1982): A169.

119. H. Buttram and E. Yazbak, "Shaken Baby Syndrome or Vaccine-Induced Encephalitis?" *ICA Review* (November–December 2000).

120. Archie Kalokerinos, MD, *Shaken Babies,* www.whale.to/a /kalokerinos_sbs.html.

121. www.rense.com/general7/onlysafe.htm.

122. Ibid.

123. K. Scott-Mumby, "Ex-vaccine developer reveals lies the vaccine industry is built upon in interview," www.Alternative-Doctor.com /vaccination/rappaport.htm.

124. J.B. Classen et al., "Association between type 1 diabetes and Hib vaccine," *BMJ (British Medical Journal)* 319 (1999): 1,133.

125. Theresa A. Deisher, Ngoc V. Doan, Angelica Omaiye, Kumiko Koyama, and Sarah Bwabye, "Impact of environmental factors on the prevalence of autistic disorder after 1979," *Journal of Public Health and Epidemiology* 6, no. 9 (September 2014): 271–84, doi:10.5897 /JPHE2014.0649.

126. "Finally the Truth," *Journal of Public Health and Epidemiology* (September 2014).

127. T. Deisher et al., op. cit.

128. Thomas E. Levy, MD, JD, *Curing the Incurable: Vitamin C, Infectious Diseases, and Toxins,* 4th edition (Henderson, NV: Livon Books, 2002).

129. Julian Winston, *The Faces of Homœopathy: An Illustrated History of the First 200 Years* (Wellington, New Zealand: Great Auk Pub, 1999), 592

130. S.S. Kim et al., "Effects of maternal and provider characteristics on up-to-date immunization status of children aged 19 to 35 months," *American Journal of Public Health* 97, no. 2 (February 2007): 259–66, doi:10.2105/AJPH.2005.076661.

CHAPTER 10

1. Marios Hadjivassiliou et al., "Gluten Sensitivity: From Gut to Brain," *Lancet Neurology* 9, no. 3 (March 2010): 318–30.

2. T. William et al., "Cognitive Impairment and Celiac Disease," *Archives of Neurology* 63, no. 10 (October 2006): 1,440–6.

3. R.P. Ford, "The Gluten Syndrome: A Neurological Disease," *Medical Hypotheses* 73, no. 3 (Sept 2009): 438–40.

4. Ibid.

5. Alan Schwarz and Cohen, Sarah, "A.D.H.D. Seen in 11% of U.S. Children as Diagnoses Rise," *New York Times,* March 31, 2013.

6. T.L. Lowe, et al., "Stimulant Medications Precipitate Tourette's Syndrome," *Journal of the American Medical Association* 247, no. 12 (March 26, 1982): 1,729–31.

7. P. Whiteley et al., "A Gluten-free Diet as an Intervention for Autism and Associated Spectrum Disorders: Preliminary Findings," *Autism* 3, no. 1 (March 1999): 45–65.

8. C. Ciacci et al., "Depressive Symptoms in Adult Coeliac Disease," *Scandinavian Journal of Gastroenterology* 33, no. 3 (March 1998): 247–50.

9. J.M. Greenblatt, "Is Gluten Making You Depressed? The Link Between Celiac Disease and Depression," *Psychology Today* (May 24, 2011).

10. J.F. Ludvigsson et al., "Coeliac Disease and Risk of Mood Disorders—A General Population-based Cohort Study," *Journal of Affective Disorders* 99, nos. 1–3 (April 2007): 117–26.

11. J.F. Ludvigsson et al., "Increased Suicide Risk in Coeliac Disease—A Swedish Nationwide Cohort Study," *Digest of Liver Disorders* 43, no. 8 (August 2011): 616–22.

12. M.G. Carta et al., "Recurrent Brief Depression in Celiac Disease," *Journal of Psychosomatic Research* 55, no. 6 (December 2003): 573–4.

13. C. Briani et al., "Neurological Complications of Celiac Disease and Autoimmune Mechanisms: A Prospective Study," *Journal of Neuroimmunology* 195, nos. 1–2 (March 2008): 171–5.

14. G. Rattue, "Schizophrenia Risk in Kids Associated with Mothers' Gluten Antibodies," *Medical News Today* (2012).

15. E. Lionetti et al., "Headache in Pediatric Patients with Celiac Disease and Its Prevalence as a Diagnostic Clue," *Journal of Pediatric Gastroenterology and Nutrition* 49, no. 2 (August 2009): 202–7.

16. L. Robberstad et al., "An unfavorable lifestyle and recurrent headaches among adolescents: the HUNT study," *Neurology* 75, no. 8 (August 24, 2010): 712–7.

17. "NIDA for Teens: Science For Starters: A Conversation with Dr. Ruben Baler," http://teens.drugabuse.gov/blog/post/science-starters-conversation-dr-ruben-baler-phd.

18. Francesca M. Filbey, Sina Aslan, Vince D. Calhoun, Jeffrey S. Spence, Eswar Damaraju, Arvind Caprihan, and Judith Segall, "Long-term effects of marijuana use on the brain," *Proceedings of the National Academy of Sciences* (November 10, 2014): doi:10.1073 /pnas.1415297111.

19. The White House Office of National Drug Control Policy, www .whitehouse.gov/ondcp/marijuana.

20. E. Silins et al., "Young adult sequelae of adolescent cannabis use: an integrative analysis," *The Lancet Psychiatry* 1, no. 4 (September 2014): 286–93.

21. K. Cousens and A. Dimascio, "Delta-9-THC as an hypnotic: An experimental study of 3 dose levels," *Psychopharmacologia* 33 (1973): 355–64.

22. A.L. Choi, G. Sun, Y. Zhang, and P. Grandjean, "Developmental fluoride neurotoxicity: a systematic review and meta-analysis," *Environmental Health Perspectives* 120 (2012): 1,362–8, http://dx.doi .org/10.1289/ehp.1104912.

23. Y. Dinga et al., "The relationships between low levels of urine fluoride on children's intelligence, dental fluorosis in endemic fluorosis areas in Hulunbuir, Inner Mongolia, China," *Journal of Hazardous Materials* 186 (2011): 1,942–6.

24. L. Valdez-Jiménez et al., "Effects of the fluoride on the central nervous system," *Neurologia* 26, no. 5 (June 2011): 297–300, e-published January 20, 2011.

25. J. Yiamouyiannis, *Fluoride: The Aging Factor,* 2nd ed. (Delaware, OH: Health Action Press, 1986).

26. Ibid.

27. K. Takahashi, K. Akiniwa, and K. Narita, Japan Epidemiological Association, "Regression analysis of cancer incidence rates and water fluoride in the U.S.A. based on IACR/IARC (WHO) data (1978-1992), International Agency for Research on Cancer," *Journal of Epidemiology* 11, no. 4 (2001): 170–9.

28. A.S. Kraus and W.F. Forbes, "Aluminum, fluoride and the prevention of Alzheimer's disease," *Canadian Journal of Public Health/Revue Canadienne de Sante Publique* 83, no. 2 (1992): 97–100.

29. D. Brownstein, *Iodine: Why You Need It* (Medical Alternative Press, 2009), 50.

30. S.K. Myun et al., "Mobile phone use and risk of tumors: a meta-analysis," *Journal of Clinical Oncology* 27, no. 33 (November 20, 2009): 5,565–72, e-published October 13, 2099, doi:10.1200 /JCO.2008.21.6366.

31. J.M. Moskowitz, "Government must inform us of cell phone risk," *San Francisco Chronicle* (April 28, 2010): www.sfgate.com/opinion /article/Government-must-inform-us-of-cell-phone-risk-3190907 .php.

32. C. Sage and D.O. Carpenter, "Public Health Implications of Wireless Technologies," *Pathophysiology* 16, nos. 2–3 (2009): 233–46, doi:10.1016/j.pathophys.2009.01.011.

33. S. Sadetzki et al., "Cellular phone use and risk of benign and malignant parotid gland tumors—a nationwide case-control study," *American Journal of Epidemiology* 167, no. 4 (February 15, 2008): 457–67, e-published December 6, 2007, doi: 10.1093/aje/kwm325.

34. Rakefet Czerninski, Avi Zini, and Harold D. Sgan-Cohen, "Risk of Parotid Malignant Tumors in Israel (19702006)," *Epidemiology* 22, no. 1 (2011): 130–1, doi:10.1097/EDE.obo13e3181feb9fo.

35. H. Eger, K. Hagen, B. Lucas et al., *"Einfluss der raumlichen Nahe von Mobilfunksendeanlagen auf die Krebsinzidenz,"* Umwelt-Medizin-Gesellschaft 17 (2004): 273–356.

36. C.M. Krause et al., "Mobile phone effects on children's event-related oscillatory EEG during an auditory memory task," *International Journal of Radiation Biology* 82, no. 6 (2006): 443–50, doi:10.1080/09553000600840922.

37. The Stewart Report, "More Reasons Children May Be at Risk," *Microwave News* 22, no. 4 (July–August 2002): 13.

38. Gaby Badre, "Excessive Mobile Phone Use Affects Sleep in Teens," *American Academy of Sleep Medicine* (May 14, 2008).

39. G. Lean, "Mobile phone radiation wrecks your sleep," *The Independent* (Sunday, January 20, 2008), www.independent.co.uk/life-style /health-and-families/health-news/mobile-phone-radiation-wrecks -your-sleep-771262.html.

40. D.K. Li et al., "Maternal Exposure to Magnetic Fields During Pregnancy in Relation to the Risk of Asthma in Offspring," *Archives of Pediatrics and Adolescent Medicine* 165, no. 10 (2011): 945–50, doi:10.1001/archpediatrics.2011.135.

41. De-Kun Li et al., "A Prospective Study of In-utero Exposure to Magnetic Fields and the Risk of Childhood Obesity," *Scientific Reports* 2, article number: 540, July 27, 2012, doi:10.1038/srep00540.

42. J.J. Mangano and J.D. Sherman, Radiation and Public Health Project (New York), "Elevated airborne beta levels in Pacific/West Coast US states and trends in hypothyroidism among newborns after the Fukushima nuclear meltdown," *Open Journal of Pediatrics* 3 (2013): 1–9, e-published March 2013: www.scirp.org/journal/ojped/ and http://dx.doi.org/10.4236/ojped.2013.31001.

43. http://enenews.com/tokyo-newspaper-60-of-fukushima-children-tested-have-diabetes-head-of-tokyo-area-medical-clinic-we-are-expecting-diabetes-in-children-because-of-fukushima-radiation-video.

44. M.E. Martinucci, G. Curradi, A. Fasulo, A. Medici, S. Toni, G. Osovik, E. Lapistkaya, and E. Sherbitskaya, "Incidence of childhood type 1 diabetes mellitus in Gomel, Belarus," *Journal of Pediatric Endocrinology and Metabolism* 15, no. 1 (January 2002): 53–7.

45. Dr. A. Zalutskaya, T. Mokhort, D. Garmaev, and S.R. Bornstein, "Did the Chernobyl incident cause an increase in Type 1 diabetes mellitus incidence in children and adolescents?" *Diabetologia* (2004): 147–8, doi:10.1007/s00125-003-1271-9.

46. N.A. Zueva, A.N. Kovalenko, T.I. Gerasimenko, B.N. Man'kovskii, T.I. Korpachova, and A.S. Efimov, "Analysis of irradiation dose, body mass index and insulin blood concentration in personnel cleaning up after the Chernobyl nuclear plant accident," *Lik Sprava* 4 (July–August 2001): 26–8.

47. C. Ito, "Trends in the prevalence of diabetes mellitus among Hiroshima atomic bomb survivors," *Diabetes Research and Clinical Practice* 24 suppl. (October 1994): S29–35.

48. Ibid.

49. R. Lorini and G. d'Annunzio, "Comment to Zalutskaya A, Bornstein SR, Mokhort T, Garmaev D (2004): did the Chernobyl incident cause an increase in type 1 diabetes mellitus incidence in children

and adolescents? *Diabetologia* 47:147–148 (letter)," *Diabetologia* 48, no. 10 (October 2005): 2,193–4, e-published August 26, 2005.

50. B.S. Alexandrov, V. Gelev, A.R. Bishop, A. Usheva, and K.O. Rasmussen, "DNA breathing dynamics in the presence of a terahertz field," *Physics Letters* A, vol. 374, no. 10 (2010), doi:10.1016/j .physleta.2009.12.077.

51. Alice Stewart and George W. Kneale, "Radiation dose effects in relation to obstetric x-rays and childhood cancer," *Lancet* 1 (1970): 1,185–7.

CHAPTER 11

1. Jeanne Fulbright, *Exploring Creation with Zoology 3: Land Animals of the Sixth Day* (Apologia Educational Ministries, Inc., 2008), 5–6.

2. J. Hollard, *Unlikely Friendships: 47 Remarkable Stories from the Animal Kingdom* (New York: Workman Publishing Company, Inc., 2011), 83.

3. Daniel Brook, "The Planet-Saving Mitzvah: Why Jews Should Consider Vegetarianism," *Tikkun Magazine,* July/August 2009.

4. Brandon Bays, *The Journey for Kids* (Novato, CA: New World Library, 2006).

5. Association for Waldorf Music Education, "About Music in Waldorf Schools," http://waldorfmusic.org/articles.html.

6. Gabriel Cousens, *Creating Peace by Being Peace* (Berkeley, CA: North Atlantic Books, 2008), 136.

7. Ibid.

8. American Music Therapy Association, www.musictherapy.org.

9. www.goodreads.com/author/quotes/113846.Raffi.

CHAPTER 12

1. F.R. Kaufman, "Type 2 diabetes in children and young adults: A new epidemic," *Clinical Diabetes* 20 (2002): 217–8.

2. Gabriel Cousens, *There Is a Cure for Diabetes: The 21-Day+ Holistic Recovery Program,* revised edition (Berkeley, CA: North Atlantic Books, 2013).

CHAPTER 13

1. P. Humphries, E. Pretorius, and H. Naudé (University of Pretoria, South Africa), "Direct and indirect cellular effects of aspartame on the brain," *European Journal of Clinical Nutrition* 62 (August 2007): 451–62, doi:10.1038/sj.ejcn.1602866.

Index

A

ADD/ADHD
  diet and, 228–29
  gluten sensitivity and, 324, 325–26
  holistic approach to, 229–30
  medication for, 325
  nature and, 208, 212
  omega 3s and, 213
  pesticides and, 97–98
  prevalence of, 290–91, 325
  sleep and, 81
  sugar intake and, 370
  vaccination and, 280, 281, 290–91
Advertising, 141, 234–36
Agar-agar
  Agar-Agar Paste, 459
  Basic Cheezecake, 458–59
Agent Orange, 104–5, 137
AGEs (advanced glycation end products), 466
Ahimsa, 155, 157, 169
Airola, Paavo, 65
Akhenaten, 156
Albo, Joseph, 158, 353
Alcohol, 236
Algae, 40–42, 133
Algood, Tammy, 33
Alive child
  creating alive environment for, 11–13
  role of, 6–7

  supporting stages of development of, 26–31, 483–84
Alive parenting
  allopathic parenting vs., 5
  creating alive environment for, 14–15
  goal of, 5–6
  governments vs., 3–4
  as spiritual work, 4–5
Allspice, 376
Almonds
  Almond Yogurt, 474–75
  Apple-Cinnamon Bread, 399
  Avocado-Collard Mini-Wraps, 418
  Basic Cheezecake, 458–59
  Bundle-It-Up Winter Salad, 438–39
  Cheeze, 442
  Rich and Creamy Steamers, 472–73
  Savory Trail Mix, 424
  Smoke-Salted Almonds, 418
Aloe vera
  Man-Go Green, 404–5
Alzheimer's disease, 53, 69, 149–50, 294
American Academy of Pediatrics (AAP), 233, 245, 246
American Dietetic Association, 38, 138
Anemia, iron-deficiency, 43–44
Angström, Johan, 134

About the Authors

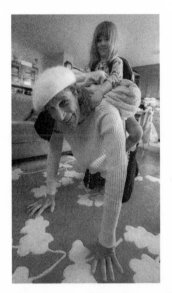

RABBI GABRIEL COUSENS, MD, is a world-recognized medical doctor and spiritual teacher. He is the founder and director of the Tree of Life Foundation, which trains spiritual counselors and coordinates international humanitarian programs benefiting disadvantaged families, children, and indigenous cultures through holistic education. A leading medical authority with forty years of success in healing diabetes naturally, he is also the founder and director of the Tree of Life Rejuvenation Center in Patagonia, Arizona, a healing center for spiritual and physical healing. A best-selling author and the creator of Dr. Cousens's Diabetes Recovery Program, he uses the modalities of diet, nutrition, naturopathy, Ayurveda, and homeopathy blended with spiritual awareness in the healing of body, mind, and spirit.

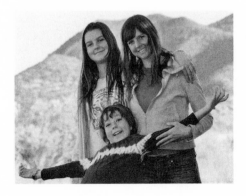

LEAH LYNN is a Montessori teacher and the author of *Baby Greens: A Live-Food Approach for Children of All Ages*. She is the founder of Mama Greens Children's Garden, a nurturing home-based daycare in Patagonia, Arizona, where her recipes were tried and perfected.